P de Silva. 4

LECTURE NOTES ON CLINICAL MEDICINE

D1273198

LECTURE NOTES ON

Clinical Medicine

DAVID RUBENSTEIN
M.D. M.R.C.P.(Lond.)
Physician, Addenbrooke's Hospital, Cambridge

DAVID WAYNE
M.A. B.M. F.R.C.P. (Ed.), M.R.C.P.(Lond.)
Physician, Northgate Hospital, Great Yarmouth

FOURTH PRINTING

Blackwell Scientific Publications
Oxford London Edinburgh Melbourne

© 1976 Blackwell Scientific Publications
Osney Mead, Oxford OX2 0EL
8 John Street, London WC1N 2ES
9 Forrest Road, Edinburgh EH1 2QH
P.O. Box 9, North Balwyn, Victoria, Australia

All rights reserved. No part of this publication may be reproduced, stored in a retrieval system or transmitted, in any form or by any means, electronic, mechanical, photocopying, recording or otherwise without the prior permission of the copyright owner

ISBN 0 632 09620 9

First published 1976
Revised reprint 1977
Second revised reprint 1977
Fourth printing 1978

Distributed in the United States of America
by J. B. Lippincott Company, Philadelphia
and in Canada by
J. B. Lippincott Company of Canada Ltd, Toronto

Set in Monotype Times

Printed and bound in Great Britain
at the Alden Press, Oxford

Contents

PART 2 ESSENTIAL BACKGROUND INFORMATION

Preface

This book is intended primarily for the junior hospital doctor in the period between qualification and the examination for Membership of the Royal Colleges of Physicians. We think that it will also be helpful to final year medical students and to clinicians reading for higher specialist qualifications in surgery and anaesthetics.

The hospital doctor must not only acquire a large amount of factual information but also use it effectively in the clinical situation. The experienced physician has acquired some clinical perspective through practice: we hope that this book imparts some of this to the relatively inexperienced. The format and contents are designed for the examination candidate but the same approach to problems should help the hospital doctor in his everyday work.

The book as a whole is not suitable as a first reader for the undergraduate because it assumes much basic knowledge and considerable detailed information has had to be omitted. It is not intended to be a complete textbook of medicine and the information it contains must be supplemented by further reading. The contents are intended only as lecture notes and the margins of the pages are intentionally large so that the reader may easily add additional material of his own.

The book is divided into two parts: *the clinical approach* and *essential background information*. In the first part we have considered the situation which a candidate meets in the clinical part of an examination or a physician in the clinic. This part of the book thus resembles a manual on techniques of physical examination, though it is more specifically intended to help the candidate carry out an examiner's request to perform a specific examination. It has been our experience in listening to candidates' performances in examinations and hearing the examiners' subsequent assessment, that it is the failure of a candidate to examine cases systematically and his failure to behave as if he were used to doing this every day of his clinical life that leads to adverse comments.

In the second part of the book a summary of basic clinical facts is given in the conventional way. We have included most common diseases but not all, and we have tried to emphasise points which are understressed in many textbooks. Accounts are given of many conditions which are relatively rare. It is necessary for the clinician to know about these and to be on the lookout for them both in the clinic and in examinations. Supplementary reading is essential to understand their basic pathology but the information we give is probably all that need be remembered by the non-specialist reader and will provide adequate working knowledge in a clinical situation. It should not be forgotten that some rare diseases are of great importance in practice because they are treatable or preventable, e.g. infective endocarditis, hepatolenticular degeneration, attacks of acute porphyria. Some conditions are important to examination candidates because patients are ambulant and appear commonly in examinations, e.g. neurosyphilis, syringomyelia, atrial and ventricular septal defects.

We have not attempted to cover the whole of medicine but by crossreferencing between the two sections of the book and giving information in summary form we have completely omitted few subjects. Some highly specialised fields such as the treatment of leukaemia were thought unsuitable for inclusion.

A short account of psychiatry is given in the section on neurology since many patients with mental illness attend general clinics and it is hoped that readers may be warned of gaps in their knowledge of this important field. The section on dermatology is incomplete but should serve for quick revision of common skin disorders.

Wherever possible we have tried to indicate the relative frequency with which various conditions are likely to be seen in hospital practice in this country and have selected those clinical features which in our view are most commonly seen and where possible have listed them in order of importance. The frequency with which a disease is encountered by any individual physician will depend upon its prevalence in the district from which his cases are drawn and also on his known special interests. Nevertheless rare conditions are rarely seen; at least in the clinic. Examinations, however, are a 'special case'.

We have used many generally accepted abbreviations, e.g. ECG, ESR, and have included them in the index instead of supplying a glossary.

Despite our best efforts, some errors of fact may have been included. As with every book and authority, question and check everything—and please write to us if you wish.

We should like to thank all those who helped us with producing this book and in particular Sir Edward Wayne and Sir Graham Bull who have kindly allowed us to benefit from their extensive experience both in medicine and in examining for the Colleges of Physicians.

David Rubenstein
David Wayne
November 1975

Part 1: The clinical approach

Nervous system

The candidate is usually asked to examine a specific area, e.g. '*Examine the cranial nerves*', '*Examine the lower limbs*', '*Examine the arms*' or '*Examine the eyes*'. By far the commonest neurological disorders suitable for a clinical examination are multiple sclerosis and the results of cerebrovascular disease. Diabetes is a common disorder which fairly frequently gives rise to neurological manifestations. Carcinomatous neuropathy should always be considered when the signs are difficult to synthesise. Neurosyphilis is becoming progressively rarer—the patient will belong to the pre-penicillin era, i.e. be over 50 years old. Parkinsonism is relatively common. Motor neurone disease, myopathies, myasthenia gravis and the neurological manifestations of vitamin B_{12} deficiency are all rare in practice but more frequently seen in examinations.

In terms of examination technique the practising physician must examine case after case, both normal and abnormal, until he has developed a system which is rapid, accurate and second nature to him. An appearance of professionalism in your neurological examination may encourage the examiner to take a less unfavourable view of minor errors than he might if you appear hesitant, clumsy or imprecise.

'Examine the cranial nerves'

Many abnormalities of the cranial nerves are the results of chronic disease and patients with them are commonly seen in examination.

The commonest disorders are disseminated sclerosis (optic atrophy, nystagmus (often ataxic), cerebellar dysarthria), stroke, and Bell's palsy. The manifestation of cerebral tumour, aneurysm, syphilis, dystrophia myotonica and myasthenia gravis are seen much less frequently. It is useful to memorise diagrams of three cross-sections of the brain-stem and one of the floor of the fourth ventricle since these may greatly improve analysis of a cranial nerve lesion. Do not spend long on the first or second cranial nerves unless there is good reason to suspect an abnormality. If the optic fundus is abnormal, the examiner is likely to ask you to look at it specifically. Eye movements must be carefully examined. Do not confuse ptosis (third nerve or sympathetic) with paresis of the orbicularis oculi (seventh nerve). Make sure you can explain clearly and concisely the difference between an upper and a lower motor neurone lesion of the seventh nerve. The corneal reflex is an essential part of the complete examination of the cranial nerves. The following approach is recommended.

Smell

'*Has there been any recent change in your sense of smell?*' If so, test formally with 'smell bottles'.

Eyes

Observe, and test when necessary, for:

— *ptosis*

Third nerve lesion (complete or partial ptosis)

Sympathetic lesion (partial ptosis) as part of Horner's syndrome

Muscle weakness. Myasthenia gravis (and rarely, dystrophia myotonica, facio-scapulo-humeral dystrophy, congenital and tabo-paresis)

NB Ptosis is not due to a seventh nerve lesion.

— *visual fields* to confrontation (second nerve) (page 5)

— *external ocular movements* (third, fourth and sixth nerves) (page 6) and *nystagmus* (page 9)

— *pupillary reactions* to light and accommodation (page 7)

— *the fundi* (second nerve) (page 22)

Face (seventh nerve)

'*Screw up your eyes very tightly.*' Compare how deeply the eyelashes are buried on the two sides. Unilateral weakness is invariably due to a lower motor neurone lesion.

'*Grin.*' Compare the nasolabial grooves.

Mouth

'*Clench your teeth*' (fifth nerve, motor). Feel the masseters and test the jaw jerk if indicated. The jaw jerk is obtained by placing one finger horizontally across the front of the jaw and tapping the finger with a tendon hammer with the jaw relaxed and the mouth just open. An increased jaw jerk occurs in upper motor neurone lesions of the fifth cranial nerve (pseudobulbar palsy, page 11).

'*Open your mouth and keep it open*' (fifth nerve, motor: pterygoids). You should not be able to force it closed. With a unilateral lesion, the jaw deviates towards the weaker side (the weak muscle cannot keep it open).

'*Say aaah*' (ninth and tenth nerves). Normally the uvula and soft palate move upwards and remain central and the posterior pharyngeal wall moves little. With a unilateral lesion the soft palate is pulled away from the weaker side (there may also be 'curtain movement' of the posterior pharyngeal wall away from the weaker side).

'*Put your tongue out*' (twelfth nerve). Look for wasting, fasciculation and whether it protrudes to one side (towards the weaker side since the weaker muscle cannot push it out).

Neck (eleventh nerve)

'*Lift your head off the pillows*' or '*Put your chin on your right (or left) shoulder*' while you resist the movement. Look at, and palpate the sternomastoids.

'*Shrug your shoulders*' while you push them down. Look at and palpate the bulk of trapezius.

Ears (eighth nerve) Test hearing with a wrist watch held at various distances from the ears (compare with your own) and perform Weber and Rinné tests. You should ask for an auriscope if indicated. The commonest cause of conductive (air conduction) deafness is wax.

Facial sensation (fifth nerve) Test the three divisions on both sides with cotton wool. Check the corneal reflexes (often the first clinical deficit in fifth nerve lesions). Ask the patient if the sensation is equally unpleasant on the two sides.

Notes

Field defects You are in principle comparing the patient's visual fields with your own. When testing his right eye, he should look straight into your left eye with his head held at arm's length. '*Keep looking at my eye and tell me when you first see my finger out of the corner of your eye.*' Then bring your finger towards the centre of the field of vision from the four main directions (right, left, up, down). It is preferable to use a white-headed hat pin if you have one. The nasal and superior fields are limited by the nose and eyebrow respectively but this is not often of clinical importance. Field defects are described by the side of the visual field which is lost, i.e. temporal field loss indicates loss of the temporal field of vision and denotes damage to the nasal retina or its connections back to the visual cortex. Perimetry will accurately define defects.

Temporal hemianopia: in one eye alone or in both eyes (bitemporal hemianopia) suggests a chiasmal compression usually from a pituitary tumour.
Homonymous hemianopia: i.e. loss of nasal field in one eye and temporal field in the other may occur with any postchiasmal lesion and usually following a posterior cerebral vascular lesion (usually with macular sparing). The side of the field loss is opposite to the side of the damaged cortex (i.e. a right-sided cerebral lesion produces a left homonymous hemianopia).
Upper outer quadrantic field loss: suggests a temporal lesion of the opposite cortex. It is homonymous.
Central scotoma: loss of vision in the centre of the visual field is detected by passing a white or red tipped pin across the front of the eyes which are held looking forward. This occurs in acute retrobulbar neuritis most commonly due to multiple sclerosis.

Blindness A history of transient blindness, total or partial (with specific field defects usually in one eye) is not uncommon in migraine. It may also follow vertebral arteriography.

Sudden blindness also occurs with
— retinal detachment
— acute glaucoma
— vitreous haemorrhage in diabetes
— temporal arteritis and retinal artery or vein obstruction

— fractures of the skull

NB The light reflex is absent except in cortical blindness.

Senile changes and *glaucoma* account for about two-thirds of blindness in this country. Diabetes is the major non-ocular (systemic) cause (7–10%) due chiefly to vitreous haemorrhage and cataract. Trachoma is a common cause on a world-wide basis.
Hysterical blindness is uncommon and should never be confidently assumed.
The blindness of *temporal arteritis* is preventable if steroid therapy is started in time.

Eye movements

These are controlled by the third, fourth and sixth nerves and conjugate movement controlled by the medial longitudinal bundle. This connects the above nuclei together and to the cerebellum and the vestibular nuclei.

Squint

Congenital squints are present from childhood and are due to a defect of one eye. The angle between the longitudinal axes of the eyes remains constant on testing extraocular movements, and there is no diplopia.
Paralytic squint is acquired and results from paralysis of one or more of the muscles which move the eye, or paralysis from proptosis. On testing external ocular movements, the angle between the eye axes varies and there is diplopia.

Rule 1 Diplopia is maximum when looking in the direction of action of the paralysed muscle.
Rule 2 The image furthest from the midline arises from the 'paralysed' eye. This may be determined by covering up each eye in turn and asking which image has disappeared.

NB It is sometimes easier to test movements in each eye separately.

'*Do you see double?*' If so, ask him in which direction it is worst, put your forefinger in that direction and then ask him if the two fingers which he sees are parallel to each other (lateral rectus palsy: sixth nerve) or at an angle (superior oblique palsy: fourth nerve). If he has not noticed diplopia, test the movements formally, right and left, up and down, and note if there is any nystagmus.

Apart from local lesions such as pressure from tumour or aneurysm, isolated external ocular palsies may result from diabetes mellitus, multiple sclerosis, polyarteritis, sarcoidosis, syphilis and meningitis (usually tuberculous or pneumococcal).

Lateral rectus palsy (sixth nerve)

This produces failure of lateral movement with convergent strabismus. It is the commonest external ocular palsy. The diplopia is maximal on looking to the affected side. The images are parallel and separated horizontally. The outermost image comes from the affected eye and disappears when that eye is covered. The palsy is produced as a false localising sign in raised intracranial pressure, by direct involvement with tumour, aneurysm, or rarely with acoustic neuroma (page 96).

Superior oblique palsy (fourth nerve)

This type is rare. Palsy produces diplopia maximal on downward gaze. The two images are then at an angle to each other when the palsied eye is abducted and one above the other when the eye is adducted. The diplopia is therefore noticed most on reading or descending stairs.

Third nerve palsy

It may not present with diplopia because there is complete ptosis. When the lid is lifted the eye is seen to be 'down and out' (divergent strabismus) and there is severe (angulated) diplopia. The pupil may be dilated. It occurs with space-occupying lesions, brain-stem vascular lesions (Weber's syndrome) and aneurysm of the posterior communicating artery.

The muscle itself is involved in myasthenia gravis and the ophthalmoplegia of thyrotoxicosis.

Pupillary reflexes

The balance between parasympathetic (constrictor) and sympathetic (dilator) tone controls pupil size. *Constriction of the pupil in response to light* is relayed via the optic nerve, optic tract, lateral geniculate nuclei, the Edinger–Westphal nucleus of the third nerve and the ciliary ganglion. The cortex is not involved.

Constriction of the pupil with accommodation. Convergence originates within the cortex and is relayed to the pupil via the third nerve nuclei. The optic nerve and tract and the lateral geniculate nucleus are not involved.

Therefore:

— if the direct light reflex is absent and the convergence reflex is present, a local lesion in the brain-stem or ciliary ganglion is implied, e.g. Argyll Robertson pupil

— if the convergence reflex is absent and the light reflex is present, a lesion of the cerebral cortex is implied, e.g. cortical blindness

Examination of the pupillary reflexes should be performed in subdued light. The pupil should be positively inspected for irregularity. A torch is flashed twice at each eye (once for direct and once for consensual responses), preferably from the side so that the patient does not focus on it (and hence have an accommodation-convergence reflex).

If the pupil is constricted consider: Argyll Robertson pupil (must also be irregular and have no light reflex); Horner's syndrome (page 8); morphine; pontine haemorrhage.

If the pupil is dilated consider: mydriatics (e.g. homatropine); a third nerve lesion; the Holmes–Adie syndrome (pupils constrict sluggishly to light, e.g. in half an hour in a bright room, and absent tendon reflexes); and congenital (ask the patient). In the unconscious patient a fixed dilated pupil (third nerve lesion) may indicate temporal lobe herniation (from raised intracranial pressure) on the same side, intracranial bleeding, tumour or abscess.

Horner's syndrome

This is rare in practice but common in examinations. The syndrome comprises unilateral
— ptosis (partial, i.e. sympathetic)
— miosis (constricted pupil) with normal reactions
— anhidrosis (decreased sweating over face)
— enophthalmos (indrawing of orbit)
i.e. everything gets smaller or contracts.

The syndrome results from lesions of the sympathetic nerves to the eye, either from their origin in the sympathetic nucleus of the brain-stem or during their passage through the cervical and upper thoracic cord, the anterior spinal first thoracic root, the sympathetic chain, stellate ganglion and carotid sympathetic plexus. It is essential to look for evidence of a T1 lesion (page 12).

Aetiology

Carcinoma of the bronchus (T1, Pancoast tumour)
Cervical node secondary deposits
Brain-stem vascular disease (lateral medullary syndrome, page 86) and demyelinating disease
Local neoplasms and trauma in the neck
Rarely carotid or aortic aneurysms
Very rarely syringomyelia and intrinsic cervical cord disease (vascular and neoplastic)

Hearing

Weber test: a vibrating tuning fork is held in the middle of the forehead. In the absence of nerve deafness, the sound is louder in the ear where air conduction is impaired, e.g. wax or otitis media. (This can easily be tested by placing a vibrating tuning fork on one's own forehead and putting a finger in one ear.)

Rinné test: air conduction is normally better than bone conduction. The vibrating tuning fork is first placed behind the ear on the mastoid process and then rapidly held with its prongs in line with the external meatus. The patient is asked 'Is it louder behind (with the tuning fork on the mastoid) or in front (with the tuning fork in line with the external meatus)?' Normally it is louder in front—this is termed Rinné positive. Negative is abnormal.

Vertigo

Vertigo refers to unsteadiness with a subjective sensation of rotation: either the patient or his surroundings appears to rotate. Vertigo results from disease of the eighth cranial nerve or its connections in the brain-stem.
Labyrinthine: Ménière's disease, acute labyrinthitis
Eighth nerve: acoustic neuroma and other posterior fossa tumours, streptomycin
Brain-stem: neoplasm, vascular disease (vertebro-basilar ischaemia, lateral medullary syndrome),

demyelination (multiple sclerosis), migraine, aneurysms, degeneration (syringobulbia)

Nystagmus

Nystagmus may result from any disturbance of either the eighth nerve and its connections in the brain-stem or the cerebellum. Its direction is named after the quick phase (of 'saw-tooth' nystagmus). Nystagmus is usually more pronounced when the patient looks in the direction of the quick phase. Nystagmoid jerks may be produced in normal eyes by errors of examination technique: either holding the object too close to the patient or too far to one side.

Horizontal nystagmus

Vestibular nystagmus occurs following damage to the eighth nerve or to its brain-stem connections and is present only in the first few weeks after the lesion because central compensation occurs. It is usually associated with vertigo and often with deafness and tinnitus. It is greater on looking *away* from the side of a destructive lesion. It may be caused by acute viral labyrinthitis, acute alcoholism, Ménière's disease, middle ear disease and surgery, multiple sclerosis, basilar artery ischaemia, and syringobulbia.

Cerebellar nystagmus usually occurs with lateral lobe lesions: central (vermis) lesions even causing severe truncal ataxia may cause no nystagmus. Since cerebellar disease is frequently bilateral, nystagmus may occur to both sides. If it is unilateral it is greater *towards* the side of the destructive lesion.

Cerebellar lesions occur in multiple sclerosis, hereditary ataxias (page 102) and vascular disease.

Nystagmus is often seen in patients who have taken high doses (though often within the therapeutic range) of sedative drugs, especially phenytoin and barbiturates.

Ataxic nystagmus The degree of nystagmus in the abducting eye is greater than in the adducting eye (and there is some failure of adduction). This is virtually pathognomonic of multiple sclerosis and is due to damage of the medial longitudinal bundle.

Vertical nystagmus

The direction of jerks is vertical. Vertical gaze usually makes it more pronounced. It may be produced by sedative drugs (especially phenytoin) but otherwise localises disease to the brain-stem (although brain-stem disorders more commonly produce horizontal nystagmus).

Pendular and rotary nystagmus

Unlike all the above, the phases of the nystagmus are equal in duration. It is secondary to an inability to fix objects and focus with one or both eyes due to a variable degree of blindness, e.g. albinism, coal miners.

Facial palsy

In unilateral upper motor neurone lesions (e.g. stroke) movements of the upper face are retained because it is represented on both sides of the cerebral cortex. The flattened forehead and sagging lower eyelid are seen in complete lower motor neurone lesions (e.g. Bell's palsy and middle ear surgery). Taste sensation from the tongue in the chorda tympani leaves the facial nerve in the middle ear, and therefore loss of taste over the anterior two-thirds of the tongue means that a facial nerve paresis must be due to a lesion above this level. Lesions in the stylomastoid foramen (Bell's palsy) and parotid gland (tumours) do not give these signs. Facial palsy is usually a late sign of acoustic neuroma. It may occur in an unusually extensive lateral medullary syndrome.

Aetiology of cranial nerve palsies

The causes of single-nerve palsies include cerebral aneurysm, diabetes mellitus, trauma, surgery, cerebral tumour and multiple sclerosis. The various eponymous vascular lesions of the brain-stem need not be separately remembered, but you should be able to discuss the localisation of such lesions with the help of diagrams: they are relatively common causes of cranial nerve palsy. Polyarteritis nodosa, sarcoidosis, meningitis, syphilis and Wernicke's encephalopathy are less common causes.

Speech disorders

'*Would you like to ask this patient some questions?*'

It is likely that the patient has a speech disorder, but there may be some degree of dementia (page 109).

Ask name, age, occupation and address
Test orientation in time (date, season) and place, for dementia
If indicated, test memory and intellectual capacity
Test ability to name familiar objects (pen, coins, watch): nominal dysphasia
Test articulation, e.g. 'baby hippopotamus', 'West Register Street'
If dysarthria is present, look in the mouth for local lesions and test the lower cranial nerves

Dysphasia (or aphasia)

A disorder of the content of speech which usually follows cerebrovascular accidents of the dominant cortex and hence is common. Test by asking patient to name familiar objects, e.g. pen, watch. Failure to name an object spontaneously but with recognition of the correct answer on prompting suggests 'nominal dysphasia' (or expressive dysphasia).

Dysarthria

Inability to articulate properly due to local lesions in the mouth or disorders of the muscles of speech or their connections. There is no disorder of the content of speech.

Stutter—relatively common
Paralysis of cranial nerves (seventh, ninth, tenth or twelfth nerves)
Cerebellar disease—'scanning' speech or staccato, seen in multiple sclerosis
Parkinson's disease: speech is slow, quiet, slurred and monotonous

TABLE 1 Clinical signs of bulbar and pseudobulbar palsies

	Pseudobulbar (UMN lesion)	*Bulbar (LMN lesion)*
Emotions	Labile	Normal
Dysarthria	Donald Duck speech	Nasal
Tongue	Spastic, small for mouth	Flaccid, fasciculating
Jaw jerk	Increased	Normal or absent
Associated findings	Bilateral upper motor neurone lesions of limbs	Sometimes other evidence of MND, e.g. fasciculation in limbs

Pseudobulbar palsy (spastic dysarthria): monotonous, high pitched 'hot potato' speech (rare)
Bulbar palsy (rare)
General paralysis of the insane (very rare nowadays)

Bulbar and pseudobulbar palsies (table 1)

Both forms are rare and unlikely to be seen in examinations. The symptoms of dysarthria, dysphagia and nasal regurgitation result from paralysis of the ninth, tenth and twelfth cranial nerves.

Pseudobulbar (upper motor neurone) palsy is commoner than bulbar palsy and is due to bilateral lesions of the internal capsule, most often the result of cerebrovascular accidents affecting both sides, usually sequentially. (It can also occur in multiple sclerosis.) Bulbar (lower motor neurone) palsy is rare because motor neurone disease, and the infective causes (poliomyelitis, Guillain-Barré) are rare.

'Examine this patient's arms (neurologically)'

You may be asked to look at a patient whose neurological syndrome involving the arm is part of a more central lesion such as a stroke or cerebral tumour (perhaps producing 'cortical' sensory or motor loss), a cerebellar lesion, brain-stem involvement or cervical cord disease (e.g. vascular disease, tumour, syringomyelia). Peripheral neuropathies affecting the hands are uncommon (cf. isolated peripheral nerve lesions).

Amongst the commonest neurological lesions of the arms are:

Carpal tunnel syndrome (median nerve palsy)
Ulnar nerve palsy (involved in the ulnar groove at the elbow—usually osteoarthritis from trauma)
Cervical spondylosis (usually of roots C5 and C6 but occasionally lower)

All three syndromes may present with motor and/or sensory signs and symptoms. A mononeuropathy is usually due to a mechanical cause or old injury and is only rarely due to polyarteritis, diabetes mellitus, sarcoidosis or underlying carcinoma. Leprosy is very rare in Britain.

In an examination the examiner may indicate that a neurological examination is required. If not, it is important to ensure that there are no obvious bone, soft tissue or joint abnormalities. Quickly look at the face for Parkinsonism or signs of a stroke. Then try to identify the problem more precisely by asking the patient 'have you any loss of strength in your arms or hands' and 'have you had any numbness or tingling in your hands'. If you suspect a specific lesion, demonstrate the complete syndrome. If not, perform a methodical examination. The following scheme is recommended.

TABLE 2 Motor root values (including reflexes)

Joint	*Movement*	*Roots*	*Muscles*	*Reflex*
Shoulder	Abduction	C4,5	Supraspinatus	
	External rotation	C4,5	Infraspinatus	
	Adduction	C6,7,8	Pectorales	+
Elbow	Flexion	C5,6	Biceps	+
	Extension	C7,8	Triceps	+
	Pronation	C6,7		
	Supination	C5,6	Biceps	+
Wrist	Flexion (palmar): radia	C6,7		
	ulnar	C8		
	Extension (dorsiflexion)	C6,7		
Fingers (long)	Flexion	C8		+
and thumb	Extension	C7		
Fingers (short)	Flexion	T1		
Hips	Flexion	L1,2,3	Iliopsoas	
	Extension	L5 S1,2	Glutei	
	Adduction	L2,3	Adductors	+
	Abduction	L4,5 S1	Glutei and tensor fasciae latae	
Knee	Flexion	L5 S1,2	Hamstrings	
	Extension	L3,4	Quadriceps	+
Ankle	Dorsiflexion	L4,5	Anterior tibial	
	Plantar flexion	S1,2	Calf	+
	Eversion	L,5 S1	Peronei	
	Inversion	L4	Anterior and posterior tibial	
Toes	Flexion	S2,3		
	Extension	L5 S1		
Anus		S2,3,4,5		+
Cremaster		L1,2		+

NB 1 A simple aide memoire for the reflexes and controlling muscle groups is:

Ankle jerk	S1, 2	Biceps jerk	C5, 6
Knee jerk	L3, 4	Triceps jerk	C7, 8

2 All muscles on the 'back' of the upper limb (triceps, wrist extensors and finger extensors) are innervated by C7.

3 T1 innervates the small muscles of the hand.

Examine motor system (page 12)

Look for obvious muscle wasting and test the strength of the appropriate muscles if it is present. If there is wasting of the small hand muscles, note whether it is generalised (ulnar) or thenar (median). Note any fasciculation or tremor (page 21).
Test muscle tone—easiest at the elbow though cogwheel rigidity may be more obvious at the wrist.
Test muscle power in groups (table 2). 'I am going to test the strength of some of your muscles'.

Shoulder: C5

'Hold both arms out in front of you and close your eyes.' Look for drifting of one arm. This test checks not only weakness of the muscles at the shoulder but also for loss of position sense (when there is no evidence of weakness) and for lesions of the cerebral cortex (when the patient will not be aware of the drift, sometimes even when his eyes are open). You should also notice any winging of the scapula (nerve to serratus anterior, C5,6,7).

Elbow flexion: C5,6: biceps

'Bend your elbow up; don't let me straighten it.'

Elbow extension: C7: triceps

'Now straighten your elbows and push me away.'

Wrist and finger extension: C7

'Keep your wrist and fingers straight, don't let me bend them.'

Ulnar nerve tests (fingers)

Abduction of fingers ('spread your fingers apart'). Try to squash them together and note how much effort this requires. Note also the bulk of the first dorsal interosseous muscle.
Adduction of fingers. Hold a piece of paper between straight fingers ('don't let me pull it out').

Median nerve tests (thumb)

Abduction of thumb. The patient places his hand down flat with the palm upwards and the thumb overlying the forefinger. Ask the patient to lift the thumb vertically against resistance.
Opposition of thumb. 'Put your thumb and little finger together and stop me pulling them apart' with your forefinger.
NB Thenar adduction is ulnar.

Examine reflexes

See table 2, page 12.

Screen sensory system

For light touch (cotton wool) and pain (pin). As a minimum, you should test once each on the front and back of the upper and lower arms and on each digit. Check vibration and position senses on a finger.

Test coordination (page 19)

Finger–nose test with eyes open and eyes closed. You are looking for:
— intention tremor (cerebellar) with the eyes open. Past-pointing may be present
— loss of position sense. These patients need vision to know accurately where their hands are and con-

sequently cannot point back to your finger with their eyes closed whilst they can with their eyes open.

Dysdiadochokinesia ('tap rapidly on the back of your hand like this . . . and now the other side'). The test is more sensitive if the patient taps alternately with the front and backs of his fingers, i.e. pronates and supinates.

'Examine this patient's legs (neurologically)'

The commonest neurological lesions affecting chiefly the legs are:

Peripheral neuropathy (particularly diabetes mellitus)
Lumbar root lesions (prolapsed intervertebral disc)
Lateral popliteal nerve palsy (local pressure at the head of the fibula causes paralysis of the peroneal muscles and foot-drop. There is no sensory loss)
Spastic paraparesis

Try to identify the problem more precisely by asking the patient about any motor or sensory deficit which he has noticed. If no obvious lesion or syndrome is noted, perform a methodical examination. The following scheme is recommended.

Examine motor system (page 12)

Look for obvious muscle wasting and test the strength of the appropriate muscles if it is present. Note any fasciculation or tremor.

Test muscle tone. Lift the knee off the bed while the patient is relaxed and let it drop: observe how stiffly it falls. Alternatively, bend the knee to and fro with an irregular rhythm (so that he cannot consistently resist the movement).

Test muscle power in groups. 'I am going to test the strength of some of your muscles.'

Hip flexion: L1,2: iliopsoas

'Lift your leg up straight'—push down on his knee.

Knee flexion: L5, S1,2: hamstrings

'Bend your knee: don't let me straighten it'—keep one hand above his patella and pull on the ankle.

Knee extension: L3,4: quadriceps

'Keep your knee straight: don't let me bend it.' Put your forearm behind his knee and push down on the ankle.

Ankle plantar flexion: S1

'Push your foot down: don't let me push it up.'

Ankle dorsiflexion: L4,5

'Pull your foot up towards you and don't let me pull it down.'

Examine knee and ankle reflexes

Also for ankle and patella clonus if these are brisk. Practise the technique.

Examine plantar response

Gently but firmly draw a key or orange stick up the outer border of the sole and across the heads of the metatarsals.

Screen sensory system (page 17)

Light touch and pinprick
— once each on the medial and lateral sides of thigh and calf

— on the dorsum of the foot, tip of the big toe and lateral border of the foot
Vibration sense at the medial malleolus and if it is absent there, progress to the knee and hip. Test position sense at the big toes.

Reduction or absence of these two modalities suggests not only dorsal column loss (now usually due to B_{12} deficiency) but also may be part of a peripheral neuropathy (now usually diabetic). However in peripheral neuropathy you expect the other modalities to be reduced (pin and touch).

Test coordination (page 19)

Heel–shin test. 'Put your heel (touching his heel) on your knee (touching his knee) and slide it down your leg (sliding your finger down his shin).' This is primarily a test for intention tremor. If present you should look for other signs of cerebellar disorders (arms, eyes, speech). Then ask the patient to stand and stand near to him (to assist him if he stumbles). Look for:

Truncal ataxia while standing with his feet together (cerebellar lesion).
Rombergism (more unsteady with the eyes closed than with them open) which indicates loss of position sense (posterior column lesion).
Ataxic gait on walking heel to toe—note direction of fall (cerebellar lesion).
Abnormalities of gait on 'normal' walking (including turning).

Abnormality of gait (excluding orthopaedic disorders)

'*Watch this patient walk*'.

Hemiplegia

The leg is rigid and describes a semicircle with the toe scraping the floor (circumduction).
Aetiology: almost invariably a stroke.

Paraplegia

Scissors or 'wading through mud' gait.
Aetiology: multiple sclerosis, cord compression; rarely spastic diplegia.

Festinant gait of Parkinsonism

The patient is rigid, stooped and the gait shuffling. The arms tend to be held flexed and characteristically do not swing. He appears to be continually about to fall forwards.

Cerebellar gait

The patient walks on a wide base with the arms held wide. He is ataxic, veering and staggering towards the side of the disease.
Aetiology: usually multiple sclerosis. Cerebellar tumour (primary or secondary), the cerebellar syndrome of carcinoma (non-metastatic), and familial degenerations should be remembered.

Sensory (dorsal column) ataxia

A stepping and stamping gait. The patient walks on a wide base and looks at the ground. He tends to fall if he closes his eyes (Rombergism).
Aetiology: tabes dorsalis, diabetic pseudotabes, subacute combined degeneration of the cord, Friedreich's ataxia. Ataxia in multiple sclerosis may very rarely be of this kind (it is usually cerebellar).

Steppage (drop-foot) gait

There is no dorsiflexion of the foot as it leaves the ground and the affected legs (or leg) are lifted high to avoid scraping the toe.
Aetiology: usually lateral popliteal nerve palsy. Less commonly poliomyelitis or peroneal muscular atrophy. Very rarely heavy metal (lead, arsenic) poisoning.

Waddling gait

The pelvis drops on each side as the leg leaves the ground.
Aetiology: wasting disorders of the muscles of the pelvic girdle and proximal lower limb muscles (page 99).

Notes

Sensory testing (touch, pain, temperature, vibration and position)

It is important that the patient understands what sensations you are testing and what is an appropriate response on his part. Two of the stimuli conventionally used (vibration and position senses) are strange ones and the patient needs quickly to be taught about them. If you already have a good and professional system the following suggested scheme will be unnecessary.

Vibration sense

Ensure that the patient can recognise vibration by placing the vibrating tuning fork on to his sternum. 'Now with your eyes closed tell me if you can feel the vibration.' Start at the medial malleoli and work proximally to the patellae and anterior superior iliac spines comparing right with left (and with yourself if necessary).

Position sense

With the patient looking, hold a big toe or a finger by its sides (holding the top and bottom introduces light touch sensation). Move the toe away from the patient—'this is down'—and then towards the patient—'this is up. Now with your eyes closed, tell me whether I move the toe (finger) up or down.'

Light touch (cotton wool) and pinprick

These stimuli should be familiar to the patient. Appropriate instructions might be: 'Say *now* every time I touch you', and/or 'Say *pin* when you feel a pinprick'.

No person is entirely consistent in sensory testing and a few discrepant responses are to be expected and ignored. Increasingly inconsistent responses are often due to wandering attention. Areas of anaesthesia are easily produced by suggestion.

Ask the patient to outline for you the extent of any numbness or tingling that he feels: you may then confirm and define the extent of sensory loss with the cotton wool or a pin.

You must have an approximate idea of the dermatomes. These are best learnt visually by reference to a standard anatomy text. The following points may be found useful.

The neighbouring dermatomes over the front of the chest at the level of the first and second ribs are: **C4** and **T2** (C5–T1 supply the upper limb)
C7 supplies the middle finger front and back
T7 supplies the 'lower ribs'
T10 supplies the umbilical region
T12 is the 'lowest' nerve of the anterior abdominal wall
L1 supplies the inguinal region
L2–3 supply the anterior thigh (lateral and medial)
L4–5 supply the anterior shin (medial and lateral)
S1 supplies the lateral border of the foot and sole, and the back of the calf up to the knee

Patterns of sensory loss in limbs

Peripheral sensory neuropathy (page 97)

All modalities tend to be lost symmetrically and the loss is more marked in the lower limbs than in the upper. This pattern is seen in diabetes mellitus, carcinomatous neuropathy, vitamin B deficiency, and drugs or chemicals.

Spinal cord lesions

Dissociated sensory loss. Classically, vibration and position sense are carried in the dorsal columns which decussate in the medulla.

All other sensations are carried in the lateral spinothalamic tracts which decussate at the level of origin in the cord, or just above it. NB Do not confuse them with the 'lateral columns' which are the pyramidal tracts.

Dorsal column loss without spinothalamic loss occurs in both legs in vitamin B_{12} deficiency. (It also occurs in the ipsilateral leg in hemisection of the cord—Brown-Séquard syndrome.)

Spinothalamic loss without dorsal column loss occurs in syringomyelia, usually in the arms. (It also occurs in the contralateral leg in hemisection of the cord.)

Cerebral cortical lesions

Stereognosis and graphaesthesia are used to determine parietal sensory loss. They are tested by asking the patient to recognise, with the eyes closed, respectively objects placed in his hands, or numbers drawn on his palm. Two-point discrimination is also a sensitive test of parietal cortical function.

Motor testing (involuntary movement, tone, power, wasting, coordination)

First look for *involuntary movements* at rest—tremor or choreoathetosis (page 21).

Then test *muscle tone* (before testing for power since this may leave the patient tense). Engage the patient in conversation so that he is relaxed. Tone is most easily assessed at the elbow (though cogwheel rigidity may be more obvious at the wrist) and at the knee. Move the joint to and fro with an irregular rhythm so that the patient cannot consistently resist the movement.

Ask the patient which movements he has found weak and then try to confirm his observations and look for related deficiencies.

Test *muscle power* in groups. 'I am going to test the strength of some of your muscles.' Then make your instructions slow and precise. Look and feel the bulk of the muscles as you test their strength.

You must have an approximate idea of the root values of at least certain movements so that you can perform a rapid 'motor root' screen. You can check the motor roots of the upper limb by testing:

shoulder abduction	C5
elbow flexion	C5,6
wrist extension	C6,7
finger flexion (terminal phalanx)	C8
opposition of thumb or splaying of fingers	T1

and of the lower limb by testing:

hip flexion	L2,3
knee extension	L3,4
foot dorsiflexion	L4,5
knee flexion	L5, S1
foot plantar flexion	S1,2

You must know the root values of the common reflexes (see table 2, page 12).

Patterns of motor loss in limbs

Lower motor neurone lesion

There is reduced or absent power with marked muscle wasting in the established lesion. The muscles are flaccid and the reflexes absent. In the foot there is no plantar response. The lesion affects the motor distribution of the spinal root or peripheral nerve.

Upper motor neurone lesion

There is reduced or absent power with relatively little wasting. The muscle tone and reflexes are increased and clonus often present. In the foot the plantar response is upgoing. There tends to be a characteristic distribution of weakness. Thus in the arms weakness is more marked in elbow extension than flexion and wrist dorsiflexion than palmar flexion. In the legs it is more marked in hip flexion, knee flexion and ankle dorsiflexion than in their antagonist movements. This is most easily remembered by recalling the posture of the limbs in the hemiplegic patient when he is walking.

Isolated peripheral nerve lesions

Median nerve lesion (carpal tunnel syndrome)

These patients may complain of tingling and numbness of the fingers and/or weakness of the thumb, worst on waking. It is often unilateral at the time of presentation.

You should examine for:
— thenar wasting and weakness of thumb abduction and opposition
— sensory loss, palmar surface only, of the thumb and two and a half fingers (i.e. to the middle of the ring finger)
— Tinel's sign. Percuss over the flexor retinaculum to elicit tingling in the same area
— evidence of pregnancy (or ask if she is on the 'pill'), myxoedema, rheumatoid arthritis and acromegaly. It is commonest in middle-aged women with none of these

NB Bilateral carpal tunnel syndrome is commonly due to rheumatoid arthritis. In the examination also consider cervical spondylosis (T1 lesion), motor neurone disease and syringomyelia if you are in doubt about the diagnosis.

Ulnar nerve lesion

The ulnar nerve supplies all the small muscles of the hand except the thenar eminence (but including adductor pollicis). These patients may complain of tingling or 'deadness' and/or weakness of the ring and little fingers. You should examine for:
— flattening of the contours of the hand due to muscle wasting. The ring and little fingers are held slightly flexed, and there is loss of power in abduction and adduction of the fingers (claw hand)
— sensory loss, back and front, over the one and a half ulnar fingers (i.e. little finger and half the ring finger)
— 'filling in' of the ulnar groove at the elbow and limitation of movement at the elbow. X-rays of the elbow may show osteoarthritis or local fracture

NB If you are in doubt about the diagnosis consider a lesion in the neck and look for restricted movements of the cervical spine (T1 lesion).

Radial nerve lesion

These are rare and result from local pressure (e.g. an arm over the back of the chair) which causes wrist-drop. Sensory loss may be very limited because the median and ulnar nerve territories overlie the radial territory.

Lateral popliteal palsy

The lateral popliteal nerve supplies the peroneal muscles which dorsiflex and evert the foot. The nerve may be damaged as it passes over the head of the fibula resulting in foot-drop. There is no sensory loss.

Incoordination

There are two chief patterns of incoordination, one dominated by a failure in controlling accurate limb movements (cerebellar) and the other dominated by an ignorance of limb position without visual or cutaneous clues (proprioceptive).

Cerebellar incoordination

'*Demonstrate some cerebellar signs.*' The signs are ipsilateral to a destructive lesion.

Finger–nose test The intention tremor is more marked when the patient has to stretch to reach your finger. If you keep your finger still and then ask the patient to repeat the test with the eyes closed, you may bring out 'past-pointing'—deviation of the patient's finger consistently to one side of your own (the same side as the cerebellar lesion). The tremor is not altered by closing the eyes. The heel–shin test has similar significance. Remember that muscular weakness alone may make the patient unsteady in these tests, and that this may resemble an intention tremor.
Dysdiadochokinesia (page 14) Rapid repetitive alternating movements of the wrists are irregular in both force and rate in cerebellar disease. Supination/pronation tests are more sensitive than flexion/extension ones.
Nystagmus (page 9) is more marked on looking towards the side of the lesion. Do not get the patient to focus on an object too far laterally or too near to the eyes.
Dysarthria Slurred and explosive, sometimes as if drunk.
Truncal ataxia The gait is reeling and staggering as if drunk with a tendency to fall to the side of the lesion. Heel–toe walking may accentuate the sign. It may be the sole cerebellar sign in midline (vermis) cerebellar lesions.

Causes of cerebellar signs

Disseminated sclerosis
Brain-stem vascular disease
Anticonvulsant therapy may produce gross nystagmus
Rarely brain-stem tumours, posterior fossa tumours (especially acoustic neuroma), degenerative disorders (e.g. alcoholism and hereditary ataxias) and the cerebellar syndrome of bronchial carcinoma

Proprioceptive incoordination (dorsal column loss)

The signs are ipsilateral to the lesion. When there is loss of proprioception, the patient can still place the limbs accurately by looking at them. Incoordination is therefore only obviously present when the eyes are closed. Tests are performed with the eyes open and the eyes closed. When the patient's coordination is worse with the eyes closed than with them open, he is said to have loss of position sense (i.e. dorsal column loss or proprioceptive loss). If there is dorsal column loss (vibration and position senses) but no spinothalamic loss (pain and temperature senses), there is said to be a 'dissociated sensory loss'. (This term also describes the rarer reverse situation of spinothalamic loss without dorsal column loss.) Dissociated sensory loss is evidence of spinal cord disease.

Finger–nose test and heel–shin test are normal when the patient can see but incoordinate when he cannot. Rombergism is present when the patient, standing with his feet together, is more unsteady with his eyes closed than when they are open.

The gait is ataxic and the patient walks on a wide base with high steps.
Muscle tone and the tendon reflexes may be diminished.

Causes of dorsal (posterior) column loss

Subacute combined degeneration of the cord. This may progress sufficiently to give dorsal column loss—peripheral neuropathy is the earliest manifestation. It is very rare in the clinic but patients treated with vitamin B_{12} may be seen in examinations (when the peripheral neuropathy may be considerably recovered though the spinal cord lesions are not).
Tabes dorsalis. This is now very rare though a few cases in older individuals may appear in the examinations.
Hemisection of the cord (page 17).

Tremor

'Look at this patient's tremor.'

There are four common tremors:

1 The resting tremor of Parkinsonism, maximal at rest and with emotion and inhibited by movement.
2 Essential tremor. This is an accentuation of physiological tremor present at rest and brought out by placing a sheet of paper on the outstretched fingers. It occurs in thyrotoxicosis when it is associated with warm moist palms, exophthalmos and tachycardia. Anxiety states may produce a similar tremor. It is occasionally familial. In alcoholics, the tremor is often reduced by ethanol and exacerbated by its withdrawal. It increases with age.
3 The intention tremor of cerebellar disease (finger–nose test). It is reduced or absent at rest and associated with past-pointing, nystagmus, and ataxia including truncal ataxia. It is rare except in multiple sclerosis.
4 Flapping tremor occurs in hepatic precoma and in the CO_2 retention of respiratory failure.

Athetosis refers to slow sinuous, writhing movements of the face and limbs, especially the distal parts. In torsion spasm (dystonia) the movements are similar but slower and affect the proximal parts of the limbs. The movements are purposeless. Both occur in lesions of the extrapyramidal system. They are rare.
Choreiform movements are non-repetitive, involuntary abrupt jerky movements of face, tongue and limbs. They may be localised or generalised (both are rare). They occur in lesions of the extrapyramidal system. Rheumatic chorea (Sydenham's chorea, page 95) is now very rare. Huntington's chorea is inherited (page 95).

Eyes

'Look at these eyes.'

Unless specifically instructed (i.e. *'Look at the pupils'* or *'Look at the fundi'*) a complete examination is required. There may be obvious exophthalmos (page 129) or squint (page 6): otherwise follow the scheme in table 3.

Optic fundus First check that the ophthalmoscope is adjusted to suit your own eyes (usually no lens) and that the

TABLE 3 Examination of the eyes

Observe	*For*	*Clinical association*
Eyelids	Xanthelasma	Diabetes, atheroma, myxoedema, primary biliary cirrhosis
	Ptosis	(page 4)
Cornea	Corneal arcus	Age and hyperlipidaemias
	Calcification	Hypercalcaemia (rare)
	Kayser–Fleisher rings	Wilson's disease (very rare)
Visual fields to confrontation (page 5)		
Eye movements (page 6)	Failure of lateral movements	Sixth nerve palsy
	Failure of down and in movement	Fourth nerve palsy
	Failure of other movements (with ptosis and fixed dilatation of pupil)	Third nerve palsy
	Failure of all movements	Usually myasthenia
	Nystagmus (page 9)	Cerebellar, vestibular or brain-stem lesion
Pupils	Dilatation	Homatropine or part of third nerve lesion, Holmes–Adie syndrome
	Constriction	Horner's syndrome, Argyll Robertson pupil Morphine
NB *Check light and accommodation reflexes (page 7). Glass eyes have neither*		
Iris (with ophthalmoscope)	Iritis (page 24)	
Lens	Lens opacities or cataract (shine light obliquely across lens); this is often missed and may make examination of the fundus difficult or impossible	Senility, diabetes, trauma. Rare causes include congenital, rubella syndrome, hypoparathyroidism, dystrophia myotonica and drugs (chloroquine and steroids)
Fundus (page 22)		

light beam is circular and bright. It is useful to start by observing the patient's eye through the ophthalmoscope from about two feet to see if there is any loss of the red light reflex (indicating opacities in the translucent media which may cause difficulty when trying to inspect the retina). You should interpret the fundal findings in the light of the patient's refractive errors (you may discover this from a rapid look at his spectacles) and you should use a similar lens in the ophthalmoscope. Short-sighted (myopic) patients have a negative (concave) lens in their spectacles (objects look smaller through them) and tend to have a deep optic cup and some temporal pallor of the disc. Long-sighted patients (hypermetropic) have a positive lens in their spectacles (convex, magnifying) and their optic disc tends to look small and have ill-defined margins. You should be able to recognise and comment on the following.

Myelinated nerve fibres A normal variant in which there are bright white streaky irregular patches, usually adjacent to the disc margin.

Diabetic fundus This is characterised by:

— microaneurysms (most frequent temporal to the macula), and blot haemorrhages

— changes secondary to vessel occlusion (ischaemia): soft exudates (cotton wool) and flame haemorrhages

— proliferative changes: new vessel formation which is followed by fibrosis and its sequelae, vitreous haemorrhage (obscuring the retina) and retinal detachment

— exudative changes: hard exudates and oedema

NB Glaucoma, cataract and optic atrophy are all commoner in diabetes.

Hypertensive fundus There are usually the changes of arteriosclerosis (grades 1 and 2 including tortuosity, arterial nipping, varying vessel calibre). Hypertension produces haemorrhages and exudates (grade 3) and more severe disease in addition produces papilloedema (grade 4, malignant hypertension). Note that the subhyaloid haemorrhage sometimes seen in subarachnoid haemorrhage may indicate underlying hypertension.

Papilloedema — raised intracranial pressure (tumour, abscess, meningitis, and the rare benign intracranial hypertension)

— malignant hypertension

— rarely, optic retrobulbar neuritis, venous obstruction, and hypercapnia of respiratory failure

Optic atrophy — secondary to papilloedema (disc edge blurred)

— primary (disc margin sharp with cup and cribriform plate well defined) occurs after retrobulbar neuritis (almost invariably multiple sclerosis) and from optic nerve pressure (e.g. pituitary tumour), in diabetes mellitus and in retinal artery thrombosis

Exudates and haemorrhages

Chiefly in hypertension and diabetes mellitus but also in uraemia, acute leukaemia, raised intracranial pressure, severe anaemia and hypercapnia.

Uveitis, iritis and choroiditis

The uveal tract comprises the choroid (posterior uvea), the ciliary body and the iris (anterior uvea). Uveitis occurs alone or as part of other generalised disease, some of which tend to involve either the iris (iritis, iridocyclitis or anterior uveitis) or the choroid (choroiditis or posterior uveitis), although virtually all may involve both. The causes are listed in table 4.

TABLE 4 Causes of iritis and choroiditis

*Iritis**	*Choroiditis*
Diabetes Sarcoid Ankylosing spondylitis Reiter's syndrome Ulcerative colitis and Crohn's disease (Rare causes include gonorrhoea, toxoplasma, brucella, tuberculosis, syphilis)	Idiopathic (i.e. unexplained), the most frequent in this country Toxoplasmosis Diabetes Sarcoid (Rare causes include toxocara, tuberculosis, syphilis)

* Recognised by vascularisation around the corneal limbus with a 'muddy' iris

Limbs (joints and peripheral vascular disease)

Legs

In the legs the usual abnormalities are neurological or vascular. Diabetes may cause both. The skin and joints should also be considered. Diabetes mellitus is very common and peripheral neuropathy its most common neurological manifestation. Many neurological diseases such as multiple sclerosis and strokes are chronic and appear in examinations. Relatively rare causes include the results of spinal injury or prolapsed intervertebral discs (cervical or lumbar), peripheral nerve damage and subacute combined degeneration. Even patients with motor neurone disease or a carcinomatous neuropathy may be well enough to be included. Syringomyelia and the myopathies are rare but have a better prognosis and are often available for examinations.

'Look at these legs'

Unless attention is directed towards a particular part of the legs such as the feet or knees, the following scheme is recommended.

Look for obvious *joint deformity*. Also note *bone deformity*, leg shortening and external rotation of fractured neck of femur, Paget's disease, previous rickets (rare except in the elderly), the results of previous poliomyelitis and syphilis (Charcot's joints).
Note if *oedema* is present.
Look at the *skin* (purpura, rash, ulcer) and note cyanosed or necrotic toes.
Peripheral vasculature: compare and assess the temperature of the dorsa of both feet, noting any interdigital infection and loss of hair. If the feet are cold, feel the dorsalis pedis and posterior tibial pulses, and if these are absent, proceed to feel for the popliteal and femoral pulses, and listen for arterial bruits. Ask the patient about a history of intermittent claudication. If there are ulcers ask the patient if they are painful. If not, there is a neuropathy, most frequently diabetic.
Then examine the legs neurologically (page 14).

Arms

In the arms the usual abnormalities seen are of the joints or the nervous system. The commonest neurological conditions in the upper limbs are the results of multiple sclerosis, stroke or peripheral nerve compression. Rarer conditions which may be seen in examinations are the results of pressure on the cord or brachial plexus (remember cervical spondylosis and cervical rib), motor neurone disease, syringomyelia and dystrophia myotonica.

***'Look at the arms'* (upper limb, hands)**

This may mean primarily the hand which should always be inspected first or the joints (including elbow or wrist). Usually it means a neurological examination, but:

Observe any tremor at rest (Parkinsonism).
Note any joint swelling (ask if they are painful before touching them) and any associated muscle wasting (often marked in rheumatoid arthritis).
Observe the skin for purpura (page 69) and signs of liver disease (liver palms, spider naevi and Dupuytren's contracture).
Look at the fingers and nails for clubbing (page 42), cyanosis, nicotine-staining, anaemia, and the splinter haemorrhages and Osler's nodes of subacute bacterial endocarditis. (Splinter haemorrhages are often occupational and not diagnostic, and Osler's nodes very rare.)
Glance at the patient's face which may provide a further clue, e.g. pallor, exophthalmos, Parkinsonian facies, spider naevi, tophi on the ears in gout.

If there is evidence of joint disease, look for:

Rheumatoid arthritis (page 116)

This is usually symmetrical, with ulnar deviation at the metacarpophalangeal joints, spindling of the fingers, muscle wasting, and swelling of the joints except the terminal interphalangeal joints. Look for the changes of psoriatic arthritis, including pitting of the nails with involvement of the terminal interphalangeal joints and psoriasis at the elbows. Rheumatoid arthritis may produce gross deformity. Nodules may present at the elbow and down the radius.

Osteoarthritis (osteoarthrosis)

Asymmetrical and most frequently seen in old people as Heberden's nodes—osteophytes around the terminal interphalangeal joints. Any joint of the hand may be involved but it involves especially the terminal interphalangeal and first carpometacarpal joints.

Gout (page 161)

May attack any joint of the body. It may be monoarticular or polyarticular. Usually the metatarsophalyngeal joint of the big toe is first involved. It becomes red, hot, shiny and tender. There is often marked soft tissue swelling and there may be superficial tophi over joints and in the cartilage of the ear. Ask about thiazide diuretics and note any polycythaemia.

NB Osteo-, rheumatoid and gouty arthritis may mimic each other but rheumatoid is usually symmetrical.

If a rapid examination as above reveals no abnormality, proceed to examine the upper limbs neurologically (page 11).

Head and neck

Head *'Look at this patient's face.'*

This somewhat unsatisfactory question usually implies either that the patient has an abnormal facies (or neck), or that he has abnormal facial movements, or poverty of movement (Parkinsonism and myxoedema). If the abnormality is not immediately obvious, the following check list of the systems which may be involved might be found useful.

Endocrine	Cushing's (iatrogenic) Myxoedema; thyrotoxicosis Acromegaly Addison's disease
Neurological	Stroke Ptosis and ocular palsies Bell's palsy Parkinsonism Cerebellar signs (eyes and speech) Myopathy (including dystrophia myotonica with cataract and baldness) Myasthenia
Cardiorespiratory	Cyanosis Mediastinal obstruction Congestive cardiac failure
Gastrointestinal	Jaundice and spider naevi Peutz-Jegher syndrome Hereditary haemorrhagic telangiectasia Anaemia (white hair and lemon yellow skin of pernicious anaemia)
Collagen disease	SLE (butterfly rash) Scleroderma (mouth, fingers) Dermatomyositis
Skin diseases	Acne vulgaris Rosacea Psoriasis

Neck *'Examine the neck.'*

This usually means either that there is enlargement of the lymph glands, or that a goitre is present, or that the jugular venous pressure is raised (page 47).

Cervical lymphadenopathy (page 74)

This is often easier to feel from behind. *Do not forget the occipital group.* If lymphadenopathy is present, check for local infection or neoplasm over the whole head and neck, and in the mouth and pharynx. Check the nose for bloody discharge and patency.

Glands in the root of the neck may be symptomatic of pulmonary, abdominal (including the testes) or breast malignancy.

Cervical glands may be the presenting symptom of a generalised lymphadenopathy. Further examination should include all lymph gland groups and palpation for enlargement of the liver and spleen. Consider malignant disease, the reticuloses, leukaemia, local sepsis, tuberculosis and infectious mononucleosis.

Enlarged thyroid

'Look at this patient's thyroid gland.'

This means that the patient has a goitre. It is unlikely that the patient is hyperthyroid but this must first be excluded by looking for the evidence such as eye signs, tachycardia or fast atrial fibrillation, quick jerky movements, hot and sweaty hands. Similarly you should check for the characteristic facies, slow movements and croaking voice of hypothyroidism, and proceed to test the ankle jerks if indicated.

Look at the patient's neck and ask him to swallow. Palpate the gland first from behind and then from the front. The patient's chin should be flexed to relax the tissues (untrained patients invariably extend the neck). If the patient has to swallow more than two or three times, you should give him a glass of water. Pay special attention to:

Character — Diffuse or nodular. In Graves disease and autoimmune thyroiditis and early simple goitre, the gland is diffusely enlarged. It is nodular in toxic nodular goitre, late simple goitre and carcinoma. Look especially for a single nodule.

Tenderness — This is unusual except in viral thyroiditis (very rare) and occasionally in autoimmune thyroiditis and carcinoma.

Mobility — Attachment to surrounding tissues suggests carcinoma.

Retrosternal extension — Feel in the suprasternal notch.

Lymph glands — An enlarged chain of lymph glands suggests papillary carcinoma.

Trachea — Central or displaced.

Thyroidectomy scar — If present you should suspect hypothyroidism or hypoparathyroidism. Perform Chvostek's sign (may be present in normal people) and Trousseau's test.

You should ask about pressure symptoms, any drugs (especially medicines containing iodine) and take a family history for inborn enzyme deficiency. If you are asked to suggest investigations you should consider:

Free thyroxine index (page 140) (or PBI)
Tests for thyroid autoantibodies
ESR
X-rays for tracheal deviation or compression
Laryngoscopy
Radioiodine tests including a scan

NB The observed incidence of simple goitre, autoimmune thyroiditis and carcinoma in one series was 89%, 10% and 1% respectively. Carcinoma is suggested by a hard fixed gland, lymph gland enlargement, pressure symptoms and evidence of metastasis to bone.

Abdomen

'*Examine this patient's abdomen.*'

The most usual abnormality seen in examinations is a palpable mass or the presence of free fluid, or both. These are relatively rare in the clinic, where the clinician more commonly elicits only areas of maximum tenderness. The commonest conditions suitable for examination purposes are diseases which are chronic and produce enlargement of the spleen or liver such as the chronic leukaemias, myelofibrosis or chronic liver disorders. Other palpable masses include renal swellings, especially polycystic kidneys. Neoplastic or inflammatory swellings may be present and it is usually not possible to distinguish between these on physical examination alone. Patients with acute abdominal disease virtually never appear in clinical examinations. Remember always to look before palpation, to have warm hands and to palpate gently so as to gain the patient's confidence and avoid hurting him. You should ask the patient to let you know if you do hurt him and look at his face periodically during palpation, especially if you elicit guarding.

A complete examination of the alimentary system involves inspection of the tongue, mouth, teeth and throat but this is rarely required in examinations. Loss of weight, clubbing, jaundice, anaemia and spider naevi should always be looked for. Hence:

Look at the hands especially for clubbing, liver palms, spider naevi and Dupuytren's contracture.
Inspect the eyes and conjunctivae for anaemia and jaundice.
Lie the patient flat (one pillow) with arms by his sides. Observe the abdomen for:
— general swelling with eversion of the umbilicus in ascites and visible enlargement of internal organs (liver, spleen, kidneys, gall bladder, stomach (in pyloric stenosis), urinary bladder and pelvic organs) on normal respiration
— abnormal veins or abnormally distended veins usually in cirrhosis with the direction of flow away from the umbilicus (portal hypertension). The flow is upwards from the groin in inferior vena cava obstruction
— scars of previous operations, striae, skin rashes and purpura
— pigmentation localised or generalised
— distribution of hair is important in endocrine disorders

— visible peristalsis suggests obstruction except in very thin patients

If general swelling is present suspect ascites and examine for shifting dullness and ballotment of the liver (dipping). A fluid thrill may be demonstrable in large effusions.

Palpate for internal organs. It is often of value to percuss the liver and spleen areas initially to avoid missing the lower border of a very large liver or spleen. It is essential to start palpation in the right iliac fossa and work upwards towards the hepatic and splenic areas.

Liver Upper border: fourth rib to fifth space on percussion. Moves down on inspiration. If enlarged the edge may be tender, regular or irregular, hard, firm or soft. Note if it is pulsatile (tricuspid incompetence).

Spleen Smooth rounded swelling in left subcostal region, usually with a distinct lower edge (as compared with the kidney). It enlarges diagonally downward and across the abdomen in line with the ninth rib. The examining hand cannot get above the swelling. Percussion over it is dull. There is a notch on the swelling. It may occasionally be more easily palpated with the patient lying on his right side.

Kidneys They are palpable in the loin bimanually, i.e. most easily felt by pushing the kidney forwards from behind on to the anterior palpating hand. They move slightly downwards on inspiration. Percussion is resonant over the kidney. The examining hand can get above the swelling. The right kidney can often be felt in thin normal persons.

Abnormal masses Palpate for abnormal masses particularly in the epigastrium (gastric carcinoma) and suprapubically (an overfilled bladder and ovarian and uterine masses are often missed) and note colonic swellings. The descending colon is commonly palpable in the left iliac fossa (faeces may be indented). The abdominal aorta which is pulsatile and bifurcates at the level of the umbilicus, is easily palpable in thin and lordotic patients. This is very seldom the only evidence of aortic aneurysm.

Complete the examination by feeling for inguinal and (if relevant) cervical glands (the drainage from the testes is to the para-aortic and cervical glands), the femoral pulses and listening for renal bruits and bowel sounds.

External genitalia It is essential to examine them in practice but rarely required in examinations.

Rectal examination Essential in practice as rectal carcinoma is common but should not be performed in examinations unless suggested by the examiner. Some examiners will expect the candidates to comment on its desirability particularly in the presence of gastrointestinal disease.

Notes

Splenomegaly

1 There are two common causes of a very large spleen:
— chronic myeloid leukaemia
— myelofibrosis
Other causes rare in this country but very common on a worldwide basis are malaria and kala-azar.
2 There are two additional causes of a moderately enlarged spleen (2–4 fingers = 4–8 cm):
— reticuloendothelial disease, e.g. Hodgkin's disease and chronic lymphatic leukaemia
— cirrhosis with portal hypertension
3 But many causes of a slightly enlarged spleen:
— any of the above
— glandular fever, brucella and infectious hepatitis (unlikely in the examination)
— subacute septicaemia including subacute bacterial endocarditis and in many infections
4 Other rare causes include amyloid (rheumatoid arthritis the commonest cause; chronic sepsis is less common), sarcoid, collagen disease and storage diseases. Other blood disorders which give splenic enlargement are idiopathic thrombocytopenia, congenital spherocytosis and polycythaemia rubra vera.

Hepatomegaly

There are three common causes:
— congestive cardiac failure
— secondary carcinomatous deposits
— cirrhosis (usually alcoholic)
Other causes include:
— infections—glandular fever, infectious hepatitis
— leukaemia and reticuloendothelial disorders
— tumours (primary hepatoma, amoebic and hydatid cysts)
— amyloid, sarcoid and storage diseases
— primary biliary cirrhosis (large regular liver in women with jaundice and xanthelasmata)
— haemochromatosis (look for pigmentation)

Hepato-splenomegaly

The list is much the same as for splenomegaly alone since the commonest causes are chronic leukaemia, cirrhosis with portal hypertension, reticuloendothelial disease and myelofibrosis but each of these is usually associated with other clinical signs.

Palpable kidneys

The left kidney is nearly always impalpable but the lower pole of a normal right kidney may be felt in thin people. *Unilateral enlargement* may result from a local lesion, e.g. carcinoma, hydronephrosis, cysts or from hypertrophy of a single functioning kidney. *Bilateral enlargement*, usually gross, occurs in polycystic disease (the liver may also be enlarged) and very rarely in bilateral hydronephrosis and amyloidosis. Following *renal transplantation* a kidney may be palpable in the iliac fossa, and the patient may be Cushingoid in appearance due to steroid therapy. Look for scars of previous renal surgery.

Mass in right subcostal region

It may be difficult or impossible to decide the nature of a mass in this region which may be derived from liver (including Riedel's lobe), colon, kidney or occasionally gall bladder. If you are uncertain, say so giving the most likely possibilities and the reasons for your conclusions. This will determine the approach to further investigation, which should start with simple studies:

Urine for haematuria and proteinuria
Stool for occult bleeding
Plain X-ray of the abdomen

Then proceed as indicated by clinical suspicion and the results of simple studies to:

IVP
Barium enema
Liver function tests, scan and needle biopsy
Cholecystogram

Laparotomy is sometimes necessary without a preliminary definite diagnosis.

Ascites

The common causes are:

— intra-abdominal neoplasms (remember gynaecological lesions)
— hepatic cirrhosis with portal hypertension (relatively late in the disease)
— congestive cardiac failure and constrictive pericarditis (rare)
— nephrotic syndrome (and other low albumin states)
— tuberculous peritonitis (rare in this country, but should be suspected in Asian and Irish patients)

Jaundice

Yellow colouration of the skin and sclerae is usually only apparent when the serum bilirubin is over 2 mg/100 ml. Keep in mind the three basic causes of jaundice (haemolytic, hepatocellular, and obstructive) but remember that the great majority of cases is due to:

Acute viral hepatitis (page 178): most of these patients are not admitted to hospital unless they are very ill or recovery is unduly prolonged
Infectious mononucleosis
Bile duct obstruction from gallstones or, more rarely, carcinoma of the head of the pancreas
Drugs (page 185)
Multiple secondary deposits of carcinoma in the liver (Clinical jaundice is not common but the bilirubin is frequently slightly raised)

Rare causes in Britain include haemolytic anaemia, congenital hyperbilirubinaemia, stricture or carcinoma of the major bile ducts or ampulla. Intrahepatic cholestasis (drugs, viral hepatitis, cholangitis and primary biliary cirrhosis) is more common.

'*Would you like to ask this (jaundiced) patient some questions?*'

Ask about

Age As a cause of jaundice, carcinoma becomes commoner and hepatitis less common as the patient grows older.
Injections or *transfusions* in the last six months (serum hepatitis). Remember drug addicts.
Contacts with jaundice and residence abroad.
Occupation Farm and sewage workers are at risk for leptospirosis.
Presence of dark urine and pale stools of biliary obstruction.
Recent drug therapy especially phenothiazines and 'the pill'.
Period of onset from first symptoms to jaundice. In general infectious hepatitis is short (1–3 weeks), carcinoma is medium (1–2 months) and cirrhosis is long. Serum hepatitis is 6 weeks to 6 months.
Alcohol consumption.
Recent abdominal pain, surgery, or a history of chronic dyspepsia may suggest cholecystitis, cholangitis, gallstones or pancreatic carcinoma. NB Halothane anaesthesia.
Family history if Gilbert's disease is suspected.

'*Would you like to examine this (jaundiced) patient?*'

Examine

Skin of the face and abdomen and assess the degree of jaundice—deep green suggests longstanding obstruction and pale lemon suggests haemolysis. The conjuctivae often show minor degrees of jaundice not evident elsewhere.
Face, upper chest and hands for spider naevi and the hands for Dupuytren's contracture, liver palms and clubbing. Note that xanthelasmata with deep jaundice in a middle-aged woman probably indicate primary biliary cirrhosis.
Neck for lymph node enlargement due to secondary spread of abdominal carcinoma.
Abdomen for:
— recent operation scars which suggest cholecystectomy or surgery for intra-abdominal carcinoma
— hepatomegaly. Irregular when infiltrated with carcinoma, tender in infectious and acute alcoholic hepatitis (and when enlarged in congestive heart failure) and sometimes with carcinoma
— splenomegaly in portal hypertension (and spherocytosis and infectious mononucleosis)
— palpable enlarged gall bladder suggesting bile duct obstruction due to carcinoma of the pancreas (rather than gallstones)
— ascites (which is probably more often due to gynaecological malignancy than to the portal hypertension of cirrhosis where it occurs late)

In obstructive jaundice the difficulty is usually to distinguish between benign causes (gallstone obstruction) and malignant causes (carcinoma of the head of the pancreas and multiple secondary deposits in the liver). Remember that infectious hepatitis often presents with the typical clinical picture of obstructive jaundice and that this may occasionally be persistent

'*What investigations would you perform?*'

The aims are:
— to discover the site of any obstruction to the outflow of bile and to determine whether operative interference is necessary
— to determine the degree of impairment of liver cell function and its cause, and to observe its course
— to eliminate rare causes such as haemolysis

Haematology

Including a reticulocyte count and Coombs test which may give evidence of haemolytic anaemia. A normal reticulocyte count virtually excludes haemolytic jaundice. A leucocytosis may indicate infection (cholangitis) or carcinoma. Abnormal mononuclear cells would suggest infectious mononucleosis (Paul Bunnell) or, possibly, viral hepatitis. Antinuclear factor (ANF) and smooth muscle antibodies may be positive in chronic aggressive hepatitis.

Urine analysis

Conjugated bilirubin renders the urine yellow and may be detected with Ehrlich's diazo reagent.
Urobilinogen is colourless but on standing the urine turns brown as urobilinogen is converted to urobilin (Ehrlich's aldehyde reagent) by oxidation.
Haemolytic jaundice is acholuric (no bilirubin in the urine) but the urine contains excess urobilinogen because excess bilirubin reaches the intestine and is re-excreted as urobilinogen.
Obstructive jaundice gives urine dark with excess bilirubin but a reduction of urinary urobilinogen because little or no bilirubin reaches the gut due to the obstruction and therefore cannot be reabsorbed or re-excreted. In the early stages of *hepatocellular jaundice* in acute viral hepatitis excess urobilinogen may sometimes be present before clinical jaundice becomes apparent. This is due to failure of the liver to take up the excess urobilinogen absorbed from the gut. With increasing severity, biliary obstruction develops and as bilirubin (conjugated) appears in the urine, it disappears from the gut and therefore urobilinogen disappears from the urine. The reciprocal effect also occurs during recovery.

Liver function tests

Protein synthesis

Serum albumin and prothrombin concentrations are reduced in longstanding liver disease. The latter is usually partially responsive to vitamin K.

Excretion of alkaline phosphatase

Serum alkaline phosphatase is characteristically more than 30 KA units in obstructive jaundice and lower in hepatocellular jaundice. A raised level in the absence of other signs of liver disease suggests the presence of malignant secondary deposits in the liver (or bone) or Pagets' disease. The normal range is higher in children.

Bilirubin metabolism Serum bilirubin is predominantly unconjugated in haemolytic jaundice and the other liver function tests usually normal. It is mainly conjugated in obstructive jaundice.

Hepatocellular damage Shown by raised serum level of aminotransferases (transaminases). Values of more than 500 international units/ml suggest viral hepatitis or toxic damage. Slight elevation is consistent with obstructive jaundice.

Mitochondrial antibodies Present in 90% of patients with primary biliary cirrhosis.

X-ray of abdomen May show gallstones and will put on record the size of the liver and spleen. *Barium swallow* and meal may show oesophageal varices or a distorted duodenal loop from pancreatic carcinoma. *Isotopic liver scans* may demonstrate 'holes' due to carcinomatous secondaries.

The following investigations may also be required:

Needle liver biopsy May provide the histological diagnosis sometimes even in focal lesions. In experienced hands it is a safe procedure provided the prothrombin concentration and platelet counts are normal. Vitamin K sometimes reverses the prolongation of the prothrombin time. Biliary obstruction is a relative contraindication because of the potential danger of causing biliary peritonitis.

Laparotomy May be the only way to distinguish between pancreatic carcinoma and gallstones.

Other investigative procedures

Pancreatic isotope scanning for carcinoma
Hypotonic duodenography for carcinoma of the pancreatic head
Percutaneous cholangiography for biliary obstruction
Peritoneoscopy
α fetoprotein estimation for hepatoma
Endoscopic retrograde cannulation of the pancreatic duct

Congenital non-haemolytic hyperbilirubinaemias These may explain persistent jaundice in the young after viral hepatitis or slight jaundice in the healthy. Up to 4% of the population may have Gilbert's syndrome in a mild form.

Gilbert's disease (autosomal dominant) Failure of uptake of bilirubin into the liver cell. The bilirubin is unconjugated and the urine acholuric. The serum bilirubin is usually less than 2 mg/100 ml. Treatment is not usually necessary.

Dubin–Johnson (autosomal dominant) Failure of excretion of bilirubin from the liver cell. Mimics obstructive jaundice. Liver biopsy and BSP tests are characteristic. It presents in adolescence and is rare compared with Gilbert's syndrome.

Crigler Najjar It is fatal in the first year of life and exceedingly rare.

'This patient is uraemic' (pages 166, 169)

'*Would you ask him some questions and examine him?*'

Ask about

Symptoms of renal failure—polyuria and nocturia, anorexia, nausea and vomiting, fatigue
Symptoms of urinary tract infection (dysuria), prostatism (poor stream), renal stone, acute nephritis (haematuria), and nephrotic syndrome (ankle oedema)
Drug therapy, especially analgesics

Past history: 'nephritis', diabetes and, in women, pelvic surgery (ureteric obstruction) and pre-eclamptic toxaemia
Family history: hypertension, polycystic kidneys and gout

Examine for

Brownish pallor of uraemic anaemia and the brown line near the ends of the finger nails. Bruising
Hypertension and its consequences, especially cardiac failure
Hypotension (especially postural) and reduced tissue turgor from dehydration
Hyperventilation from acidosis
Palpable kidneys (polycystic disease and hydronephrosis)
Ankle (or sacral) oedema of nephrotic syndrome or congestive failure
Signs of dialysis (abdominal scars, vascular shunts)
Peripheral neuropathy
Pericarditis is usually a late event in uraemia
Muscular twitching and uraemic frost are terminal manifestations
NB Urine for specific gravity, microscopy, protein and sugar.
Rectal examination for prostatic hypertrophy or carcinoma

Dysphagia

'*This patient complains of dysphagia; please question and examine him.*'

This term includes both difficulty with swallowing and pain on swallowing. The former symptom is more prominent in obstruction and the latter with inflammatory lesions. The patient can sometimes point to the site of the obstruction.

The history should be taken of the commoner causes remembering that previous reflux oesophagitis suggests peptic stricture and that recurrent chest infections occur with achalasia, bronchial carcinoma or pharyngeal pouches.

Examine the mouth and pharynx (pallor, carcinoma, neurological abnormalities), neck (goitre, and glands from carcinoma) and abdomen (carcinoma) with an initial glance at the hands for koilonychia.

Commonest causes

Carcinoma of the oesophagus and gastric fundus usually give a history of increasing painless difficulty with swallowing foods for the previous 2–3 months. The patient is frequently reduced to taking only soups and drinks by the time of presentation.
Peptic oesophagitis (with pain) proceeds to stricture with difficulty in swallowing.

Rarer causes

Achalasia of the cardia, mainly in the relatively young. Food 'sticks' and is regurgitated unchanged a short while later (without acid); 25% present with recurrent pulmonary infection.
External pressure. The oesophagus is slippery and symptoms of pressure from outside masses (especially carcinoma of the bronchus) are very seldom presenting ones. A retrosternal goitre large enough to produce dysphagia is usually obvious.

Very rare causes

Neurological diseases: myasthenia gravis (page 100) and bulbar palsies (page 11).
Plummer–Vinson syndrome (Paterson–Kelly–Brown). Sideropenic dysphagia usually occurs in middle-aged women who have iron deficiency anaemia, koilonychia and glossitis (perhaps due to a combination of iron and vitamin B deficiency). It may be associated with a postcricoid web which is precancerous.

NB Globus hystericus is diagnosed only after full investigation and when positive evidence of psychological stress exists.

Investigation

If you are asked to discuss investigation, suggest:

Radiology

Barium swallow
NB The postcricoid web occurs in the anterior oesophageal wall and appears on barium swallow as an anterior indentation at the top of the oesophagus at the level of the cricoid cartilage.

Oesophagoscopy and biopsy

May differentiate between benign peptic stricture and carcinoma.

Diarrhoea

Acute gastroenteritis with diarrhoea and vomiting is the second most common group of disorders affecting the community (second only to acute respiratory infections).

Aetiology

Infectious diarrhoea

Non-bacterial gastroenteritis, e.g. winter vomiting disease, travellers' diarrhoea and infant diarrhoea. The aetiology of these syndromes remains unknown with the exception of some outbreaks of infant diarrhoea due to specific serotypes of *E. coli*. They may be caused by viruses but none of the common enteroviruses (Coxsackie, polio, echoviruses) can be confidently incriminated. The vast majority of patients is successfully treated symptomatically.

Food poisoning. *Salmonella typhimurium* is responsible for 75% of bacterial food poisoning. Staphylococcal food poisoning results from eating precooked meats and is produced by the bacterial toxin.

Enteric fevers. Typhoid and paratyphoid must also be considered in patients returning from endemic areas.

Dysentery. Results from ingestion of organisms of the genus shigella (bacillary dysentery). Amoebic dysentery and giardiasis should also be considered in patients recently returned from the tropics.

Non-infectious diarrhoea

The following conditions must be considered:

Drugs, including purgatives (common), antibiotics and digoxin (both rare)
Diverticulitis (common)
Colonic carcinoma sometimes with spurious diarrhoea secondary to partial obstruction
'Spastic colon'/'nervous diarrhoea' (common)
Ulcerative colitis and Crohn's disease
Malabsorption syndromes post-vagotomy
Diabetes, thyrotoxicosis (rare)

'*This patient has developed diarrhoea. Would you question and examine him.*'

In hospital practice, the acute diarrhoeas are seen less frequently than in general practice. It is important to determine whether the recent attack is an isolated one, or part of a chronic or recurrent history. If it is isolated and acute, ask about travel and residence abroad, contact history, and if food poisoning is suspected, the time relationship to previous food and its effect on other eaters. If the diarrhoea is recurrent or chronic, ask about appetite, weight loss, abdominal pain, blood or mucus in the stools and drug ingestion including purgatives.

Examination

In practice a complete medical examination is required. In examinations note particularly weight loss, anaemia and clubbing (Crohn's disease). Look for abnormal abdominal masses (usually carcinoma but Crohn's disease should be suspected in young patients). Rectal examination and sigmoidoscopy should invariably be performed in chronic and recurrent diarrhoeas but these should not be attempted in examinations (though the examiner should be told of their necessity).

Investigation

'*How would you investigate this patient?*'

If it is a single episode of acute diarrhoea, perform:

Full blood count for anaemia and blood cultures for *S. typhi* and *S. paratyphi* particularly in travellers from abroad.
Stool to laboratory for examination for cysts, ova

and parasites and for culture (amoeba, typhoid and paratyphoid, and giardia).
Sigmoidoscopy particularly in suspected ulcerative colitis or carcinoma (or amoebic colitis). Biopsy and histology of local lesions seen on sigmoidoscopy may be diagnostic.

If acute diarrhoea remains undiagnosed or fails to respond to simple symptomatic remedies within a few days or in chronic diarrhoea, it is usually necessary (if not previously indicated) to proceed to further investigation, including:

Barium enema and, if necessary, barium meal and 'follow through.'
Investigation of 'non-infectious diarrhoea' (page 39).

NB Dysentery (bacillary and amoebic), typhoid and paratyphoid, and cholera are notifiable to the Public Health Authorities.

Bloody diarrhoea suggests:
— colonic carcinoma
— diverticular disease
— ulcerative colitis
— dysentery
— ischaemic colitis
but the most common cause of rectal bleeding is haemorrhoids.

Respiratory system

The most usual types of clinical case seen in examinations are those secondary to carcinoma of the bronchus or due to longstanding chronic disease. Asthma and chronic bronchitis are very common chronic disabilities. Bronchiectasis is still sufficiently common to appear in examinations. Pleural effusions are usually secondary to underlying carcinoma (primary or secondary) or infection. There are still many patients with chronic tuberculosis and fibrosis (mainly of the upper lobes) with mediastinal shift.

'*Examine the chest*' or '*Examine the lungs*'. This means '*Examine the respiratory system*' unless otherwise specified.

Observation

On approaching the patient note dyspnoea and cyanosis and any evidence of loss of weight.
Examine the hands for clubbing, tobacco-staining and feel for the bounding pulse of carbon dioxide retention if you suspect respiratory failure. Ask the patient his age and occupation (for occupational lung diseases) and assess hoarseness.
Quickly check the height of the jugular venous pressure, and the tongue for cyanosis.
Remove all clothes above the waist and observe the chest movements for symmetry and expansion (subtle differences are best seen from the end of the bed), and the use of accessory muscles in the neck and shoulders.

Palpation

Palpate for chest expansion comparing movements on both sides. *Diminished movements means pathology on that side.*
Palpate the trachea in the suprasternal notch (easier with the head partially extended). Deviation denotes fibrosis or collapse of the upper lobe or whole lung in the direction of deviation, or pneumothorax (or very rarely a large pleural effusion) on the other side.
NB Local causes may produce deviation in the absence of lung disease, e.g. goitre and spinal asymmetry. The position of the apex beat is rarely of use except in checking mediastinal shift.
Palpate for cervical lymphadenopathy.

Percussion

Percuss by moving down the chest comparing both sides. Stony dullness in the axilla usually indicates pleural effusion. Pleural thickening and collapse, consolidation, or fibrosis of the lung also give dullness.
NB Upper lobe fibrosis in an otherwise fit elderly patient is probably due to old tuberculosis.

Diminished movement with resonance usually means pneumothorax (or occasionally a large bulla).

Auscultation

Bronchial breathing occurs in consolidation including that at the top of effusions. Diminished breath sounds occur overlying an effusion, pleural thickening, pneumothorax and, in the obese, due to interposition of abnormal features between the lung surface and the stethoscope. Diminished breath sounds also occur with obstructed airways.

Added sounds are either *rhonchi* (wheezes) or *crepitations* (crackles). Wheezing is common in asthma and bronchitis but sometimes occurs in left ventricular failure. Crepitations are fine in pulmonary congestion and fibrosing alveolitis and coarse in the presence of excess bronchial secretions. *Tactile fremitus* and *vocal resonance* are both increased over areas of consolidation. Friction rubs occur with pleurisy.

NB Forced expiratory time can be measured by listening over the trachea (normally the vital capacity is expired in 3–4 seconds).

If allowed to question the patient, enquire about occupation, dyspnoea, chest pain, cough, sputum, and haemoptysis, allergy, family history of allergy and past history of mining. The diagnosis of chronic bronchitis is made on the history of 3 months productive cough in 2 consecutive years.

Notes

Clubbing

Associated with diseases in the lungs, heart and abdomen.

Carcinoma of bronchus
Pus in the pleura (empyema)
lung (abscess)
bronchi (bronchiectasis)
Fibrosing alveolitis

Cyanotic congenital heart disease
Subacute bacterial endocarditis

Crohn's disease (less commonly ulcerative colitis and cirrhosis)

Pleural effusion

Aetiology

Carcinoma: primary bronchus (the effusion implies pleural involvement) or secondary (commonly breast)
Cardiac failure
Pulmonary embolus and infarction
Tuberculosis
Other infections (pneumonia)
Rarely, lymphomas, systemic lupus erythematosus, rheumatoid arthritis and transdiaphragmatic spread of ascites including Meig's syndrome and peritoneal dialysis

NB Aspiration of the fluid is usually necessary both

for treatment and to assist diagnosis. A pleural biopsy should be performed at the same time. The fluid is routinely examined:
— microscopically for cells (including malignant cells) and bacteria including acid-fast bacilli
— bacterial culture
— protein content (3 g/100 ml approximately divides exudates from transudates)

Cyanosis

'Cyanosis' is a clinical description and refers to the blue colour of a patient. It is almost always due to the presence of an excess of reduced haemoglobin in the capillaries. Over 5 g/100 ml must be present before cyanosis is apparent. Thus in anaemia severe hypoxaemia may be present without cyanosis. Cyanosis may be central or peripheral.

'*Look at this (cyanosed) patient.*'
It is often difficult to tell whether cyanosis is present or not. Comparison of the colour of the patient's tongue or nail beds with your own nail beds (presumed to be normal) may help if both hands are warm.

'*Look at the patient's tongue.*'
If it is cyanosed, the cyanosis is central in origin and secondary to:
— chronic bronchitis and emphysema often with cor pulmonale
— congenital heart disease (cyanosis may be present only after exercise)
— polycythaemia
— massive pulmonary embolism
In central cyanosis there is always cyanosis at the periphery.

If the tongue is not cyanosed but the fingers, toes or ear lobes are, the cyanosis is peripheral and:
— physiological due to cold
— pathological in peripheral vascular disease (the cyanosed parts feel cold)

NB Left ventricular failure may produce cyanosis which is partly central (pulmonary) and partly peripheral (poor peripheral circulation).

Two rare causes of cyanosis which are not due to increased circulating reduced haemoglobin are the presence of methaemoglobin (and/or sulphaemoglobin) and methylene blue (from cardiac investigation—dye curves). These patients are relatively well and not dyspnoeic.

Methaemoglobinaemia and *sulphaemoglobinaemia* are usually the result of taking certain drugs, the commonest of which is phenacetin. Sulphonamides and primaquine (an 8-amino quinoline) may also be responsible.

Remember that cyanosis is an unreliable guide to the degree of hypoxaemia.

Blood gases

'Comment on these blood gases.'

The normal arterial values are:

$P\text{O}_2$	90–105 mmHg
$P\text{CO}_2$	36–44 mmHg
pH	7·36–7·44
Standard HCO_3^-	21–28 mEq/1

Look at the pH for acidosis or alkalosis.
Look at the $P\text{CO}_2$. If it is raised this may account for an acidosis of respiratory origin (respiratory failure). If it is reduced this may account for an alkalosis due to hyperventilation (pain, stiff lungs, anxiety and hysterical hyperventilation or artificial ventilation).
Look at 'standard HCO_3^-' (measured at $P\text{CO}_2$ of 40 mmHg, i.e. with simulated normal ventilation). If it is raised this accounts for a metabolic alkalosis. If it is reduced it accounts for a metabolic acidosis (usually renal or ketotic).
Look at $P\text{O}_2$. If it is high the patient is on added O_2. If low the patient has lung disease (the $P\text{CO}_2$ is usually high) or a right to left shunt.

Interpretation

$P\text{CO}_2$ reflects ventilation
$P\text{O}_2$ reflects gas transfer or shunts

Gas patterns

High $P\text{CO}_2$, low $P\text{O}_2$ Respiratory failure of chronic bronchitis.
Normal or *low $P\text{CO}_2$, low $P\text{O}_2$* Anoxia due to parenchymal lung disease with normal airways. These patients hyperventilate and hence lower the $P\text{CO}_2$ because of anoxia (and 'stiff lungs'), e.g. pulmonary embolism, fibrosing alveolitis. Another cause is 'venous admixture' from right to left shunts (e.g. Fallot).
Low $P\text{CO}_2$, normal $P\text{O}_2$ A common pattern seen usually after painful arterial puncture (causing hyperventilation), and in hysterical hyperventilation.

Ventilatory function tests (FEV$_1$, FVC, PEFR)

The simplest tests of lung function are spirometric. If a patient exhales as fast and as long as possible from a full inspiration into a spirometer, the volume expired in the first second is the FEV$_1$ (forced expiratory volume in one second) and the total expired is the FVC (forced vital capacity). Constriction of the major airways (e.g. asthma) reduces the FEV$_1$ more than the FVC. Restriction of the lungs (e.g. by fibrosis) reduces the FVC and, to a lesser degree, the FEV$_1$. The ratio of FEV$_1$ to FVC (FEV %) thus tends to be low in obstructive airways disease (e.g. chronic bronchitis and asthma) and normal or high in fibrosing alveolitis (page 219). It is best to see the shape of the actual curve as well as the figures derived from it.

The PEFR (peak expiratory flow rate) measures the rate of flow of exhaled air at the start of a forced expiration. It gives similar information to the FEV$_1$.

Normal values for all these tests vary with age, sex, size and race, and suitable nomograms should be consulted unless the changes observed are gross.

Cardiovascular system

There is no shortage of patients with cardiovascular disease who are suitable for inclusion in examinations. Patients with ischaemic heart disease have few physical signs and a diagnosis of angina of effort may have to be made on symptoms alone. Valvular disease, whether acquired or congenital, and septal defects often give rise to murmurs which may be diagnostic. The penalties for failing to elicit and describe and interpret these correctly are often disproportionate to their real importance in diagnosis and treatment. A cardiologist rarely reaches a final decision on physical signs alone unsupported by an electrocardiogram and chest X-ray. Patients with congestive heart failure and cases of myocardial infarction are very common in hospital and during the recovery phase may be sufficiently well to be included in an examination list.

Arterial pulse

'*Examine the (arterial) pulse.*'

If you are asked this, there is frequently an arrhythmia (often atrial fibrillation or multiple ectopic beats). Less commonly you may feel the very slow pulse of complete heart block or there may be a tachycardia such as that associated with thyrotoxicosis, the clinical features of which you may notice on approaching the patient (though not necessarily in the elderly).

Do not attempt to estimate the blood pressure from the pulse.

Examine either a radial or a brachial pulse—whichever you are familiar with assessing. Describe:

Approximate rate

Glance at the jugular venous pressure whilst counting, since this may give valuable additional information about cardiac rhythm and failure (see below).

Rhythm

Regular, basically regular with extra or dropped beats, or completely irregular. If it is clinically atrial fibrillation, remember that the pulse rate is different from the heart rate; you should listen at the apex.

Character (table 5)

These abnormalities fall into three categories:

Useful to confirm or assess other findings in the cardiovascular system (plateau, collapsing, small volume)
Rare and/or difficult (alternans, bisferiens and paradoxus)
Examination 'catch' (absent radial)

TABLE 5 Special pulses

Type	*Character*	*Seen in*
Plateau	Low amplitude, slow rise, slow fall	Aortic stenosis (relatively rare)
Collapsing (waterhammer)	Large amplitude, rapid rise and rapid fall	Aortic incompetence. Also severe anaemia, hyperthyroidism, AV shunt, heart block
Small volume	Thready	Low cardiac output due to obstruction: valve stenosis (TS, PS, MS, AS) or pulmonary hypertension Shock
Alternans	Alternate large and small amplitude beats rarely noted in pulse; usually on taking blood pressure (note doubling in rate as mercury falls)	Left ventricular failure
Bisferiens	Double-topped	AS with AI (rare)
Paradoxus	Pulse volume decreases excessively with inspiration (of little diagnostic value)	Cardiac tamponade, constrictive pericarditis, severe inspiratory airways obstruction (chronic bronchitis)
Absent radial		Congenital anomaly (check brachials and BPs) Tied off at bypass surgery Blalock shunt Arterial embolism (usually AF)

Notes

The state of the vessel wall does not necessarily correlate with the state of the arteries elsewhere.

It takes little time to check if the left radial (or brachial) pulse is present.

If you think the patient may have hypertension, you should look for radio-femoral delay (aortic coarctation).

If the character of the pulse is abnormal you should ask whether you may take the blood pressure, to estimate the pulse pressure (and to check alternans).

NB The rate and rhythm are relatively easy to assess, but the character of the pulse extremely difficult.

Neck veins

'*Look at the veins of the neck*' ('*Examine the jugular venous pressure*', table 6).

You should comment on the *vertical* height of the top of the column of blood above the sternal angle. The patient will usually be lying at 45° and the neck should be relaxed. The deep venous pulse is seen as a welling up between the heads of sternomastoid in the front of the neck on expiration, and is a better guide to right atrial pressure than the superficial venous pulse which may be obstructed by the soft tissues of the neck. If you can find neither:

Look at the other side of the neck.

TABLE 6 Jugular venous pressure

Character	Compression of neck	Conclusion
Non-pulsatile	No change in jugular venous pressure	Superior mediastinal obstruction (usually carcinoma of bronchus) or platysmal compression
Pulsatile	Jugular vein fills and empties	Right heart failure Expiratory airways obstruction (asthma and bronchitis) Cardiac tamponade (very rare)

Notes
Large 'a' wave (corresponds with atrial systole) occurs in tricuspid stenosis, pulmonary stenosis, in complete heart block (cannon wave) and rarely in pulmonary hypertension.
Large 'v' wave (corresponds with ventricular systole) and occurs in tricuspid incompetence, usually secondary to cardiac failure.
There is no 'a' wave in atrial fibrillation.

Suspect a low level and press on the abdomen firmly (unless the liver is tender) in order to raise the column. A positive reflux may have no pathophysiological significance. The sole purpose of this manoeuvre is to demonstrate the vein and to show that it can be filled (i.e. the pressure is not high).
Suspect a high level with distension of the veins (not easily seen) with the top of the column above the neck. Check if the ear lobes move with the cardiac cycle and sit the patient vertical to get a greater length of visible jugular vein above the right atrium. The venous pressure can sometimes be demonstrated in dilated veins of an arm or hand held at a suitable height above the right atrium. The level at which pulsation occurs should be determined.

If the jugular venous pressure is raised (especially if more than 10 cm):

Look for a large 'v' wave indicating tricuspid incompetence (a murmur may be audible on auscultation of the heart).
Examine the abdomen for an enlarged tender pulsatile liver.
Check the ankles for oedema and then sit the patient up and examine the back of the chest for crepitations and for pleural effusions (unilateral or bilateral) and for sacral oedema. These should be done even if the jugular venous pressure is not raised since oedema may persist after the jugular venous pressure has been reduced by treatment of cardiac failure.

Heart '*Examine the heart.*'

Most 'heart cases' in an examination have a murmur. Such patients make it easy for an examiner to assess the candidate's ability to elicit and describe accurately the physical signs which are present. You may be watched throughout your examination and you must therefore have devised a system of examination which is second nature to you even in this stressful situation.

A full examination of the heart is not advisable without examining the arterial and venous pulses and this is usually done first. It is important to know not only the auscultatory features of the various heart abnormalities but also know which of them are found in association with each other and to examine for these with particular care. Thus every patient in whom you have diagnosed mitral stenosis should be examined with special attention to the aortic valve.

Chronic rheumatic heart disease is still the commonest type of 'heart' case in examinations, though many of them have had cardiac surgery. You may see patients with ventricular septal defects; the smaller lesions may not require surgery and often produce loud murmurs (maladie de Roger). For similar reasons you may be shown a patient with an atrial septal defect (often not diagnosed until middle age) but the auscultatory findings may be difficult to elicit. Beware of coarctation of the aorta where loud murmurs may originate in collateral vessels over the chest wall.

On approaching the patient note any cyanosis, dyspnoea or malar flush.

Examine the arterial pulses and look for clubbing (page 42).

Examine the jugular venous pulse.

Examine the front of the chest. First look for the localised thrusting apex beat of left ventricular hypertrophy and the parasternal lift of right ventricular hypertrophy. Then palpate for these phenomena and for thrills (palpable murmurs). Note that a tapping apex is thought to be an accentuated mitral first sound and in the subsequent examination you will be trying to substantiate a diagnosis of mitral stenosis. Finally listen to the heart starting at the apex. It may be difficult to establish the timing of the sounds, but an experienced clinician recognises them by their quality.

Examine each part of the cardiac cycle for murmurs. (Remember to listen for a friction rub of pericarditis and a triple rhythm of cardiac failure. These are easily missed.) There is no alternative to experience for this and it is essential to know the character of the murmurs of the commoner cardiac lesions. Their description is formalised and stereotyped so that if you say there is a rumbling diastolic murmur at the apex you have diagnosed mitral stenosis. You should attempt to make whatever you hear fit one of the known patterns (table 7).

Listen to the lungs especially at the bases posteriorly for fine crepitations. Look for sacral and ankle oedema.

NB The signs of left ventricular failure are tachycardia, triple rhythm, fine basal creptitations of

TABLE 7 Characteristics of murmurs

Lesion	*Murmur and position*	*Radiation and notes*
Aortic stenosis (often with aortic incompetence)	Basal mid-systolic, usually loud and with a thrill	Maximal in 2nd RICS and radiating into neck. Also at apex
Pulmonary stenosis (may be part of Fallot's tetralogy)	Basal mid-systolic	Maximal in 2nd LICS. Increase on inspiration (with increased blood flow). Pulmonary component of 2nd sound is quiet
Aortic incompetence (often accompanying mitral stenosis in this country because syphilis is now rare)	Early immediate blowing diastolic murmur	Usually maximal in 3rd LICS or less often in 2nd RICS. Radiation between right carotid and cardiac apex. Look for Argyll Robertson pupils
Pulmonary incompetence (rare except as congenital lesion)	Early immediate blowing diastolic murmur	Maximal in 2nd and 3rd LICS
Mitral stenosis	Mid or late rumbling diastolic murmur at apex	Loud mitral 1st sound. Opening snap. Turn patient on left side (and exercise) to accentuate murmur. Presystolic accentuation if in sinus rhythm
Mitral incompetence (usually mitral stenosis is present as well)	Pan-systolic at apex	Radiation to axilla (but often heard parasternally)
VSD (slight degrees are common, severe are rare)	Rough, loud and pan-systolic Maximal at 3rd-4th LICS parasternally	
ASD	Pulmonary systolic murmur with fixed split 2nd sound. (There is no murmur due to blood flow through the defect)	Possible diastolic murmur from tricuspid valve
PDA	Machinery murmur, maximal in late systole and extending into diastole. Maximal in 2nd-3rd LICS in mid-clavicular line	Audible also posteriorly
Coarctation	Loud rough murmur in systole, maximum over apex of left lung both posteriorly and anteriorly	Murmurs of scapular and internal mammary shunt collaterals. Radio-femoral delay. Hypertension in arms
Friction rub	Scratchy noise usually in systole and diastole	Varies with posture and breathing

Notes
'Base' denotes the 1st and 2nd intercostal spaces.
'RICS' and 'LICS' refer to right and left intercostal spaces

pulmonary oedema and pleural effusion usually associated with signs of right ventricular failure (raised jugular venous pressure, hepatomegaly, ankle and sacral oedema). If right ventricular failure is secondary to lung disease (cor pulmonale), there is evidence of this—usually of chronic bronchitis (page 200). Treatment is with digitalis, diuretics (i.v. in acute pulmonary oedema plus oxygen), potassium chloride supplements and salt restriction.

Hypertension

'This man has hypertension—would you examine him?'

Slight or moderate hypertension usually gives no abnormalities detectable on physical examination. In longstanding or severe hypertension there will usually be left ventricular hypertrophy and a loud aortic second sound. The other consequences of sustained hypertension should be looked for, i.e. hypertensive retinopathy, heart failure, renal failure, cerebrovascular disease. It is essential to think of the less common causes of hypertension and therefore to examine:

— for aortic coarctation (radio-femoral delay, weak femoral pulses and the bruits of the coarctation and of the scapular anastomoses and visible pulsation of the anastomoses)

— a renal artery bruit may be present in the epigastrium in renal artery stenosis

— the kidneys are palpable in polycystic disease

— observe the facies for evidence of Cushing's syndrome—usually due to steroid or ACTH administration

— think also of the chronic renal diseases (test the urine), of phaeochromocytoma (rare), and of primary hyperaldosteronism (very rare)

Myocardial infarct

'This patient has had a myocardial infarction, would you ask him some questions?'

The patient will be in the recovery stage. The history is more important than the physical signs. Symptoms (pain or fatigue) are often present in the preceding week.

Ask about

Pain Onset (rest or exercise), quality (compressing), distribution (including radiation), duration (usually over half an hour). Interscapular pain suggests dissecting aneurysm.

NB Intensity is not a reliable guide to the extent of the infarct.

Breathlessness About a quarter of all cases describe an acute attack of dyspnoea as a feature of the attack.

Cold sweat Also common, and often associated with nausea and vomiting.

Pallor Normally reported by witnesses.

Previous attacks or angina If they have had a previous infarct or angina their new pain will usually resemble that which they have had previously.

Past history of hypertension, strokes, symptoms of peripheral vascular disease and, in young women, whether they have diabetes mellitus or are on the contraceptive pill.

Family history of heart attacks, especially if young; diabetes; hypertension; gout.

Examination — *'Would you like to examine him?'*

Evidence of a low cardiac output (hypotension and small volume pulse).
Signs of cardiac failure including crepitations at the lung bases.
Arrhythmias, tachycardia, bradycardia.
Evidence of a cardiac aneurysm (double impulse, rocking apex).
Pericardial friction (immediate and post-infarction syndrome).
Evidence of mitral incompetence (papillary muscle dysfunction).
Deep venous thrombosis—a complication of immobilisation.
Evidence of hyperlipidaemia, especially xanthelasmata and tendon xanthomata.
Evidence of the relevant alternatives in the differential diagnosis, especially pulmonary embolism, pericarditis, dissecting aneurysm, pleurisy, cholecystitis, reflux oesophagitis, radicular pain.

Investigation — *'What investigations would you perform?'*

Ask for an ECG series and an SGOT series. You may note rises in the white cell count, ESR and temperature. A chest X-ray is necessary in all cardiac investigations.

Management — *'Discuss the management.'*

The following aspects should be considered (see page 221):

Bed rest
Analgesia and sedation
Oxygen therapy
Cardiac failure and shock
Anticoagulants
Complications (arrhythmias, rupture of septum, papillary muscle dysfunction and cardiac aneurysm)
Smoking
Obesity
Hyperlipidaemia (page 151)
Advice on discharge from hospital

Cardiac arrhythmias (table 8)

Digitalis may cause almost any arrhythmia if serum potassium is low, e.g. patients in cardiac failure on diuretics.
Consider thyrotoxicosis in any tachyarrhythmia, especially atrial fibrillation.
Confirm the rhythm with an ECG.

Electrocardiograms

Many physicians approach the interpretation of ECGs with a feeling of insecurity. There are, however, a relatively small number of common patterns (page 54) and these become easily recognisable with experience. Complex dysrhythmias are virtually never shown to examination candidates. Under examination conditions determination of the mean frontal QRS

TABLE 8 Cardiac arrhythmias

Rhythm	Rate: Atrial	Rate: Ventricular	Diagnosis
Regular	90+	90+	Sinus tachycardia
	120–200	120–200	Paroxysmal atrial tachycardia
	200–400	100–200	Atrial flutter with block
	80+	30–45	Complete heart block with cannon 'a' waves in JVP, variable intensity 1st sound, high pulse pressure
	40–50	40–50	Sinus bradycardia
Irregular			Multiple ectopics (including coupled beats) ECG basically regular
		60–100 treated, 100+ untreated	Atrial flutter with varying block; Atrial fibrillation (apex rate is only guide to true heart rate. ECG essential)
		120–200	Ventricular tachycardia
Cardiac arrest		No peripheral pulse	Ventricular fibrillation; Ventricular asystole

axis (page 64) does not give information commensurate with the time taken to determine it. It should be attempted only if specifically requested.

'Look at this ECG.'
Make sure that you understand the layout of the leads. Little is lost by ignoring AVr and AVl.

AVf is useful in inferior ('posterior') myocardial infarction.

Whatever your final diagnosis, you should initially comment on the rate and rhythm.

Rate Assess the rate by counting the large squares between two QRS complexes (and dividing into 300).

R–R interval		*Rate*
2 squares	=	150/min
3 squares	=	100/min
4 squares	=	75/min
5 squares	=	60/min

Rhythm Quickly scan *all* the QRS complexes. Check if there is a P wave before every QRS complex.

1 *If the rate is fast and rhythm regular*, consider:

— paroxysmal atrial tachycardia (a rate of 150—two big squares—should make you suspect this)

Underlying diseases	*Therapy* (treat underlying disease)
Anxiety, cardiac failure, thyrotoxicosis, fever, anaemia	Underlying disease
None (60%), thyrotoxicosis, digitalis, tobacco, caffeine, Wolff–Parkinson–White syndrome	Vagal stimulation (pressure on the carotid sinus)
Ischaemic heart disease, thyrotoxicosis, (digitalis)	Digoxin, DC cardioversion
Post-infarction, idiopathic, digitalis, cardiomyopathy	Nil if idiopathic and asymptomatic. Atropine or cardiac pacemaker after myocardial infarction (see page 221). Stokes–Adams attacks may be diagnosed as epileptic
Athletes, myocardial infarction, myxoedema, hypothermia	As heart block if following infarction (see page 223)
Ischaemia, digitalis, thyrotoxicosis, cardiomyopathy	Stop digitalis and give potassium if necessary. β-blockade (e.g. practolol)
Digitalis, ischaemia, thyrotoxicosis	
Ischaemia, rheumatic heart disease (MS), thyrotoxicosis. Rarely pulmonary embolism, constrictive pericarditis, cardiomyopathy or bronchial carcinoma	Digoxin, or DC cardioversion following myocardial infarction (see page 221) and following treated MS and thyrotoxicosis
Myocardial infarction and ischaemia	See page 221
Myocardial infarction	

— atrial flutter ('sawtooth baseline'). F (flutter) waves in leads II and V_1
— pulmonary embolism (page 215)
— ventricular tachycardia (page 223)

2 *If the rate is fast and rhythm irregular*, consider:
— atrial fibrillation (total irregularity) with a ragged baseline and absent P waves
— atrial flutter with varying block
— multiple ectopic beats

3 *If the rate is slow and rhythm regular*, consider:
— complete heart block
— myxoedema (low voltage QRS and flat T waves)
— hypothermia (low voltage and J waves)

NB It is sometimes difficult to determine whether the complexes are completely regular or not, especially with an unusually regular atrial fibrillation. The easiest and most accurate way to determine this is to put a piece of paper with its edge along the trace and to mark every QRS complex for about five beats. If you then move the paper up by one or two beats, the marks on the paper will still coincide accurately with QRS complexes only if the rhythm is regular. Total irregularity is almost always diagnostic of atrial fibrillation. The same procedure is useful for checking on P waves in suspected supraventricular extra beats; it demonstrates the compensatory pause well.

4 *Extra beats* with:
— normal QRS complexes (supraventricular or 'atrial')
— wide QRS complexes (ventricular or supraventricular with aberration)

5 *Prolonged PR interval*
— partial heart block (look for Wenckebach)
Now that you have scanned the total ECG trace, you may have found an obvious abnormality such as the changes of an extensive acute anteroseptal myocardial infarction or one of the special patterns (page 54). If not, check the trace for abnormal QRS complexes.

Myocardial infarction

Anterior or inferior, old or new. Look for pathological Q waves, convex ST elevation and T inversion. Remember that Q waves in leads III and AVf should be accompanied by Q in II before making a firm diagnosis of inferior myocardial infarction. They may otherwise reflect a change of axis or represent a pulmonary embolus.

Ventricular hypertrophy (right or left)

Large R waves occur over the appropriate ventricle in the chest leads (right ventricle, R in V_{1-2}; left ventricle, R in V_{5-6}). There tend to be large negative (S) waves in the reciprocal leads, e.g. S in V_{1-2} in left ventricular hypertrophy.
NB If SV_1 plus RV_5 is more than 35 mm it denotes left ventricular hypertrophy.

Bundle branch block (right or left)

This is present if the QRS is over 0·12 seconds and is not present if it is less. The diagnosis is as easy as counting small squares. Characteristic patterns are shown (page 58). Right bundle branch block may or may not be pathological; left bundle branch block invariably is.

If you have not yet made a diagnosis, methodically work through the cardiac cycle using as many leads as you need for each component.

P wave

Usually most easily seen in leads V_1 and V_2 though the significant shape of it may be best seen in II and the lateral chest leads (V_{4-6}).
The P wave is bifid in left atrial hypertrophy (P mitrale) in leads II and V_{4-6} and biphasic in leads V_{1-2}.
The P wave is peaked in right atrial hypertrophy including 'cor pulmonale' (P pulmonale).
The P wave may be 'lost' in nodal rhythm, i.e. when it coincides with the QRS complex.
The P wave may be inverted in nodal rhythm and precede or follow the QRS complex.

PR interval

For first, second or third degree heart block (usually due to ischaemic heart disease).
NB A short PR interval occurs in nodal rhythm, and in the Wolff–Parkinson–White syndrome (note the delta wave.)

QRS complex It may now be worth making a rough estimate of the mean frontal QRS axis (page 64).

ST segment It is raised convexly (domed) in myocardial infarction and raised concavely in pericarditis.
It is depressed, especially leads V_{5-6}, in digitalis intoxication, left ventricular hypertrophy and in ischaemic heart disease (plane depression), particularly on effort.

T wave It is ‘peaked’ in hyperkalaemia and sometimes acutely after myocardial infarction.
It is inverted in:
— bundle branch block (T always in the reverse direction to the main QRS complex)
— digitalis effect (‘reversed tick’ \/)
— ventricular hypertrophy
— ischaemia (arrowhead)
Roughly check the Q–T interval (from the beginning of the QRS complex to the end of the T wave). It varies as a function of the square root of the R–R interval (rate). The upper limit of normal is approximately

Rate	*Q-T*
60	0·43
75	0·39
100	0·34

This may be exceeded in hypocalcaemia, myocardial disease (ischaemic and rheumatic) and with anti-arrhythmic drugs (e.g. procaine amide and quinidine).

U wave It can be normally present, and is maximal in leads V_{3-4}. It is increased in hypokalaemia and may be inverted in ischaemia.

If you have still failed to find any abnormality recheck quickly for the following special patterns:

ST segments for pericarditis, especially in leads II and V_{2-5}—concave elevation of the ST segment in all leads
QT interval for hypocalcaemia (long) and hypercalcaemia (short). The QT_c is the QT corrected for rate (to a standard of 60)
S_1, Q_3, T_3 pattern of pulmonary embolism
General voltage decrease of myxoedema, hypothermia, pericardial effusion and obesity
Changes of *hypokalaemia* and *hyperkalaemia*
Digitalis effect, ‘reversed tick’ depression of ST segment and depression of T
NB Some ECGs ‘tell a story’
for example:
— ECG changes of hypokalaemia with ‘digitalis effect’—pattern of ‘digitalis and diuretics without potassium’
— ECG changes with hypokalaemia and LV hypertrophy—usually hypertensive heart disease treated with diuretics without potassium, but remember Conn’s syndrome and Cushing’s disease

— atrial tachycardia with AV block—digitalis intoxication (especially with hypokalaemia)

Digitalis can produce almost any arrhythmia particularly in potassium depletion (thiazide diuretics)

Sample electrocardiograms

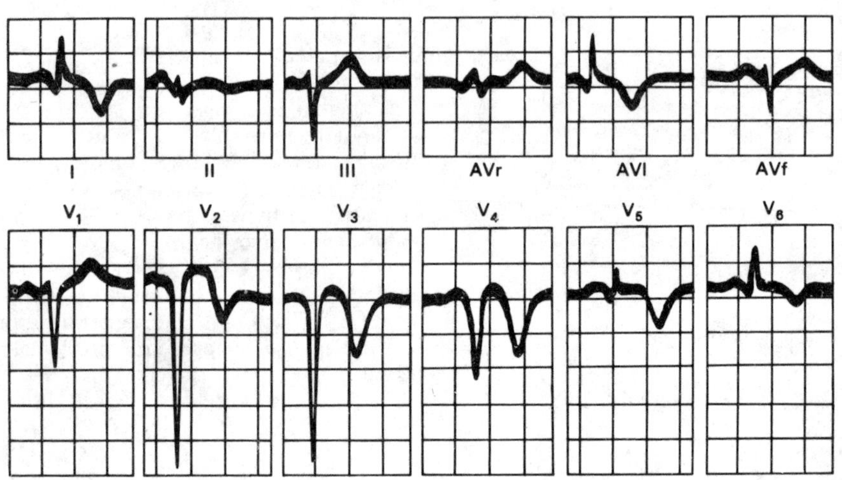

FIGURE 1 Anterior myocardial infarction. The main Q and STT changes are in the anteroseptal leads V_{2-4}.

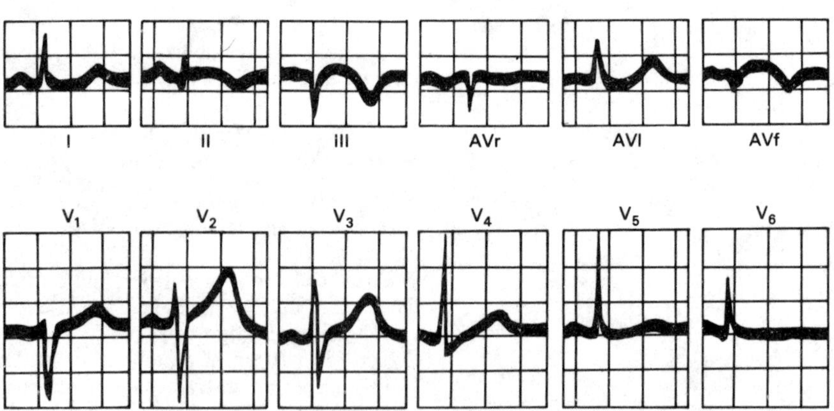

FIGURE 2 Inferior myocardial infarction. The main changes are in II, III and AVf. T wave changes in V_{5-6} suggest inferolateral infarction.

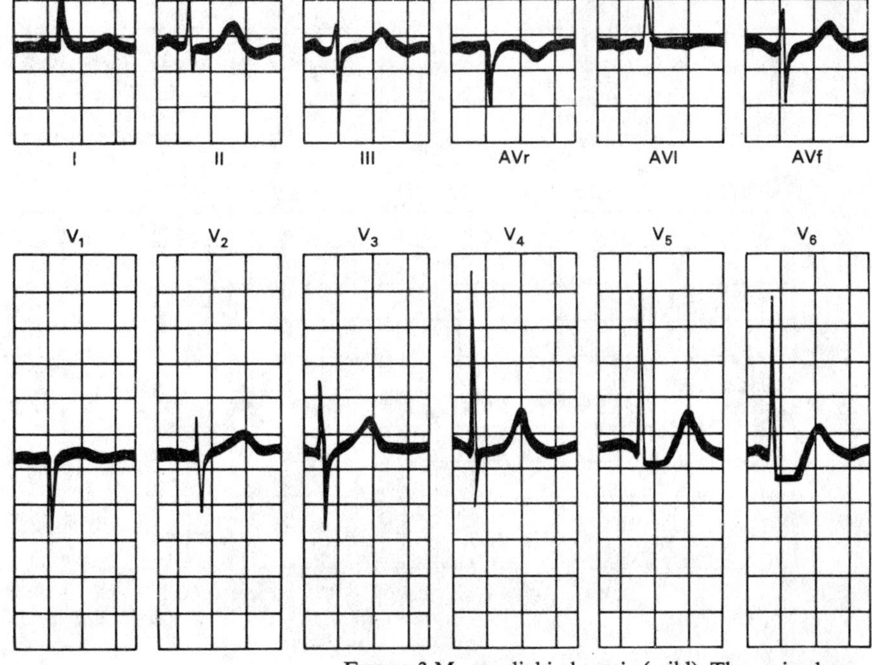

FIGURE 3 Myocardial ischaemia (mild). The main characteristic is a flat ST segment in leads standard II and V_6. Also note inverted U waves in II, III, AVf and V_{4-6}.

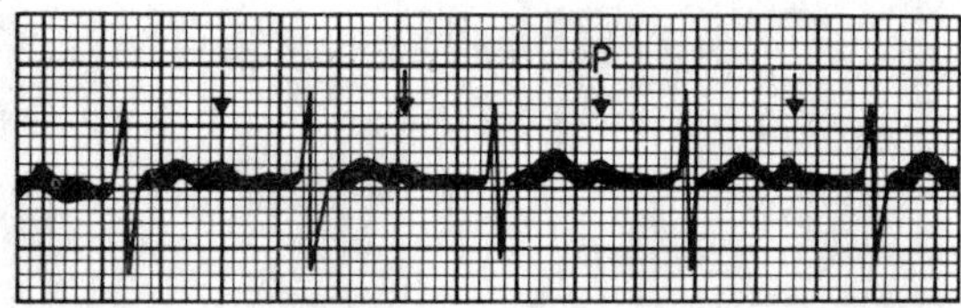

FIGURE 4 Heart block grade I. PR interval 0·30 seconds.

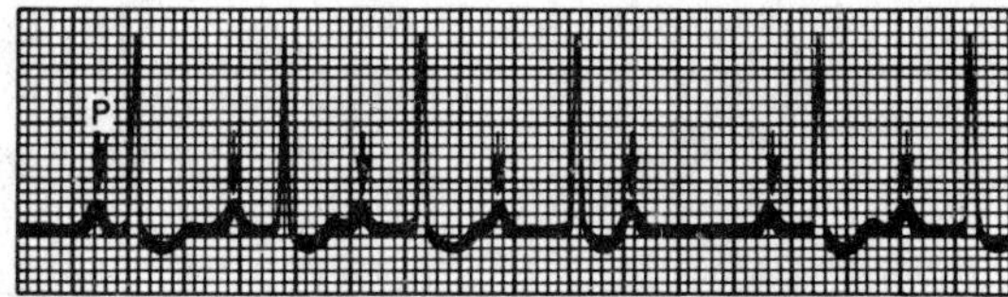

FIGURE 5 Heart block grade II (Wenkebach).

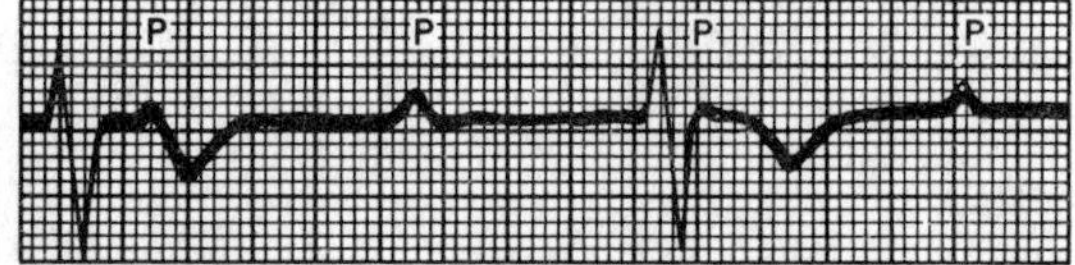

FIGURE 6 Heart block grade III (complete). A–V dissociation.

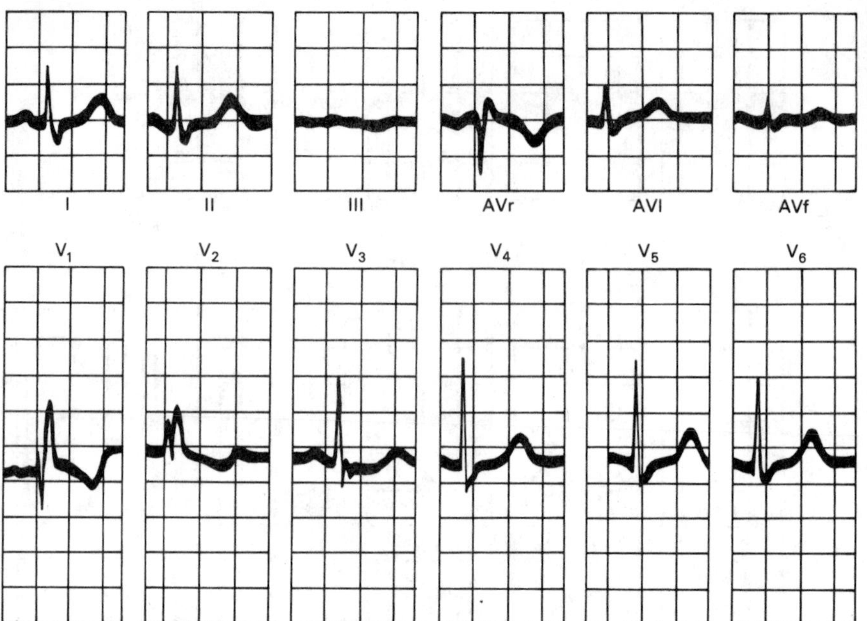

FIGURE 7 Right bundle branch block. 'M complexes' in the right ventricular leads V_{1-2} and slurred S waves in the left ventricular leads I, AV1 and V_{4-6}.

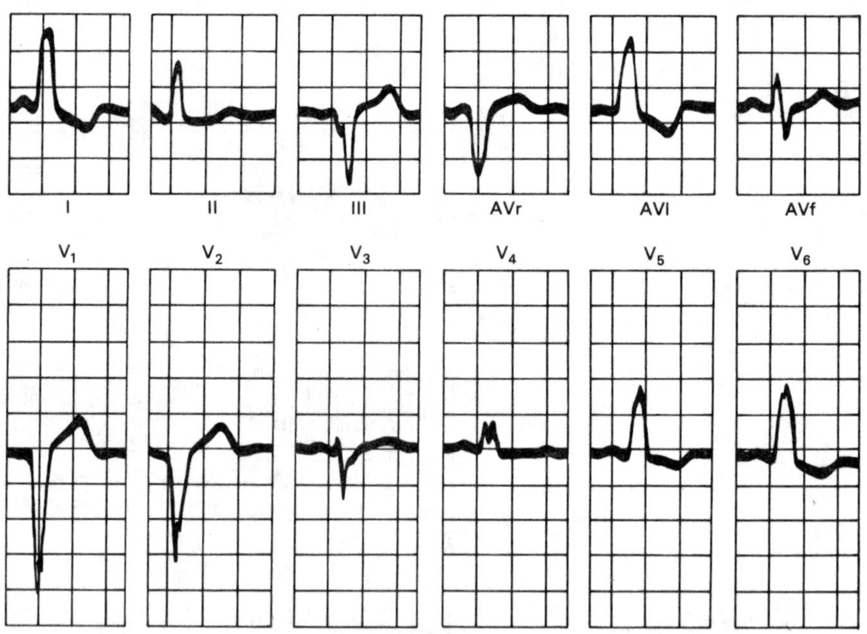

FIGURE 8 Left bundle branch block. 'M complexes' are visible in some of the left ventricular leads, I, AV1 and V_{4-6}; and notched QS complexes in the right ventricular leads, V_{1-2}.

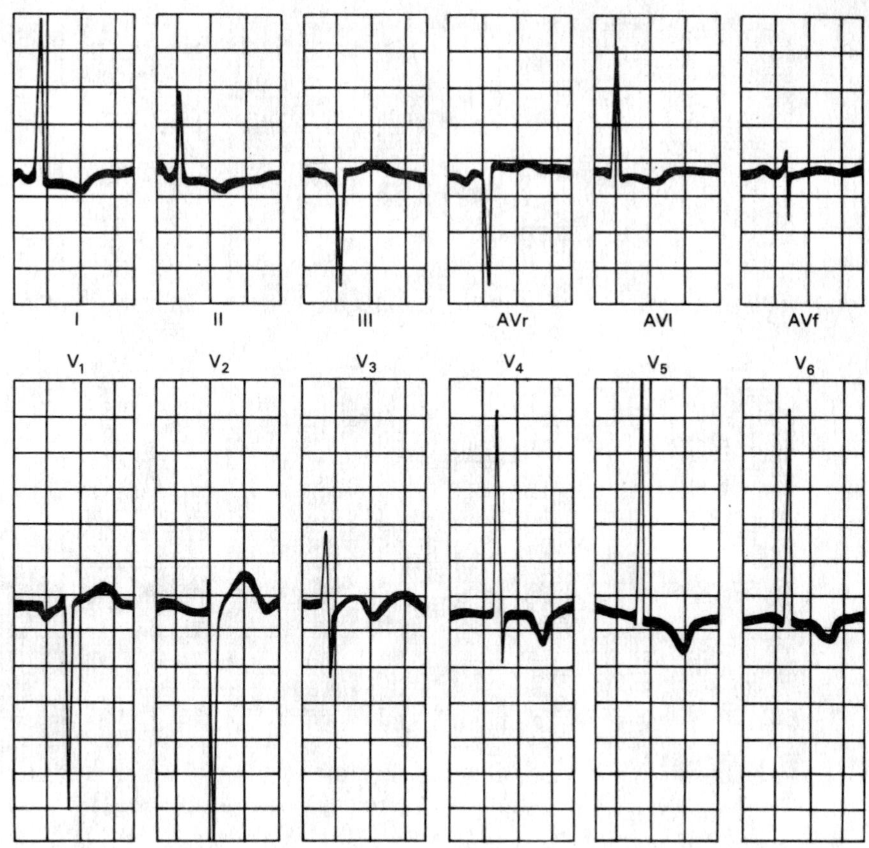

FIGURE 9 Left ventricular hypertrophy. Sv_1 and $Rv_{5 or 6}$ > 35 mm and STT 'strain' changes in the left ventricular leads, I, AV1 and V_{4-6}.

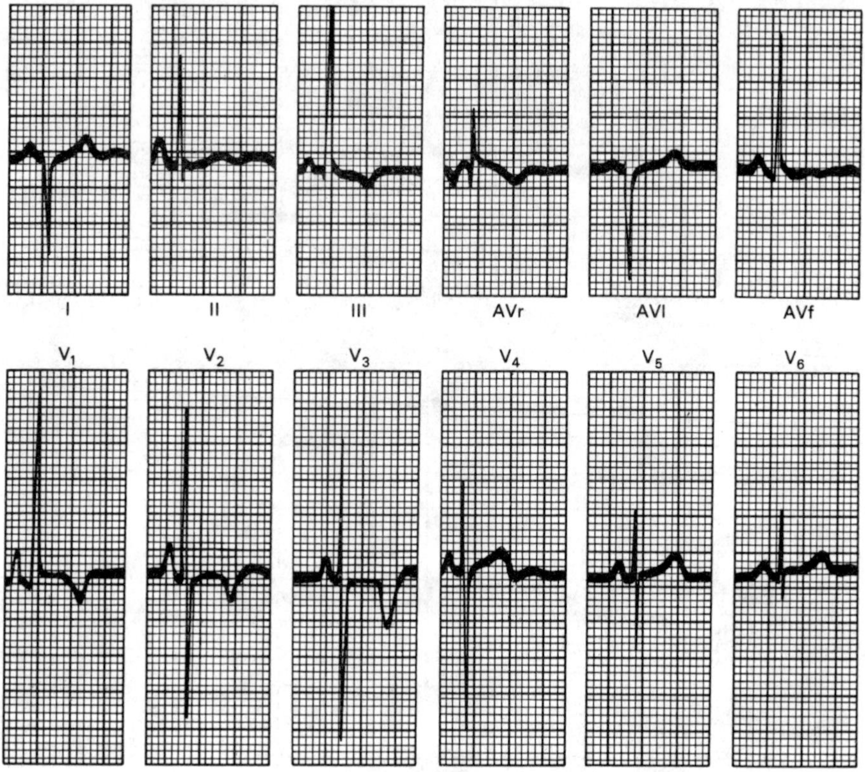

I II III AVr AVl AVf

V_1 V_2 V_3 V_4 V_5 V_6

FIGURE 10 Right ventricular hypertrophy. Tall R waves and STT 'strain' changes in the right ventricular leads V_{1-3} and a mean frontal QRS axis to the right (+120°)

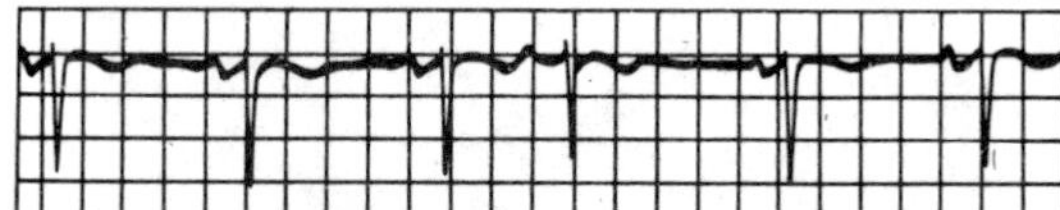

FIGURE 11 Atrial extrasystole.

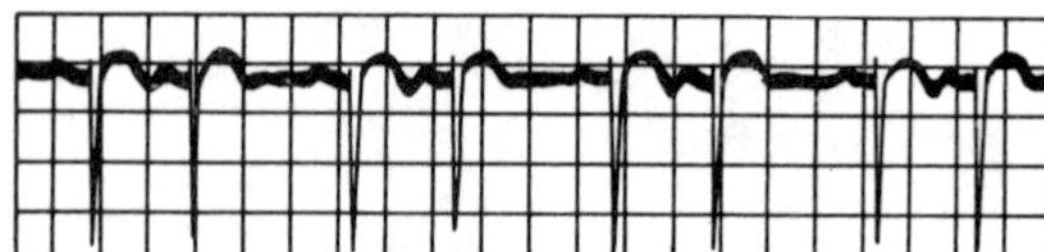

FIGURE 12 Atrial coupling or bigeminy: alternate atrial extrasystoles.

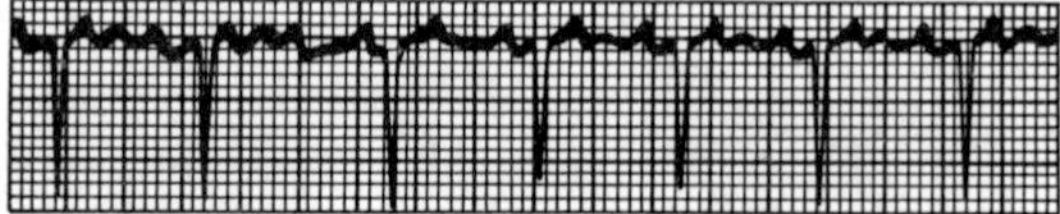

FIGURE 13 Supraventricular tachycardia with varying A–V block.

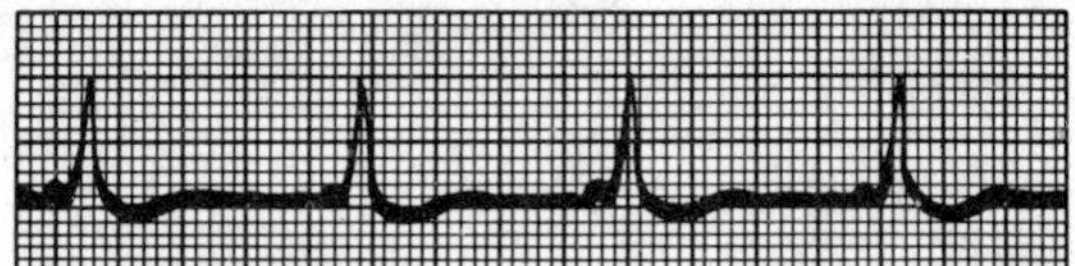

FIGURE 14 Wolff–Parkinson–White syndrome. Short PR interval and delta waves.

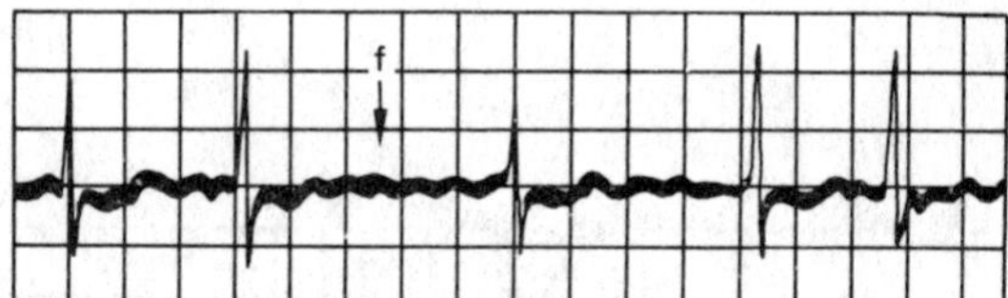

FIGURE 15 Atrial fibrillation.

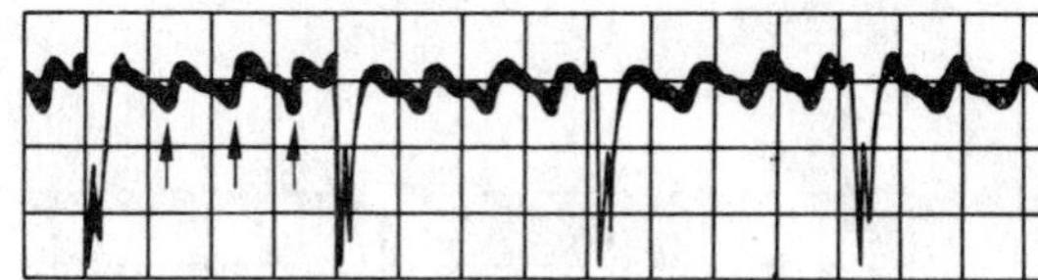

FIGURE 16 Atrial flutter with 'saw-tooth' atrial waves.

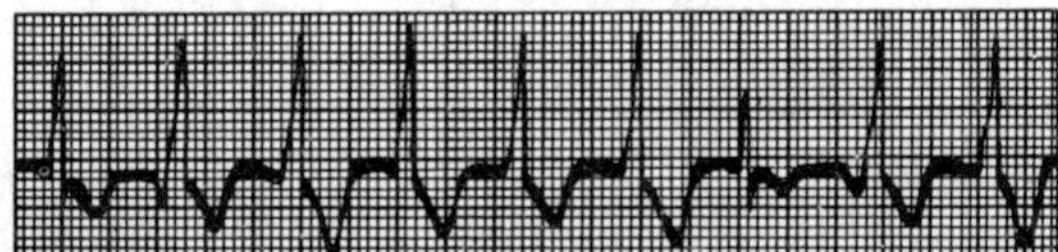

FIGURE 17 Ventricular tachycardia with slightly irregular 'ventricular' QRS complexes and variable T waves due to dissociated superimposed P waves.

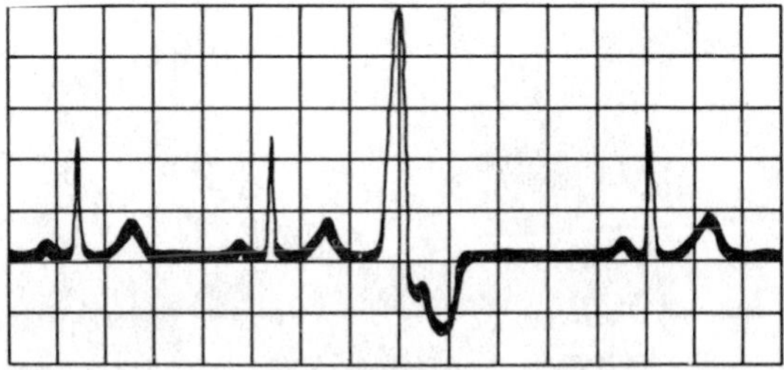

FIGURE 18 Ventricular ectopic. A 'ventricular' bizarre QRS complex. These are more ominous if multifocal, i.e. QRS of varying shape.

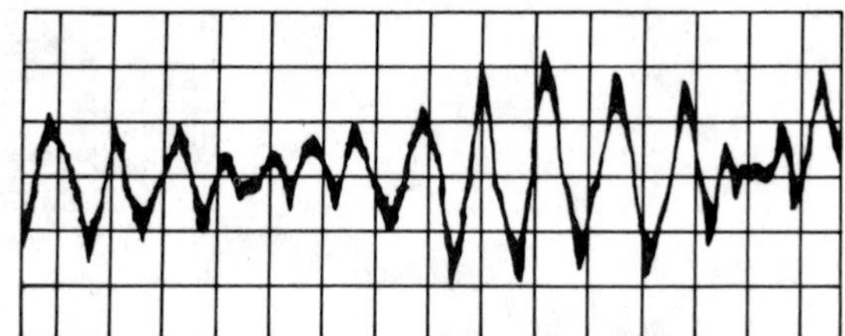

FIGURE 19 Ventricular fibrillation. This is often seen in 'cardiac arrest' and may be irreversible. It may sometimes alternate with ventricular tachycardia (and sinus rhythm).

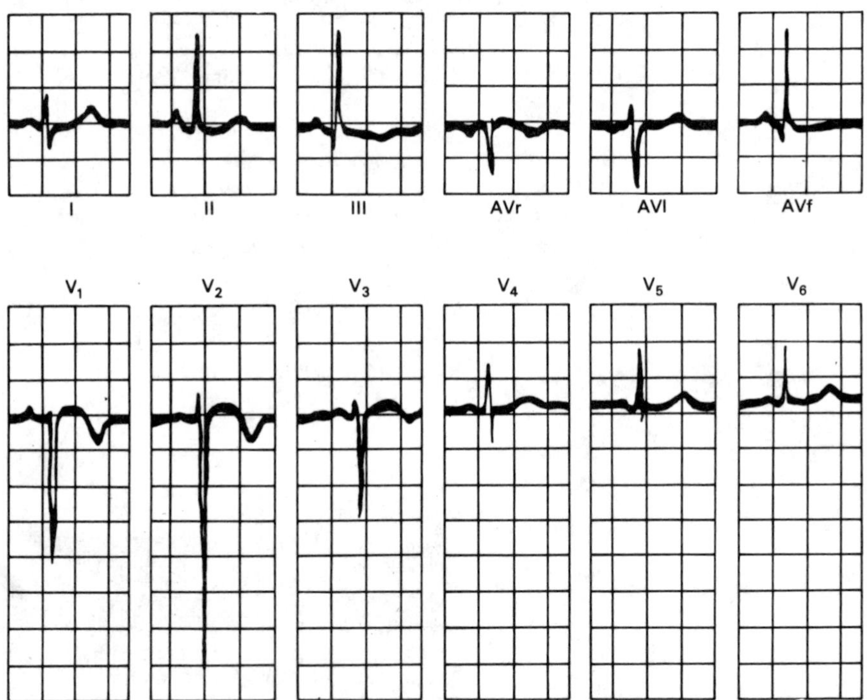

FIGURE 20 Acute pulmonary embolism with S_1, Q_3, T_3 pattern, a mean frontal QRS axis towards the right (+90°) and 'RV strain' pattern in leads V_{1-3}.

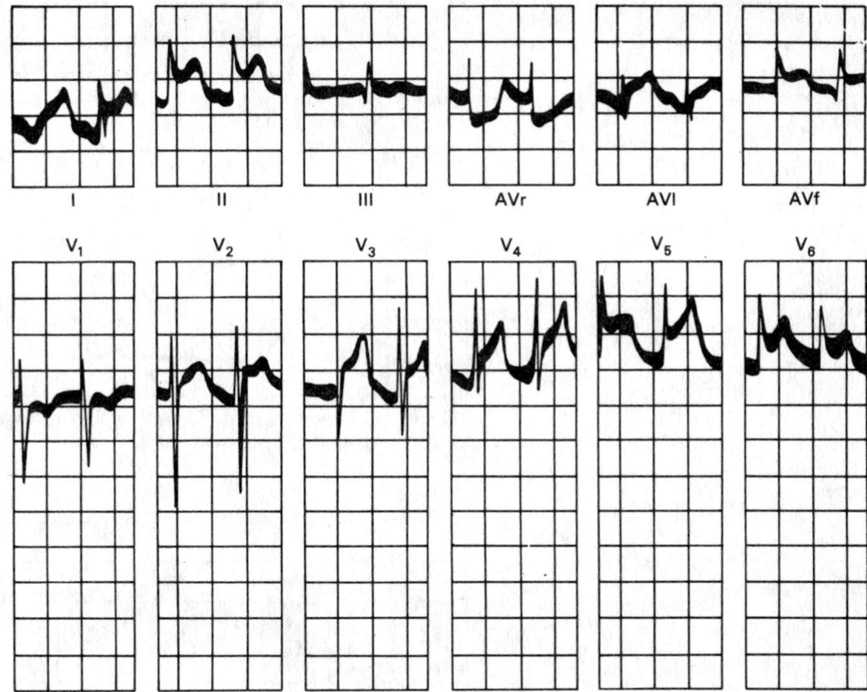

FIGURE 21 Acute pericarditis. Raised concave-upwards ST segments in most leads, maximal in lead II and V_{5-6}.

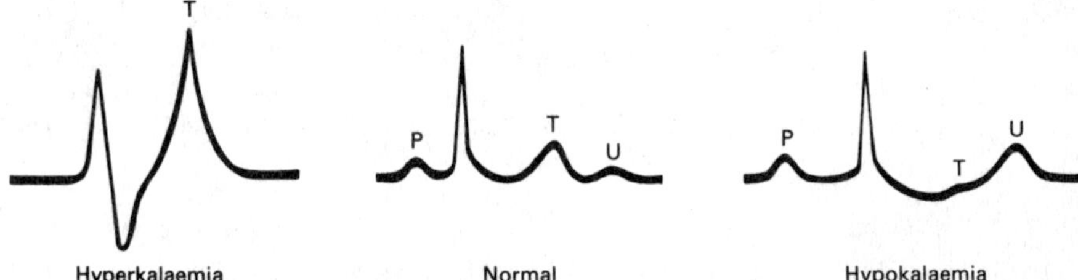

FIGURE 22 Hyperkalaemia and hypokalaemia. The T wave amplitude varies directly with the serum potassium and the U wave inversely (it is often normally present in V_{3-4}). In hyperkalaemia the P waves become smaller and the QRS complex widens into the ST segment. In hypokalaemia the PR interval lengthens and the ST segment becomes depressed.

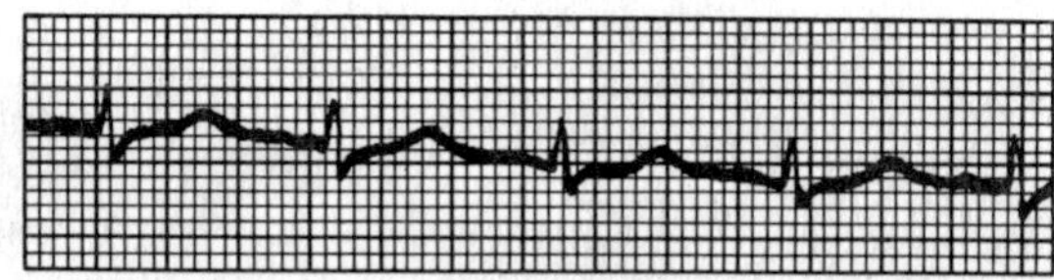

FIGURE 23 Hypocalcaemia. Normal complexes apart from a prolonged QT_c. (Rate 95/min, QT 0·40, QT_c 0·50.)

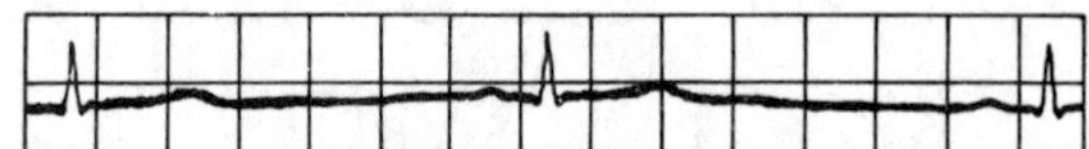

FIGURE 24 Myxoedema. Sinus bradycardia of 44/min and reduced amplitude of P, QRS and T waves which is present in all leads.

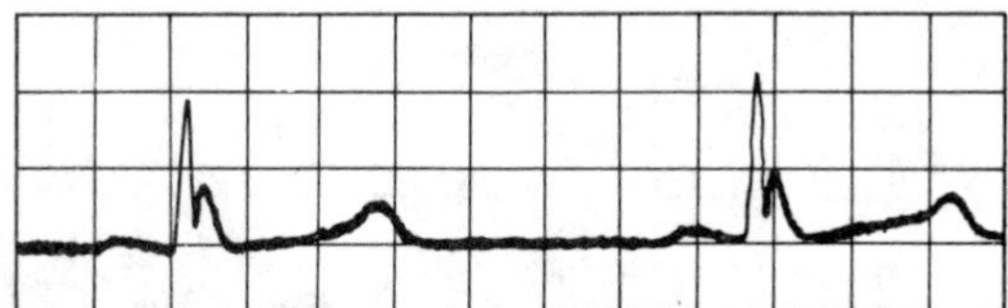

FIGURE 25 Hypothermia. Sinus bradycardia and J waves (Junction of QRS with ST segment).

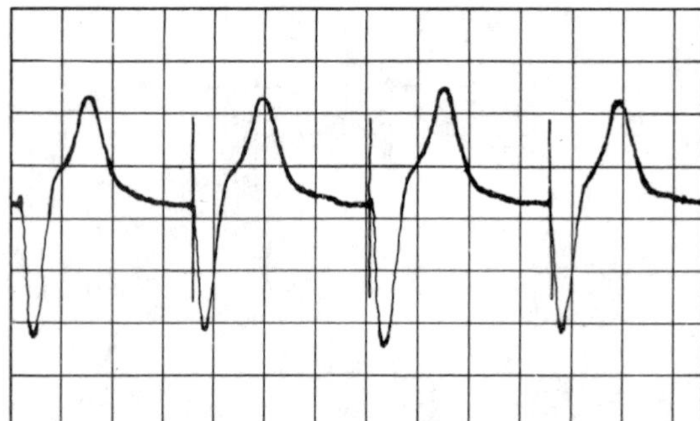

FIGURE 26 Ventricular pacemaker. Linear pacing artefact immediately preceding the widened 'ventricular' QRS complex.

Mean frontal QRS axis

If you have a system which is quick and which works, don't read any further.

The QRS axis seldom gives information which is diagnostically helpful. Use leads I, II and III only (i.e. a triaxial reference system) and practise drawing the axes (60° between each). Label them as in figure 27 at the positive ends. The other ends of the axes represent negative QRS deflections.

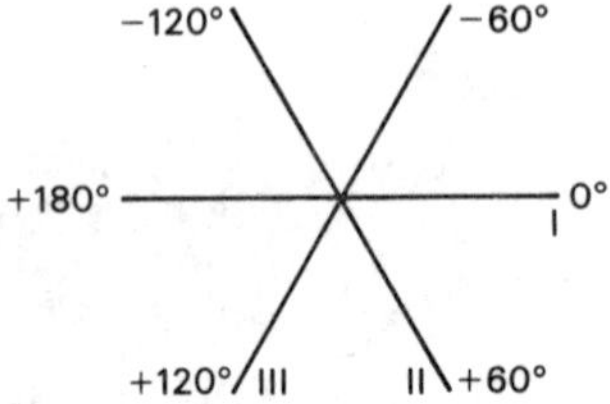

FIGURE 27 Main QRS axes for leads I, II and III.

Look at the three standard leads on your ECG and decide which one has the biggest net deflection (positive or negative). The QRS axis must be lying closer to this lead than any other. If the net deflections in two leads are equally large (e.g. I and II) the QRS axis will be pointing midway between them.

Thus, so far, you should be able to determine the axes shown in figure 28.

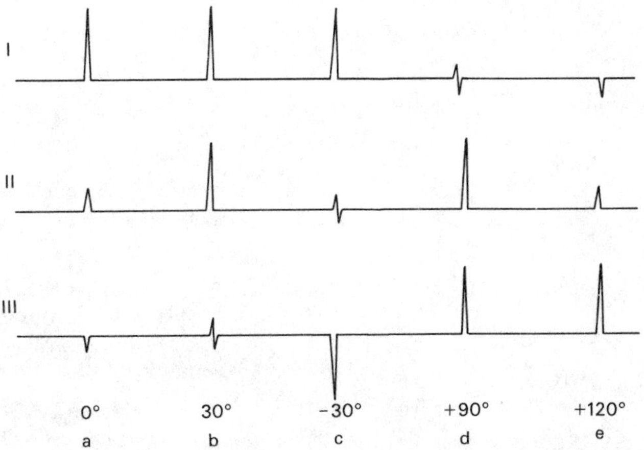

FIGURE 28 Determination of main deflection patterns in leads I, II and III.

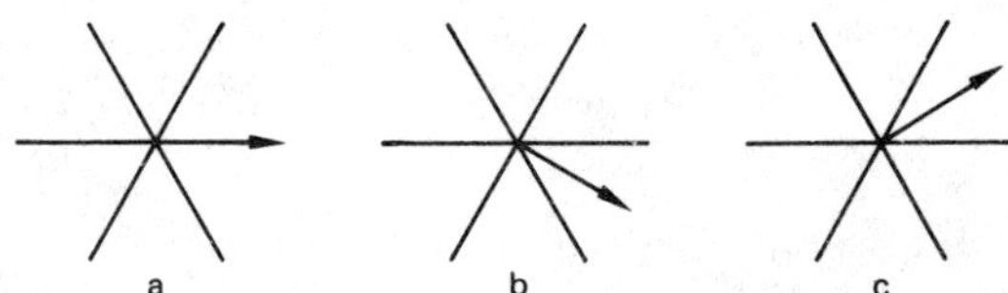

FIGURE 29 QRS axes plotted for deflection patterns shown in figure 28a, b and c.

You will now have noticed that when a QRS axis is perpendicular to a lead (e.g. a QRS axis of +90° is perpendicular to lead I), there is no net deflection in that lead. Examples b, c and d in figure 28 demonstrate this.

Now draw your own reference system and plot the examples given in figure 28 (figure 29).

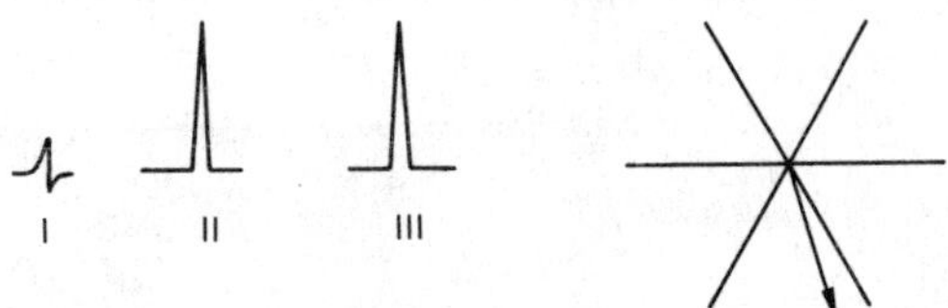

FIGURE 30 Fine adjustment of deflection patterns in leads I, II and III.

You can regard the 'biggest deflection' procedure as a rough assessment (to within 60°). The 'smallest deflection' then becomes the 'fine adjustment' (to about 10–15°). Thus if the smallest deflection (in, say, lead I in figure 30) is slightly net positive, the QRS axis must be slightly to the positive side of perpendicular in that lead (say 75° in this example) (compare with d in figure 28).

Now you should be able to determine the axis shown in figure 31.

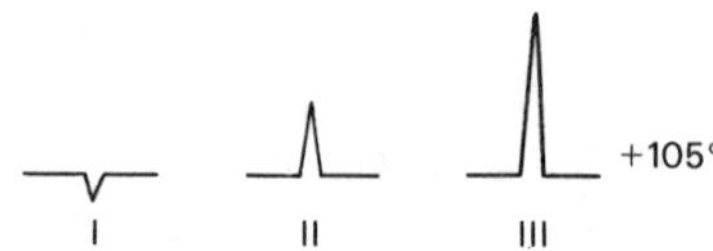

FIGURE 31 Sample deflection patterns in leads I, II and III.

The normal range is 0° to +90° though significant left axis deviation is usually more negative than −30°. For 'instant' diagnoses you can use the mnemonic:

> in significant LAD the QRS is negative in II
> in significant RAD the QRS is negative in I

Right axis deviation occurs in right ventricular hypertrophy (e.g. cor pulmonale and pulmonary stenosis). It is present in almost all cyanotic congenital heart disease.
Left axis deviation results from block of the superior branch of the left bundle (anterior hemiblock) and is usually due to ischaemic heart disease but also occurs in left ventricular hypertrophy.
In atrial septal defect, the ostium primum type tend to have a left axis deviation (despite a right bundle branch block) due to involvement of the left branch of the bundle in the lesion. Ostium secundum defects have a right axis deviation (with a right bundle branch block).

Haematology

Anaemia

It is essential to distinguish between pallor and anaemia. Pallor may be due to a deep-lying venous system and opaque skin. In Britain the commonest cause of anaemia is iron deficiency due to chronic blood loss especially in women during the child-bearing period. The second commonest cause is probably megaloblastic anaemia and most of these are due to intrinsic factor deficiency. The malabsorption syndrome including the postgastrectomy syndrome can give rise to deficiency in iron, vitamin B_{12} or folic acid. Chronic uraemia may present with a chronic anaemia. Anaemia may be a feature of many conditions in which other clinical features are usually more obvious. These include the leukaemias, reticuloses and rheumatoid arthritis. In tropical countries chronic infections, especially chronic malaria and hookworm infestation, are common and the haemoglobinopathies should be considered.

'*Examine this anaemic patient.*'

Observe and assess degree of anaemia

Face and conjuctiva: note the white hair and pale lemon yellow skin of pernicious anaemia.
Tongue: for glossitis of vitamin B_{12} or folate deficiency and angular stomatitis of iron deficiency.
Nails and nail beds: brittle nails and koilonychia of iron deficiency and the splinter haemorrhages (sometimes with clubbing) of infective endocarditis.
Note purpura (aplastic anaemia, leukaemia), mouth ulcer in neutropenia and the leg ulceration of the haemoglobinopathies.
Note rheumatoid arthritis and consider uraemia.
Note racial origin: thalassaemia and 'sickle cell' anaemia.

Ask patient

Blood loss: menstrual loss, pregnancy, haemorrhoids, indigestion and melaena, salicylate ingestion.
History of drugs: aplastic anaemia, and folate deficiency (anticonvulsants).
History of gastric surgery, colitis or malabsorption.
Paraesthesiae and sore tongue of pernicious anaemia.
Diet: the elderly pensioner may suffer from iron and/or ascorbic acid deficiency. Vegans may develop B_{12} deficiency and alcoholics folate deficiency.

Examine

Neck for lymph nodes, which may be enlarged in chronic lymphatic leukaemia and reticuloendothelial diseases or be secondaries from carcinoma.
Abdomen for splenomegaly, hepatomegaly and neoplasms (especially of the stomach, colon and uterus).

NB In the clinic rectal examination is essential, and sigmoidoscopy should be performed for haemorrhoids, carcinoma and colitis in patients with a history of rectal bleeding.

There may be congestive cardiac failure in severe anaemia.

If you suspect pernicious anaemia, examine for peripheral neuropathy and subacute combined degeneration of the cord.

Retinal haemorrhage may occur in leukaemia and B_{12} deficiency (severe anaemia).

'*What investigation (of anaemia) would you perform?*'

Do a full blood count and film to confirm the diagnosis or to define the type of anaemia. If the anaemia is:

Hypochromic

Perform serum iron, iron binding capacity, faecal occult blood, and proceed, if indicated, to sigmoidoscopy, barium enema, barium meal and follow-through. A gynaecological examination may be indicated from the clinical history at the outset. Check other possible causes which normally produce normochromic but sometimes hypochromic anaemia (see below).

Exclude thalassaemia and sickle cell anaemia if indicated (haemoglobin electrophoresis and sickling tests).

Macrocytic

Perform a serum B_{12} and folate (or red cell folate). A bone marrow examination shows megaloblastic change in vitamin B_{12} and folate deficiencies. In pernicious anaemia there will be a pentagastrin-fast achlorhydria. Parietal cell and intrinsic factor antibodies may be present. An abnormal Schilling test ($< 6\%$ in 24 hours) is corrected by intrinsic factor in pernicious anaemia.

Other causes of vitamin B_{12} and folate deficiencies, e.g. alcoholism, blind loops and ileal disease (Crohn's) are all rare. In ileal disease, the Schilling test is not corrected by intrinsic factor.

Investigate causes other than vitamin B_{12} and folate deficiencies. Aplastic and haemolytic anaemias are sometimes macrocytic but not megaloblastic.

Normocytic

These are usually anaemias secondary to other severe disease such as rheumatoid arthritis, carcinoma, renal failure and chronic infection.

Notes

Hypochromic anaemia, unresponsive to oral iron therapy, occurs in:

— patients who do not take their tablets
— continued bleeding (reticulocytosis persists)
— rheumatoid arthritis, SLE, infections (and other chronic illness)
— malabsorption
— thalassaemia
— sideroblastic anaemia (marrow stores are full of iron which cannot be utilised)

Megaloblasts are found in the marrow and only

rarely in the peripheral blood. They are characterised by a large and inactive nucleus (maturation arrest) in a relatively hypermature, and even haemoglobinised, cytoplasm. They are not present in normal marrow and their presence denotes vitamin B_{12} or folate deficiency.

Patients with pernicious anaemia which has been treated with vitamin B_{12} usually have normal peripheral blood, normal marrow (within 24 hours) and normal serum folates and B_{12}. They may still be investigated with pentagastrin and the Schilling test and antibodies are still present.

Vitamin B_{12} and folate deficiencies produce (if sufficiently severe) depression of all the marrow elements including neutrophils and platelets. The polymorph nuclei appear hypersegmented. There is usually some haemolysis with a raised unconjugated serum bilirubin.

In folic acid deficiency consider pregnancy, dietary intake (vegans), malabsorption, drugs (phenytoin), alcoholism and haemolytic anaemia.

In haemolytic anaemia the serum bilirubin (unconjugated) is raised. There is no bile pigment in the urine (acholuric) but urobilinogen is present in the urine in excess. Reticulocytosis is present and its degree is a measure of the rate of haemolysis. The rate of disappearance of chromium-tagged red cells gives a more accurate measure of the rate of haemolysis Splenomegaly and pigment stones may occur.

Haemolytic anaemias are rare in Britain. They are usually classified as:

1 Intracorpuscular defects (Coombs negative) Thalassaemia, sickle cell anaemia, hereditary spherocytosis, glucose-6-phosphatase deficiency.

2 Extracorpuscular defects

a Autoimmune haemolytic anaemias (Coombs positive) are either primary, or secondary to drugs (methyl-dopa), leukaemia or reticuloses.

b Rhesus incompatibility (and mismatched transfusion) is an immune but not autoimmune disorder since the antibody is extrinsic (fetal).

c Non-immune, e.g. burns, malaria.

Primary aplastic anaemia. A pancytopenia with reduction in all the formed elements is rare.

Secondary bone marrow failure. Toxic factors acting on the marrow may affect one or all of the formed elements of the blood, red cells, white cells or platelets. Important recognised causes include drugs (gold, phenylbutazone, chloramphenicol, carbimazole), radiation and leukaemias.

Skin haemorrhage

'*Purpura*' refers to small (pin head) cutaneous bleeding. '*Ecchymosis*' refers to larger lesions (bruises). Bruising is very common, purpura is rare. Bleeding into the skin results from:

— increased capillary fragility (senile purpura and, rarely, steroids)

— thrombocytopenia (increased destruction or decreased production)
— disorders of clotting constituents

'*Examine this patient's skin*' (showing purpura or ecchymosis).

Quickly note

Patient's age (senile purpura).
If he is anaemic (marrow infiltration, aplasia and leukaemia).
If he has rheumatoid arthritis (purpura usually due to drugs, steroids, phenylbutazone, gold).
Henoch–Schönlein purpura (rare). This 'purpura' is actually a vasculitis and often most obvious around the buttocks, and upper thighs. The rash is polymorphic and may be extensive simulating a skin disease. It is associated with acute nephritic syndrome, arthralgia and abdominal pain.
Ecchymoses of the lower limbs in the elderly may be due to scurvy. This is seen in persons living alone and on 'ulcer' diet. Potatoes are the usual source of vitamin C in those who cannot afford citrus fruits.

If invited to question the patient ask about drugs (phenylbutazone, carbimazole, chloramphenicol, anticoagulants, steroids) and about a family history of bleeding (haemophilia and Christmas disease), and about anticoagulant therapy.

Examination

Mouth and pharynx for the ulceration of neutropenia (marrow depression from leukaemia or drugs).
For anaemia and lymphadenopathy (marrow aplasia and leukaemia).
For splenomegaly (leukaemia and idiopathic thrombocytopenic purpura).

NB Platelet deficiency tends to result in multiple small bleeds (purpura, microscopic haematuria) and clotting-factor deficiency in isolated larger bleeds (haemarthrosis, haematemesis, stroke, haematomata in muscles).

Blood count (table 9)

'*Comment on this blood count.*'

TABLE 9 Normal values

Hb (*men*)	13–17	g/100 ml
Hb (*women*)	12–16	g/100 ml
RBC (*men*)	4·5–6·4	M/mm^3
RBC (*women*)	3·9–5·6	M/mm^3
PCV (*men*)	40–50	%
PCV (*women*)	36–47	%
MCV	80–96	$c\mu$ (PCV/RBC)
MCH	27–32	$\mu\mu g$ (Hb/RBC)
MCHC	32–36	% (Hb/PCV)
Reticulocytes	0–2	% (of red cells)
WBC	4000–11,000	mm^3
Platelets	150,000–400,000	mm^3

Check the haemoglobin for anaemia or polycythaemia.

NB A normal white cell and platelet count virtually excludes leukaemia and marrow aplasia.

Check the indices for hypochromia (MCH and MCHC) and microcytosis (MCV). If present suggest iron deficiency.

Check the indices for macrocytes (MCV and MCH). In pernicious anaemia there is usually an associated low WBC and low platelet count.

If the indices are normal, consider uraemia, rheumatoid arthritis, carcinoma, chronic infection and myxoedema as causes of an anaemia.

If the reticulocyte count is raised this denotes marrow hyperactivity and usually (*a*) haemolytic anaemia, (*b*) response to vitamin B_{12}, folate or occasionally iron therapy, or (*c*) continued bleeding.

If the WBC and/or platelet counts are low and there is anaemia, this suggests marrow aplasia, usually secondary to drugs (and rarely toxic chemicals) or marrow infiltration (leukaemia, myelofibrosis, multiple myeloma, carcinoma).

Primitive white cells (blast) in the peripheral film indicate an acute leukaemia or occasionally a leukaemoid response to acute infection. The total WBC count is usually raised. The differential film may indicate whether the leukaemia is myeloid or lymphatic.

Eosinophilia suggests drug sensitivity, intestinal worms, allergy (e.g. asthma), polyarteritis nodosa, allergic aspergillosis, Loeffler's syndrome and, rarely, reticulosis such as Hodgkin's disease.

In polycythaemia rubra vera, the RBC, WBC and platelet counts are usually raised. There is an increase in red cell mass. In secondary polycythaemia (secondary to hypoxia) only the RBC count is raised. Polycythaemia is also associated with renal carcinoma and cerebellar haemangioblastoma.

A very high ESR (over 100 mm/h) suggests (*a*) multiple myeloma, (*b*) systemic lupus erythematosus or temporal arteritis, (*c*) rarely carcinoma or chronic infection, (*d*) polymyalgia rheumatica.

TABLE 10 Normal values

Blood film	Check for anaemia and leukaemia
Platelets	150,000–400,000 per mm^3
Prothrombin time	Not more than 2 s longer than control
Control time	11–13 s
Partial thromboplastin time	Not more than 7 s longer than control
Control time	30–45 s
Bleeding time	Up to 6 min
Hess (tourniquet) test (80 mmHg for 5 min)	Not more than 3 spots in a square inch
Clotting time	Up to 10 min
Fibrinogen	200–400 mg/100 ml

Coagulation defects

'Comment on this coagulation screen.'

A good history from the patient is essential. A patient who has a convincing history of considerable haemorrhage and who is a special risk in surgery or biopsy procedures, may nevertheless have a normal coagulation screen (table 10). These simple tests cannot always exclude a bleeding abnormality and factors (table 11) may have to be

TABLE 11 Coagulation mechanism

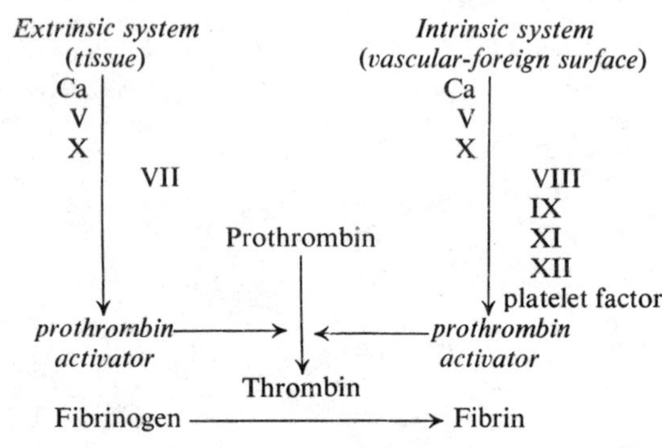

reduced to 10% of their normal level before they can be detected by them. Thus a patient with a bleeding history but a normal coagulation screen will require more detailed investigation including assays of the individual factors.

Apart from those due to anticoagulant administration, 95% of serious coagulation defects are due to von Willebrand's disease and the haemophilias.

Notes

The important factors to remember by *number* are shown in table 12.

TABLE 12 Important coagulation factors

Factor	*Deficiency states*
V	Very rare
VII	Warfarin therapy and liver disease
VIII = AHG	Haemophilia A and von Willebrand's disease
IX = Christmas factor	Haemophilia B, warfarin therapy and liver disease

Prothrombin time

Measures the *extrinsic system*. It is the time taken for the patient's citrated plasma to clot when a tissue factor (brain extract) and calcium are added. In a coagulation screen it is important because it measures deficiencies of V, VII, X, prothrombin and fibrinogen. It is normal in the haemophilias. It is relatively insensitive to reduction in prothrombin.

Partial thromboplastin time

Measures the *intrinsic system*. It is the time taken for the patient's citrated plasma to clot when kaolin (activates XI and XII), platelet substitute and calcium are added. In a coagulation screen it is important because it measures deficiencies of factors V, VIII to XII prothrombin and fibrinogen.

A normal control is necessary because of the variable potency of the tissue factor.

Thromboplastin generation test

In difficult cases the thromboplastin generation test is used. In this test three components of the clotting mechanism, i, ii, and iii are mixed together. Of these three, either i or ii is obtained from the patient. The other two components are either from a normal individual or are laboratory reagents.

i *Absorbed plasma*: V and VIII are normally present (VII and IX were removed by absorption)
ii *Serum*: VII and IX (and X) are normally present (V and VIII were removed because used up in the clot)
iii *Platelets* (or platelet substitute) and *calcium*

In classical haemophilia (factor VIII deficiency or haemophilia A) for instance, the mix containing the patient's absorbed plasma (i) with normal serum (ii) would have an abnormal prolonged test.

von Willebrand's disease

Autosomal dominant. May be due to two abnormalities:
— increased capillary fragility
— variable degree of factor VIII (AHG) deficiency or of a precursor (von Willebrand factor)
It presents with excessive bleeding, particularly from mucous membranes. There is usually a prolonged bleeding time.

Vitamin K and anticoagulants

Low levels of vitamin K and administration of coumarins (e.g. warfarin) or indandiones (e.g. phenindione) affect the synthesis of prothrombin and factor X plus:
— VII in the extrinsic system
— IX in the intrinsic system
Similar deficiencies occur in cirrhosis due to hepatocellular failure (often unresponsive to vitamin K). In addition in cirrhosis with portal hypertension, bleeding may be exacerbated by the thrombocytopenia of hypersplenism.

Defibrination syndrome

Synonyms: consumption coagulopathy, disseminated intravascular coagulation. This occurs in obstetric practice, thoracic surgery and pulmonary embolism, and in shock, especially when associated with infection or bleeding, and following mismatched blood transfusion.

The syndrome may present more chronically as a disorder with intravascular coagulation rather than excessive bleeding. The thrombophlebitis migrans of malignancy may be an example.

Platelets and factor V and VIII are consumed in the pathological coagulation as well as fibrinogen.

Fibrinolysis takes place and produces fibrin degeneration products which can be measured in the serum and urine.

Treatment is by replacement of the deficient factors by fresh (12 hours) whole blood or frozen fresh plasma and fibrinogen concentrates. Heparin may be given in normal (or lower) doses, progress being monitored by changes in the fibrinogen level.

Haemophilia therapy

In the treatment of the haemophilias A and B (VIII and IX deficiencies respectively), fresh frozen plasma which contains all factors may be given. Cryoprecipitate is used in haemophilia A but not haemophilia B (Christmas disease) because it does not contain IX. AHG concentrate (purified factor VIII) is now the preferred treatment when it is available and may be used to raise factor VIII in von Willebrand's disease.

Thrombocytopenia

May result from decreased production (idiopathic thrombocytopenic purpura or marrow aplasia, leukaemia or infiltration) or increased destruction (hypersplenism and consumption coagulopathy).

Osler's disease

Hereditary haemorrhagic telangiectasia: autosomal dominant. May present as intermittent bleeding, usually gastrointestinal. There are small capillary angiectases throughout the gastrointestinal tract including the buccal mucosa and tongue.

Multiple myelomatosis

This is a rare malignant disorder of plasma cells in the bone marrow which produce an excessive amount of an immunoglobulin, usually IgG (but also IgA or IgD) and often including light chains from this molecule (present as Bence-Jones protein). The clinical features are due to:

—the abnormal protein: greatly raised ESR, renal failure, infections

—bone involvement: bone pain, fractures, hypercalcaemia

—marrow replacement: anaemia, leucopenia, thrombocytopenia

Treatment is with radiotherapy to local bone lesions and by intermittent (4 days every 6 weeks) combination therapy with melphalan (0·25 mg/kg/day) and prednisolone (2·0 mg/kg/day).

Lymphadenopathy

Localised

Usually results from:

— local infection (any age)

— carcinoma (usually over 45 years old)

— Hodgkin's disease (usually young patients under 35 years)

NB Tuberculosis must be considered in all cervical lymphadenopathy. This is also a common site for stage I Hodgkin's disease, and also for neoplastic secondary deposits from the lung and nasopharyngeal carcinomas (ENT examination should be performed before biopsy).

Generalised

Usually results from:
— reticuloendothelial disorders
— chronic lymphatic leukaemia
— other less common causes include toxoplasmosis, tuberculosis, sarcoidosis, glandular fever and brucellosis.

NB A biopsy usually supplies the diagnosis (though a non-specific histology report does not exclude Hodgkin's disease). A blood count is essential in all cases particularly to confirm or exclude leukaemia.

Hodgkin's disease

The choice of therapy in Hodgkin's disease depends upon the clinical staging. In terms of prognosis it is important to know whether the disease has spread beyond the clinically observed regions, and lymphangiography (for para-aortic nodes) and in some centres laparotomy with splenectomy and liver biopsy are routine staging procedures.

Staging

I A single region (usually one side of the neck)
II Two regions involved
III Disease above and below diaphragm but limited to the reticuloendothelial system (nodes, spleen)
IV Widespread disease involving bone marrow, liver, and lung

Subclasses of each stage indicate the presence—class A—or absence—class B—of symptoms of weight loss, fever and pruritis.

Stages I, II and IIIA are treated by radical radiotherapy. Multiple chemotherapy is given to patients in stage IV. The best treatment of stages IIIA and IIIB, i.e. radiotherapy or chemotherapy, or both, is uncertain. About 80% of patients so treated survive 5 years and 60% of the original number are 'disease free'. Overall, women fare better than men, the presence of symptoms worsens the prognosis, and the absence or deficiency of lymphocytes in the histological section indicates a very poor outlook, whereas the outlook is good if lymphocytes are the predominant cell type.

Diabetes

'*This patient has diabetes mellitus; would you ask him some questions*' (also page 143).

A similar approach is advised in the clinic. You should ask his age and occupation and notice if he is under- or over-weight. Ask when the diabetes was first diagnosed. Ask about the common presenting symptoms of thirst, polyuria, fatigue and pruritus vulvae. In the young there is often loss of weight even when the appetite is well preserved.

NB This combination also occurs in thyrotoxicosis (common), some malabsorption states, some tumours early in their course (e.g. carcinoma of the bronchus), some hyperkatabolic states (e.g. leukaemia), and, to all appearances, in anorexia nervosa.

You should take:

— family history for diabetes

— obstetric history (big babies, stillbirths)

— drug history (corticosteroids and ACTH, thiazide diuretics)

Go quickly over the systems which can be involved in diabetes, asking questions about relevant symptoms.

Cardiovascular — Angina and myocardial infarcts. Intermittent claudication, cold feet, gangrene.

Nervous (pages 97 and 144) — *Legs, feet* Numbness, pain or paraesthesiae, painless ulcers.
Eyes (page 144) Failing vision (transitory with poor control), retinopathy, cataract.
Brain Ischaemic attacks or strokes.
Autonomic Impotence, postural hypotension. Diarrhoea (especially at night).

Respiratory — Cough, usually due to chronic bronchitis but tuberculosis is commoner in diabetics than in the general population.

Renal (page 144) — Polyuria (glycosuria, renal failure). Frequency and/or dysuria of infection.

Skin (page 145) — Sepsis e.g. boils. Xanthelasma (page 152). Necrobiosis lipoidica (very rare). Vaginitis (usually monilial).

Management — Define the outlines of his treatment and assess the adequacy of control (page 77).

Diet — The carbohydrate content (CHO) is usually expressed in grams. 120 g is average: a manual worker may need 200 g or more.

NB The calorie content is numerically about ten times this.

Drugs

Insulin — Ask about the type (PZ, soluble, lente etc), strength and frequency of injection. Do not confuse units of insulin with the number of marks on the syringe (the patient often does). Standard strength insulin is 20 units/ml: the standard insulin syringe has 20 marks per ml, i.e there is 1 unit of '20' insulin per mark. With 'double strength' insulin (40 units/ml), units taken = marks × 2. With '80 strength' insulin, units taken = marks × 4.

Oral therapy — Try to determine the name, tablet size and frequency of administration. You should know whether they are sulphonylureas or biguanides.

Urine testing results — Ask for his routine charts (e.g. Clinitest). Note that persistent blue tests without hypoglycaemic symptoms suggest that the patient has a high renal threshold for glucose and that the charts may be meaningless for the control of his diabetes. Check the blood sugars.

Symptoms of poor control

Hyperglycaemia — Polyuria (with nocturia) and thirst. Hospital admissions with ketoacidosis. Intermittent blurring of vision. Weight loss.

Hypoglycaemia — 'Hypo's' or 'reactions'. Determine at what time of day (in relation to food, exercise and insulin) they occur. Weight gain.

Examination — '*Would you examine him.*'
You will probably be directed by the history. Otherwise, examination should include:

Obesity — In the clinic perform routine height and weight measurements.

Injection sites — For fat atrophy.

Eyes — Dilate pupil if possible. Cataract and retinopathy (microaneurysms, exudates, retinal vessel proliferation, arteriosclerosis).

Legs and feet — Peripheral neuropathy (chiefly sensory). Test the tendon reflexes and for light touch and vibration sense.
Peripheral vascular disease. Check the arterial pulses and temperature of the feet. Even if the pulses are present, the toes may be blue and cold due to 'small vessel disease'.

Remember necrobiosis (very rare).
Quadriceps wasting (amyotrophy).
Infection.

Chest The history may indicate infection.

Abdomen Feel for the liver which may often be palpable in the longstanding insulin-dependent diabetic due to fatty infiltration.
(NB Haemochromatosis is very rare.)

Ask if you may (*a*) take the blood pressure; (*b*) test the urine for sugar, protein and ketones.
Ask if you may see (*a*) the result of a recent blood sugar (or series), and be told its relationship to the last main meal and to therapy; (*b*) a recent chest X-ray; (*c*) the result of an MSU if there is a history of dysuria.
NB Management of diabetes, see page 145.

Diabetes and pregnancy The risks to the fetus are considerable with a high perinatal mortality. Large babies are sometimes delivered with difficulty. Fetal mortality is related to the degree of diabetic control. The aims should be a patient without symptoms of diabetes or hypoglycaemia and without ketosis. The 2-hour postprandial blood sugar should not exceed 180 mg/100 ml. or the preprandial 120 mg/100 ml. Fetal loss should be under 5% if this is achieved but it is often 10% or more. Urine testing may not be useful because of the fall in renal glucose threshold. Insulin requirements tend to fall in the first trimester, stabilise in the second trimester, and rise again in the last trimester only to fall abruptly on delivery. The patient is usually admitted for elective Caesarean section at about the thirty-sixth week (see *Diabetes and surgery* below).

Diabetes and surgery The main danger is that the patient becomes hypoglycaemic whilst anaesthetised. Long-acting hypoglycaemic drugs (e.g. PZI and chlorpropamide) should be discontinued 24–48 hours before surgery, and soluble insulin bd substituted if necessary. The patient should be first on the operating list. No food or insulin is given on the morning of operation. The blood sugar can be checked during surgery if necessary and should be performed again within 2 hours of recovery. Catheterisation is not indicated for diabetic control. The evening dose of insulin can be given if required, but often the patient can wait until the next morning. If surgery is prolonged and i.v. glucose required, about 20 g per hour may be necessary (e.g. 400 ml of 5% dextrose or 40 ml of 50% dextrose).

Part 2: Essential background information

Neurology

'Headaches' and 'giddiness' constitute the most commonly presenting neurological symptoms. Cerebrovascular accidents are the most common neurological cause for hospital admission. In the Membership examination these are not commonly seen and frequently eliminated on the grounds of being too easy. Nonetheless it is often difficult to decide when to investigate in depth patients with headache and giddiness, and the management of 'strokes' may not only be difficult but present a major clinical challenge in terms of numbers of patients alone.

Headache

This is perhaps one of the most common of all presenting symptoms. The aims are to exclude treatable underlying intra- or extra-cranial disease and to make a definitive diagnosis (e.g. migraine). There are seldom any useful physical signs and the diagnosis is usually made on the history. Commonly the patient's history will correspond with one of the following:

Unilateral facial pain

Including migraine (see below).

Psychogenic headache

This is characteristically a severe continuous pressure felt bilaterally over the vertex, occiput or eyes. It may be band-like or non-specific in character and of variable intensity. It is commonest in middle-aged women but may occur at any age in association with stress or depression (ask about family, work, money and for symptoms of depression). The headache may be described with considerable drama and standard analgesics are almost invariably ineffective. Occasionally it may be symptomatic of worry about a brain tumour and relieved by definite reassurance.

Post-concussion headache

The pain has many of the features of psychogenic headache but is usually associated with dizziness (not vertigo) and loss of concentration. There is often a history of inadequate recovery following the head injury and of impending litigation.

Raised intracranial pressure

Intracranial tumour, haematoma or abscess. The pain is worst after lying down and is then associated with vomiting. It improves 1–2 hours after rising in the morning and is exacerbated by coughing, sneezing or straining. Visual defects may not occur despite severe papilloedema. The patient usually presents within 6 weeks of the onset of symptoms and these usually respond to standard analgesics.

Patients whose histories do not fit into one of these categories usually have either an obvious diagnosis (meningitis, subarachnoid haemorrhage, sinusitis, otitis media) or a less obvious local cause (teeth, cervical spine, skull, orbits). Benign hypertension, defects in visual acuity, glaucoma and ocular muscle imbalance seldom present as headache.

Investigation and management

In addition to the physical examination, a few investigations are commonly performed (chest and skull X-rays, WR and blood urea). If suspicion of organic disease is fairly high the 'non-invasive' investigations of brain scan and EEG may be added. The patient may need to be admitted for observation, lumbar puncture and even angiography or air studies.

Preliminary investigation

Patients with a headache of more than 6 weeks' duration and without abnormal clinical signs probably do not require investigation. Most hospital physicians, when seeing the patient referred from a family practitioner would request:

— full blood count including an ESR (to exclude temporal arteritis in the over fifties)

— chest X-ray for bronchial carcinoma

— possibly skull X-ray to detect (*a*) evidence of raised intracranial pressure; (*b*) shift of the midline if the pineal is calcified; (*c*) calcification within tumours (meningiomas and craniopharyngiomas)

In case of doubt it is usually reasonable to see the patient in the clinic at intervals to observe changing symptoms, the development of physical signs or increasing anxiety or depression.

Further investigation

This is rarely necessary but is probably indicated in the presence of:

— frontal headache on waking with nausea, i.e. symptoms suggestive of raised intracranial pressure

— occipital headache of sudden onset (subarachnoid haemorrhage)

— abnormal, and in particular progressive, neurological signs including confusion and dementia

It should include serological studies for syphilis (VDRL); isotope brain scan may reveal space occupying lesion; EEG; lumbar puncture; carotid arteriography and/or air encephalography (both have a distinct morbidity and mortality and should only be performed after careful consideration).

NB Patients with headache and facial pain may not give histories which fit conveniently into any well-recognised category. They should be seen at intervals to determine:

— symptoms of increasing anxiety or depression

— symptoms of changing pain patterns

— developing abnormal clinical signs

In the absence of these treatment is with simple analgesics.

Unilateral facial pain

Migraine

Migraine is episodic. It usually begins about puberty and continues intermittently to middle age. It is commoner in females than males and there is often a family history. There may have been episodes of unexplained abdominal pain in childhood. It may be associated with periods and 'the pill', with various foods and emotions, and with various times of the day or week. A characteristic attack starts with a sense of ill-health and is followed by a visual *aura* (shimmering lights, fortification spectra, scotomas) usually in the field opposite to the side of the succeeding headache. The throbbing *unilateral headache* is associated with anorexia, nausea, vomiting photophobia and withdrawal. There may be transient hemiparesis or sensory symptoms. It is very rarely associated with organic disease and angiography is only indicated if abnormal physical signs persist or progress.

Management

Precipitating causes should be identified and removed. Drugs may be used either to abort an attack if given early enough by an appropriate route (ergotamine by injection, buccal absorption, aerosol or suppository) or prophylactically (clonidine 25–75 μg bd indefinitely, or methysergide 1 mg bd for not more than 3 months). Phenobarbitone, promethazine and prochlorperazine have also been used.

Cluster headaches (migrainous neuralgia)

These appear to be a form of migraine. Attacks occur in clusters every 12 to 18 months and consist of very severe pain around an eye occurring often at night for 1–3 weeks. The eye becomes injected and watery and the nostril of the same side blocked up. It often responds to ergotamine.

Neuralgias

Neuralgias are intermittent, brief, severe, lancinating pains occurring along the distribution of a nerve.

Trigeminal neuralgia

Occurs almost only in the elderly. (If the syndrome occurs in a patient under 50 years old it may be symptomatic of multiple sclerosis.) The agonising pain is usually triggered from a place on the lips or the side of the nose. It tends to get worse with age but may be specifically relieved by carbamazepine (Tegretol). Phenytoin may also be useful. Eventually the patient may need section of the sensory root of the fifth nerve. Suicide is a definite risk.

Glossopharyngeal neuralgia

Precipitated by swallowing which produces pain in the pharynx.

Auriculotemporal neuralgia (Costen's syndrome) Precipitated by swallowing and may be treated by correcting a malocclusion.

Post-herpetic neuralgia Occurs in patients with a history of herpes zoster and the scars of the healed disease are usually obvious. The pain may be almost impossible to relieve.

Temporal arteritis (giant cell arteritis) Temporal arteritis is a local expression of a connective tissue disease (page 115). The pain is felt in the temples or over the entire scalp and the affected artery is usually dilated and tender. The patient usually feels ill and the ESR is greatly raised. Biopsy is performed if it can be done rapidly and the patient given steroids before sudden blindness supervenes.

Atypical facial pain This refers to a syndrome with episodes of constant ache in the jaw and cheek lasting several hours occurring usually in young to middle-aged women who frequently are depressed. It is often bilateral. Treatment is difficult but patients may respond to antidepressants or antihistamines.

Unilateral pain Local pathologies involving the eyes, sinuses, teeth or ears may give unilateral pain, as may tumours involving the fifth nerve (cerebellopontine angle tumours). Pain from herpes zoster may occur before the rash appears.

Cerebrovascular disease

Intracerebral haemorrhage, thrombosis and embolism These give rise to a 'stroke' which may be of any degree of severity. It is impossible to distinguish clinically between the three except that embolism is more likely if atrial fibrillation is present, after a myocardial infarction, or in infective endocarditis. The commonest presentation is with hemiplegia and dysphasia but there are numerous variants and slight weakness of a hand or confusion may be the only evidence of an attack.

Management During the unconscious phase evidence of continued one-sided haemorrhage is shown by a rising blood pressure, falling pulse rate and papilloedema. An enlarging ipsilateral pupil which finally becomes fixed and dilated indicates ipsilateral pressure of the third cranial nerve as it passes over the tentorium cerebelli. (Surgical evacuation of the blood clot may prevent pressure damage to the contralateral cortex.)

In any one patient it is impossible to assess how much recovery will occur, and attention must be paid to hydration and caloric intake during the unconscious phase. The patient must be turned regularly to prevent sores and catheterisation is usually necessary. Care in clinical management during the unconscious phase cannot be overemphasised. Passive and active physiotherapy must be started immediately and full support should be requested from specialists in rehabilitation. Hypertension is treated in the usual way.

Extracerebral haemorrhage

Extradural

This results from traumatic damage to the middle meningeal artery as it passes upward on the inside of the temporal bone. Classically, momentary loss of consciousness is followed by apparent recovery and death 1–7 days later. Not every fracture of the temporal bone results in middle meningeal haemorrhage but suspicion alone warrants skull X-rays and admission of the patient to observe his conscious level. Should signs of local haemorrhage ensue, burr holes are performed, the clot removed and the vessel tied.

Subdural

This occurs most frequently in the elderly, the alcoholic with vitamin deficiency, and children. It often follows trauma. A small haemorrhage occurs and the clot slowly enlarges in size by absorbing fluid osmotically from the CSF.

Clinical presentation: The symptoms may develop over a period of weeks to months. Confusion and progressive loss of conscious level occur and there may be fluctuation of consciousness with 'lucid' intervals. The other signs are of a one-sided intracranial mass with contralateral weakness and hemiplegia, possibly with signs of raised intracranial pressure (falling pulse rate, rising blood pressure and papilloedema).

Management: Full recovery may follow removal of the haematoma, irrespective of the patient's age. Subdural haematomas may be bilateral.

Subarachnoid

This usually results from rupture of a berry aneurysm from the vessels of the circle of Willis. Rupture is more common in the presence of hypertension. Subarachnoid haemorrhage may result from rupture of an angioma and severe intracerebral haemorrhage may spread into the subarachnoid space.

Clinical presentation: Consciousness may or may not be lost. If not, a history of headache described as 'a severe blow in the back of the neck' may be obtained. There may be associated nausea and vomiting.

On examination, photophobia and neck stiffness are present. The level of consciousness progressively decreases if haemorrhage continues, with signs of rising intracranial pressure (rising blood pressure, falling pulse rate, papilloedema). There may be localising signs in the cranial nerves.

Lumbar puncture shows raised pressure and uniform blood staining and later, xanthochromia. Proteinuria and glycosuria may occur.

Management: Arteriography is indicated to determine the site of haemorrhage (25% show multiple aneurysm and 10% are negative). The optimum time after haemorrhage to perform arteriography is not agreed though it is usually delayed until the patient has recovered consciousness. When haemorrhage has stopped spontaneously, some surgeons prefer to delay arteriography for 7–10 days to allow arterial spasm to subside. Immediate radiology may be indicated if progressive cerebral deterioration is observed since clipping the artery at this stage may prevent further damage.

Prognosis: This can be considered 'in thirds'. One-third of the patients die in the first attack. Another third have a recurrence (normally between the first and second weeks), and a third of these survive. Of those who survive a year, about half remain well and symptom-free.

Ischaemic cerebrovascular disease

Internal carotid artery stenosis

Platelet emboli dislodge from the damaged intima of the carotid artery and lodge in the cerebral arteries. This may result in a typical hemiplegic stroke (middle cerebral artery) or transient syncopal attacks and transient blindness (ophthalmic artery). The thrombi tend to break up where they lodge and symptoms tend to be transient but recurrent (transient ischaemic attacks). Platelet emboli may, very occasionally, be seen in the optic fundi.

Management: Surgical removal of the atheromatous plaque identified on carotid arteriography has been curative. However, there is usually atheroma in all of the cerebral vessels and surgery is ineffective. Anticoagulant therapy may improve symptoms in individual patients without improving life expectancy.

Vertebrobasilar insufficiency

This presents as transient episodes of vertigo with nystagmus and occasionally 'drop attacks'. This results from decreased blood supply through narrowed arteries to the brain-stem and is itself often the result of nipping of the vertebral arteries by osteoarthritic cervical vertebrae in the presence of an 'incompetent' circle of Willis. It carries a relatively good prognosis compared with disease of the internal carotid arteries. Anticoagulants may improve symptoms. Thrombosis in the same area often affects the upper medulla and cerebellum and causes cranial nerve paralyses (page 3), e.g. lateral medullary syndrome.

Epilepsy

Many patients who present following a 'fit' have only had an episode of unconsciousness. It is important to consider and exclude other conditions which are commonly confused with epilepsy, e.g. syncope and metabolic disorders.

Syncope

Vaso-vagal fainting attacks
Cerebral arterial disease—carotid artery stenosis and vertebrobasilar ischaemia
Low cardiac output—Stokes–Adams attacks in heart block, and aortic stenosis
Micturition and cough syncope. Syncope of emotional distress and carotid sinus syncope
Postural hypotension may be due to hypotensive or sedative drugs, particularly in the elderly

Metabolic disorders

Hypoglycaemia, renal or hepatic failure, and drug poisoning

Apart from vaso-vagal attacks and emotional syncope, each of these syncopal and metabolic situations can be followed by true epilepsy.

Aetiology of epilepsy

Usually no cause can be demonstrated, though the following should be considered:

Cerebral tumour, abscess or angioma
Sequel of severe head injury and birth injury
Cerebral atherosclerosis
Other rare causes include toxoplasmosis, cysticercosis, syphilis and systemic lupus erythematosus
Falciparum malaria should be considered in travellers (examine blood film)

Clinical presentation

Grand mal

In over 50% of cases, a fit is preceded by an aura. This is followed by coma and the tonic phase. This lasts up to 30 seconds and cyanosis may occur as the respiratory muscles are also tonically contracted. The clonic phase follows in all limbs and micturition and tongue biting occur in this stage, which is followed by sleep for 1–3 hours. During sleep the corneal and limb reflexes may be absent and the plantar responses up-going.

Management of acute phase Protect the patient from injury during convulsion and wedge the jaw open. Intravenous diazepam (10–50 mg) and/or phenobarbitone intramuscularly (200 mg) will control most fits. Status epilepticus may require continued diazepam, phenobarbitone and intravenous phenytoin.

Long-term therapy The object is to decrease the number and intensity of fits and if possible to abolish them with the least side-effects (chiefly sedation). The standard drugs usually used alone or together are: phenobarbitone 30–60 mg bd or tds, phenytoin (Epanutin) 50–100 mg bd or tds.

Other drugs include primidone (Mysoline) which is substituted for phenobarbitone, sulthiame (Ospolot), carbamazepine (Tegretol), clonazepam (Rivotril) and sodium valproate (Epilim).

NB Sometimes it is not possible to stop all fits

without unacceptable sedation. Epileptics are allowed to drive if they have not had a fit for three years whether on or off therapy or if all fits have been nocturnal for 3 years.

Petit mal

This presents in childhood and is characterised by moments of absence, and occasionally akinetic seizures and myoclonic jerks of the limbs. The EEG shows typical spike and wave complexes at 3 per second. It virtually never continues beyond adolescence but may be superseded by adult epilepsy. Management: Normal schooling. Ethosuximide (Zarontin) is the drug of first choice. Phenytoin, sodium valproate and troxidone are also used.

Temporal lobe epilepsy

This is characterised by temporary disturbances of the content of consciousness. Hallucinations may occur (déjà vu phenomenon) as may visual disturbances such as macropsia and micropsia. Unreasoning fear or depersonalisation may be present. Olfactory or gustatory auras may be the only symptom and are related to abnormal foci in the uncinate lobe (uncinate attacks). Automatism may follow the aura. In these, patients perform a complex movement pattern, repeated with each attack (psychomotor epilepsy). Treatment is similar to that of grand mal.

Jacksonian (focal) epilepsy

Convulsions originate in one part of the precentral motor cortex. Fits begin in one part of the body (e.g. the thumb) and may proceed to involve that side of the body and then the whole body. Subsequent paresis of the affected limb may last up to 3 days (Todd's paralysis). Sensory epilepsy is a parallel condition originating in the sensory cortex. Treatment is similar to that of grand mal.

Investigation of 'fits'

The object is to detect treatable underlying brain disease.

A full history and clinical examination is taken to exclude other causes of loss of consciousness (see above).

All patients should have skull and chest X-rays. An EEG may be helpful by demonstrating the site of an epileptic focus (slow activity may suggest the presence of a tumour).

After a single isolated fit and in the absence of neurological signs, no further investigation is usually necessary. The patient is seen at regular intervals and if he has a further fit or develops neurological signs (particularly if they are progressive) detailed investigations are indicated. Investigations should include a brain scan and examination of the cerebrospinal fluid. Carotid angiography or air encephalography may become necessary.

Transmission of epileptic tendency

The presence of cortical dysrhythmia on EEG does not mean epileptic attacks will definitely occur. In 35% of cases both parents have EEG dysrhythmias, whereas only in 5% of cases both parents have normal EEGs.

Meningitis

Aetiology

TABLE 13 Bacterial and viral causes of meningitis

Bacterial	*Viral*
Meningococcus	Mumps
Haemophilus influenzae	Echovirus } enterovirus
Pneumococcus	Coxsackie } enterovirus
	Lymphocytic choriomeningitis (LCM)
Rare causes	
Tuberculosis	Herpes simplex
Staphylococcus	Poliovirus (enterovirus)
Leptospira	Arboviruses
Listeria	
Toxoplasma	
Cryptococcus (in immunosuppressed patients)	
E. coli (in neonates)	

Besides the bacterial and viral causes listed in table 13, the following points should be considered:

Tuberculous meningitis is easily missed and should be considered in the differential diagnosis of all cases of viral meningitis.

Cerebral tumours, abscesses and venous sinus thrombosis may produce a lymphocytosis and raised protein in the CSF.

Neck stiffness and headache without more severe signs may follow a small subarachnoid haemorrhage.

Diabetics may be precipitated into coma by meningitis.

The confident diagnosis of 'meningism' may mean failure to diagnose meningitis. If in doubt lumbar puncture should be performed.

Pneumococcal meningitis is often secondary to underlying pneumococcal infection in the lung, sinuses or ear.

Clinical features

These are:
— of infection
— of meningism (±mild encephalitic features)
— of raised intracranial pressure

Meningococcal meningitis

The meningitis is part of a septicaemia. The meningococcus is carried in the nasopharynx often asymptomatically (carriers) and tends to produce epidemics of infection. These occur in conditions of overcrowding and in closed communities. After a short incubation period of 1 to 3 days the disease begins abruptly with fever, headache, nausea, vomiting and neck stiffness. Mental confusion and coma may follow. There may be a characteristic rash with widespread irregular petechiae of variable size.

Lumbar puncture — The CSF is purulent and shows a raised protein (100–300 mg/100 ml), 1000–3000 polymorphs and a low or almost absent sugar. Intracellular and extracellular Gram-negative diplococci are present. The organism can also be isolated in blood culture.

Treatment — *Drug of choice* Benzylpenicillin initially 12–20 mega-units intravenously per day in divided doses. Sulphonamides (sulphadimidine 8–12 g daily) may be given in addition when indicated by bacterial sensitivities, but are not recommended alone because sulphonamide-resistant organisms are becoming more frequent.
Secondline treatment (when the patient is allergic to penicillins) Chloramphenicol 1 g 6-hourly.

Pneumococcal meningitis — Infection may be secondary to pneumococcal pneumonia or it may spread from infected sinuses or ears or through fractures of the base of the skull. It is commoner in paediatric and geriatric practice. Symptoms develop rapidly, sometimes within hours, and fever, headache, nausea and vomiting may quickly proceed to coma.

Lumbar puncture — The CSF is purulent with a raised protein, high polymorph count and low sugar. Gram-positive diplococci are present. Blood culture is often positive (as it is in pneumococcal pneumonia).

Treatment — *Drug of choice* Benzylpenicillin as for meningococcal meningitis. The dose can be reduced after about 3–4 days provided the fever has fallen and there is clinical improvement. Treatment should continue for 10 days.
Secondline treatment Chloramphenicol as for meningococcal meningitis.
Pneumococcal meningitis is extremely serious and especially so if the patient is in coma before therapy is started. The overall mortality is high (20–30%).

Haemophilus influenza meningitis — This usually occurs in children under 5 years old and may be insidious in onset with a longer incubation period than in the meningitides described above (5 days). It usually follows an influenzal-type illness and presents with fever, nausea and vomiting.

Lumbar puncture — The CSF is purulent with a high protein and polymorph count and low sugar. Gram-negative bacilli can be seen, and grown on culture.

Treatment — *Drug of choice* Chloramphenicol 3–5 g daily (children 50–100 mg/kg/day for 10 days though a lower dose is required in the neonate).
Secondline treatment Ampicillin intravenously 15–30 g daily.
The overall mortality is 5–10%.

Intrathecal penicillin therapy — There is little evidence to support the use of intrathecal therapy but most physicians would give one dose of intrathecal benzylpenicillin (10,000–20,000 units in adults) through the lumbar puncture needle on finding a purulent CSF. Some physicians consider daily intrathecal therapy of value particularly in pneumococcal meningitis. There is no evidence that this improves the outlook.

Bacterial meningitis of unknown cause

This problem occurs when a purulent CSF is obtained from a patient with meningitis but no organisms are seen with Gram staining. This is most frequently due to preadmission antibiotic therapy. There is no time to wait for the results of culture and antibiotics should be started immediately. In adults there are a number of recommended courses of action, all of which should treat effectively the common organisms found (i.e. pneumococcus, meningococcus, *Haemophilus influenzae*):

Chloramphenicol alone
Ampicillin alone
Ampicillin with penicillin

The drugs are to be given in the doses mentioned above. The use of chloramphenicol with penicillin, although theoretically inadvisable (bacteriostatic drug with a bactericidal one respectively), is used in some centres with considerable success.

Multiple sclerosis (MS) [Disseminated sclerosis (DS)]

A disease characterised by acute episodes of neurological deficit appearing irregularly throughout the central nervous system both in place and time, with spontaneous but partial remission. It is a demyelinating disease with first episodes occurring in young adulthood. The aetiology is unknown; currently 'slow viruses' have been postulated, on the 'kuru', Jakob–Creutzfeldt, and scrapie models. The patches of demyelination occur in the white matter of the brain and spinal cord, especially in
— optic nerves
— brain-stem
— cerebellar peduncles
— dorsal and pyramidal (lateral) tracts

Clinical presentation

Retrobulbar neuritis with ocular pain and dimming of vision. After recovery 'optic atrophy' or temporal pallor of the disc are characteristic. Only about 25% of patients with retrobulbar neuritis subsequently develop multiple sclerosis.
Diplopia due to an oculomotor (III, IV or VI) or internuclear paralysis. After recovery, ataxic nystagmus (i.e. with nystagmus greater in the abducting eye than in the adducting eye) is characteristic.
Acute vertigo and vomiting.
Cerebellar signs with intention tremor, nystagmus and dysarthria.
Sensory deficit with paraesthesiae and proprioceptive loss in a limb or half of the body.
Upper motor neurone motor deficit with weakness, as a paraparesis, hemiparesis, or monoparesis.
Disturbed micturition. Precipitancy is common.

Eventually there is remaining evidence of optic atrophy, cerebellar lesions, and spastic paraparesis, frequently with posterior column loss. There is some dementia with change of mood and euphoria is characteristic.

NB Multiple sclerosis may present differently in middle age as a slowly-progressive spastic paraparesis, with or without some posterior column loss, i.e. as spinal cord disease.

Diagnosis

The clinical diagnosis is made on the basis of a minimum of two characteristic episodes. Other causes of spastic paraparesis may have to be excluded, particularly in patients presenting in middle age. Lumbar puncture is usually sufficient to establish a diagnosis. The CSF protein may be normal or raised, the Lange curve show an early zone rise, and immunoelectrophoresis may demonstrate a high γ-globulin.

Prognosis

When multiple sclerosis presents in the young, it is an intermittent disease and usually, but not always, progresses over 20–30 years. The last few years are marked by complete invalidism, the patients being confined to bed or a chair.

In the middle-aged, multiple sclerosis progresses more slowly but is less intermittent. The patient may never be seriously incapacitated.

Management

Psychological support is essential throughout the illness. Patients usually remain surprisingly euphoric but not infrequently there is marked depression.

Physiotherapy and occupational therapy to maintain mobility of joints and allow mobilisation. This is particularly important in later stages of the disease.

ACTH (ACTH gel 80 units daily with gradual dose reduction over 6 weeks) helps to shorten the acute episodes of demyelination, but probably has no effect on the degree of residual disability.

Parkinson's disease and extrapyramidal disorders

Parkinsonism

James Parkinson, 1755–1824, London.

Clinical presentation

This is a disturbance of voluntary motor function characterised by the triad of rigidity, tremor and bradykinesia (slow movements).

The classical picture of Parkinsonism is of immobile flexion at all joints except the interphalangeal (neck, trunk, shoulders, elbows, wrists and metacarpophalangeal joints). On walking, even in the early case, the arms do not swing fully and later the gait is shuffling and the patient may show festination. The face is expressionless and unblinking, and speech slurred and monotonous. In the long-standing case, a number of other symptoms is commonly present: difficulty in initiating movement (rising from a chair or turning in bed), poor balance with a tendency to fall because of slow correcting movements, small handwriting, rarely increased salivation (which, with dysphagia, may give rise to drooling), and a soft unintelligible voice (dysarthria). Oculogyric crises (forced upward deviation of the eyes) occur characteristically in drug-induced and post-encephalitic Parkinsonism. These patients may also have symptoms of the side-effects of treatment (see below).

The tremor (4–6 per second) is usually most obvious in the hands ('pill-rolling'), improved by voluntary movement and made worse by anxiety. Titubation refers to tremor involving the head. The rigidity may be leadpipe or, with the tremor superimposed, cogwheel. The patient may demonstrate a glabellar tap. Parkinsonism is usually asymmetrical. Patients are frequently, and understandably, depressed.

Aetiology

Idiopathic (paralysis agitans) This is of slow onset and inexorably progressive. It presents in the 50–60 year age group and in males more often than females. It appears to result from an imbalance or defect of transmitter substances (dopamine and acetylcholine) in the extrapyramidal cells. It may be familial.
Atherosclerosis This is often associated with other manifestations of vascular disease (stroke, dementia, ischaemic heart disease, intermittent claudication and hypertension). There tends to be less tremor and more festination than in idiopathic Parkinsonism.
Drugs Phenothiazines (e.g. chlorpromazine) and, less commonly, reserpine, may produce Parkinsonism. The high doses used in psychiatry make it relatively common in schizophrenics. Dystonic movements—facial grimacing, involuntary movements of the tongue and oculogyric crises—are more common than in idiopathic Parkinsonism.
Poisoning Rarely, Parkinson-like disorders may result from poisoning with heavy metals—manganese and copper (NB Wilson's disease, page 94)—and after carbon monoxide poisoning.
Post-encephalitic Parkinsonism occurred following outbreaks of encephalitis lethargica (between 1917 and 1925) and still occurs sporadically.

Management

The object is to reduce each of the symptoms—rigidity, tremor and bradykinesia.
Physiotherapy
Anticholinergic drugs (a relative excess of acetylcholine may be responsible for symptoms). Standard atropine-like drugs should be used first, e.g. benzhexol (Artane 2 mg bd increasing to 5 mg bd), benztropine (Cogentin) and orphenadrine (Disipal). They are useful in over 60% of patients, and are more effective in treating rigidity than tremor and least in bradykinesia. Side-effects include blurred

vision, dry mouth, tachycardia, urinary retention, constipation and glaucoma. There may be confusion and loss of concentration, especially in the elderly. *Levodopa* (250 mg bd increasing to 2–8 g daily in divided doses) should be used in addition to anticholinergic drugs. It is effective in 75% of patients (excellent in 20%), particularly in those with bradykinesia, less so in those with tremor. It is not used in drug-induced Parkinsonism. Side-effects are common (40%) and include anorexia, nausea and vomiting (which respond to cyclizine: preferably not pyridoxine which antagonises levodopa or metoclopramide which may give dystonic movements), choreiform movements, cardiac arrhythmias and hypotension. The extracerebral side-effects are reduced by concomitant administration of a decarboxylase inhibitor (e.g. carbidopa in Sinemet).
Amantidine may be added to the other two groups of drugs.
Stereotactic surgery—ablation of the ventrolateral nucleus of the thalamus—is less used since the advent of levodopa. It is most effective in cases of tremor, less so in patients with rigidity. It may produce a stroke of variable severity and is therefore often reserved for the non-dominant side. Parkinsonism tends to recur after a year or two.
Depression is easy to overlook in Parkinsonism due to reduced emotional expression. It should be treated with tricyclic antidepressants but not with monoamine oxidase inhibitors since the combination with levodopa may induce acute hypertension.

The remaining extrapyramidal disorders are very uncommon.

Hepatolenticular degeneration

(Kinnier Wilson's disease) (page 185)

Aetiology

It is a Mendelian recessive disorder producing a deficiency of the copper-carrying globulin, caeruloplasmin. Copper is deposited in the putamen, cornea, lens and liver.

Clinical presentation

Onset aged 10–25. The extrapyramidal disorder presents with tremor (often an intention tremor, *cf.* paralysis agitans), rigidity and, occasionally, athetoid movements of the limbs. The face may be mask-like and loss of emotional control with frank dementia occurs. Kayser–Fleischer corneal rings result from copper deposition. Cirrhosis may finally result from deposition of copper in the liver.

Management

Is aimed at decreasing intestinal copper absorption with a low copper diet, and increasing urinary excretion with D-penicillamine.

Chorea

This term describes disorderly involuntary movements, usually of the face and/or arms which appear pseudo-purposive unless very marked. They may interfere with voluntary movements of limbs and with speech, eating and respiration. They cease during sleep.

Sydenham's chorea (seventeenth century English)

A child of 5–15 years (female more often than male) is described as restless, clumsy or fidgety. There is proximal chorea of the arms (and less so, the legs) and grimacing. It is associated with rheumatic fever and usually recovers completely in 2–3 months. It must be differentiated from a nervous tic. It is very rare.

Huntington's chorea (1851–1916, American)

This is a Mendelian dominant disorder and there is usually a family history. The symptoms usually start between 30 and 45 years of age. The chorea is distal initially and involves the legs (with ataxia), arms (with clumsiness) and face. The movements are rapid and jerky. Mental changes develop gradually, usually without insight and progress to dementia and death in about 10–15 years. The chorea reponds to tetrabenazine. It is rarely seen outside mental hospitals.

Chorea may follow a stroke or kernicterus. It may be congenital.

Cerebral tumours

May be primary (80%) or secondary (20% from bronchus, breasts, kidney, colon, ovary, prostate or thyroid). Primary tumours originate from:
— nervous tissue (very rare)
— supporting tissues (relatively common) such as gliomas (or astrocytomas), oligodendrogliomas and ependymomas (both benign)
— meninges producing meningiomas
— blood vessels—angiomas and angioblastomas

Symptoms and signs

Due to raised intracranial pressure

Headache, classically frontal and early morning associated with nausea, vomiting and later papilloedema.
Mental confusion, drowsiness and dementia.
Sixth nerve palsy results from pressure on the nerve somewhere along its long intracranial path (a 'false localising sign').

Epilepsy

Occurs in 30% of tumours, particularly of the frontal or temporal lobe.

Progressive focal signs

These depend upon the site of the tumour.
Prefrontal Progressive dementia with loss of affect and social responsibility. Anosmia may be present and the grasp reflex and palmar-mental reflexes present in the contralateral hand.
Precentral Contralateral hemiplegia and Jacksonian epilepsy.
Parietal The chief parietal signs are falling away of the contralateral outstretched arm, astereognosis

and tactile inattention. Apraxia and spatial disorientation may occur. Low-sited tumours may produce upper quadrantic homonymous hemianopia rather than complete homonymous hemianopia (or visual inattention). Dysphasia occurs with lesions in the dominant temporoparietal region.

Temporal lobe Symptoms of temporal lobe epilepsy with aphasia (if on the dominant side) and an upper quadrantic homonymous hemianopia.

Occipital lobe Lesions produce homonymous hemianopia either complete or quadrantic with macular sparing.

Acoustic neuroma

A neurofibroma of the acoustic (eighth) nerve. It is more common in neurofibromatosis. It is relatively rare.

Clinical presentation

Typically, symptoms begin at 35–45 years with progressive deafness and diminished reaction on caloric testing, sometimes with tinnitus and mild vertigo. Pressure on other nerves and the brainstem of the same side produce:

Seventh nerve: facial palsy
Fifth nerve: weakness of mastication, loss of corneal reflex and facial sensory loss
Sixth nerve: lateral rectus palsy
Cerebellar syndrome

Investigation

Skull radiology reveals erosion of the internal auditory meatus and/or petrous temporal bone. CSF protein is usually considerably raised (above 100 mg/100 ml).

Benign intracranial hypertension

This mimics cerebral tumour with headaches and papilloedema, but is probably due to thrombosis of the venous sinuses. It may follow infection (e.g. otitis media), head injury and pregnancy. It is commoner in obese young women. It tends to recover in a few months spontaneously, but if vision is endangered, high-dose steroids may be used to decrease intracranial pressure.

Motor neurone disease

This disease involves degeneration of:
— anterior horn cells in the spinal cord
— cells of the lower cranial motor nuclei
— pyramidal tracts

Clinical presentation

Motor neurone disease normally presents in patients over 35 years of age with the clinical features of one of the above groups but usually progresses to produce features of the other two as well. It is rare in all its forms. It is characterised by:
— muscular weakness and fasciculation
— absence of sensory signs

There are three classical forms of clinical presentation:

1 Patients may present with lower motor neurone weakness, wasting and fasciculation of the small muscles of the hand. This is followed by wasting of the upper and then lower limb muscles. This lower motor neurone wasting and fasciculation is termed 'progressive muscular atrophy' and, characteristically, tendon reflexes are lost early.

2 Patients may present with lower motor neurone weakness and wasting of the tongue and pharynx producing dysarthria, dysphagia, choking and nasal regurgitation ('progressive bulbar palsy').

3 Patients may present with upper motor neurone spastic weakness starting in the legs, and later spreading to the arms ('amyotrophic lateral sclerosis').

Any combination of the above three groups can occur. In most cases upper and lower motor neurone lesions are combined at the time of presentation. The reflexes may be absent or exaggerated depending upon the balance between upper and lower motor disease. Lower limb lesions are usually of upper motor neurone type, and the upper limb lesions of lower motor neurone type. The upper limbs may demonstrate marked muscular wasting but still have exaggerated reflexes. The abdominal reflexes are usually preserved until late in the disease. Pseudobulbar palsy (page 11) may occur but is very uncommon.

Differential diagnosis

The syndrome may be the presenting feature of underlying carcinoma but in these cases sensory changes are usually also present.

Prognosis

Death occurs within 2–3 years of presentation.

Peripheral neuropathy

Definition

A disorder of peripheral nerves, either sensory, motor or mixed, usually symmetrical and affecting distal more than proximal parts of the limbs. By convention isolated cranial nerve palsies and isolated and multiple peripheral nerve lesions (median, ulnar, lateral popliteal palsies, and mononeuritis multiplex) are excluded.

Aetiology

In general medical practice four disorders must be considered: diabetes mellitus, carcinomatous neuropathy, vitamin B deficiency (including B_{12}) and drugs or chemicals. Only the first is common.

Diabetic neuropathy

Apart from causing isolated cranial and peripheral nerve lesions (including mononeuritis multiplex), diabetes causes a distal, predominantly sensory, neuropathy affecting commonly the distal lower limbs in the 'stocking' distribution. Symptoms of numbness, paraesthesiae and sometimes pain in the feet are associated with loss of vibration and position sense. Characteristically the ankle reflex is also lost (see page 144).

Carcinomatous neuropathy Carcinoma may be associated with either a sensory neuropathy affecting the 'glove' and 'stocking' regions or motor neuropathy in which there is muscle weakness and wasting usually of the proximal limb muscles. The neuropathy may be mixed. If distal muscles are affected, the neuropathy may be indistinguishable from any motor neurone disease.

Vitamin B deficiency Sensory neuropathy characterises deficiency of vitamin B_1. Patients, often alcoholics, present with numbness ('walking on cotton wool') and paraesthesiae. Pain and soreness of the feet may be a feature. In vitamin B_{12} deficiency the peripheral neuropathy may be associated with subacute combined degeneration of the cord (page 105) and megaloblastic anaemia (page 68).

Drugs Peripheral neuropathy may result from treatment for tuberculosis with INAH which is pyridoxine-dependent and occurs in 'slow acetylators' (page 214). Other drugs include vincristine, vinblastine, phenytoin and nitrofurantoin.

Other rare causes Uraemia, myxoedema, polyarteritis nodosa, heavy metal and industrial poisoning (e.g. lead, triorthocresyl phosphate), infectious disorders (leprosy, diphtheria, Guillain–Barré syndrome), amyloidosis, sarcoidosis and porphyria.

NB Investigation of patients with peripheral neuropathy is aimed at excluding underlying carcinoma and confirming the other common and treatable disorders. In about 50% of cases the aetiology remains unknown.

Mononeuritis multiplex A disorder affecting two or more peripheral nerves at one time, producing symptoms of numbness, paraesthesiae and sometimes pain in their sensory distribution with associated muscle weakness and wasting. The lower limbs are more commonly affected and the neuropathy is asymmetrical. This uncommon syndrome occurs in diabetes mellitus, polyarteritis nodosa and less commonly in other collagen diseases.

Polymyositis and allied disorders A rare disorder presenting with progressive weakness in the proximal limb muscles, usually more marked in the lower limbs. The disease merges with dermatomyositis in which skin manifestations are an obvious feature, and with the other collagen disorders in which muscle weakness may be a marked or dominant feature. In the over fifties there is a high incidence (40–50%) of underlying carcinoma as with dermatomyositis.

Clinical presentation The disorder presents at any age, but more commonly in the over thirties with muscle pain and tenderness with progressive weakness and diplegia (50% of cases). Proximal muscles are affected more than distal ones, and patients may first notice difficulty climbing or standing from a sitting position, and difficulty lifting objects above their heads. Neck muscles are frequently involved (60%) but the facial and ocular muscles rarely (*cf.* myasthenia gravis). Arthralgia occurs in about 25% of cases. Raynaud's phenomenon is common in the young and may proceed to scleroderma. Skin rashes are common (60%) and range from diffuse erythema to the manifestations of dermatomyositis (page 113).

Prognosis

This is variable but generally worse in older patients. The disease may remit spontaneously, particularly in the young (under 30), but may recur and/or progress to a more diffuse systemic collagen disorder (30–50 years). In the over fifties the prognosis depends on the underlying carcinoma if present. The overall mortality of untreated cases is about 50%.

Treatment

Corticosteroids (prednisone 40–60 mg daily) are given initially, and the dose reduced gradually depending upon the patient's clinical state and the serum creatine phosphokinase level. This is high during active disease but falls rapidly if therapy is successful. Steroid therapy is usually needed for 1–3 years before being gradually withdrawn.

Differential diagnosis

Trichinella spiralis infection of muscles may produce acute myositis. Proximal muscle wasting and weakness also occur in carcinomatous neuromyopathy, hereditary muscular dystrophies, Cushing's disease and with steroid therapy, thyrotoxicosis, osteomalacia and diabetes (amyotrophy, see page 145). NB Polymyalgia rheumatica usually presents with pain and stiffness. Wasting is not a characteristic feature (page 115). All these conditions are relatively rare.

Investigation

Serum aldolase and creatine phosphokinase

These enzymes are greatly elevated in the muscular dystrophies during the most active stage of muscle degeneration (in the second and third decades of life). In polymyositis, the level of the enzymes gives a measure of active muscle destruction and should decline rapidly on corticosteroids coincident with improvement in muscle strength.

Electromyography

In the muscular dystrophies, evidence of decrease in active muscle is shown by the presence of short duration, low amplitude polyphasic action potentials. Polymyositis produces a similar picture but also with evidence of spontaneous fibrillation, possibly evidence of muscular irritability. Spontaneous fibrillation is characteristic of degenerated muscle undergoing active degeneration, and is associated with evidence of a decrease in the number of motor units on voluntary movement. EMG findings often do not fit neatly into the above patterns as the distribution of muscle involvement is patchy and as the EMG recording depends upon the particular region of muscle sampled.

Myasthenia gravis

A disorder of muscle weakness resulting from failure of neuromuscular transmission.

Aetiology

The disease may present as an isolated entity but the clinical picture also occurs in association with:
— thymoma in 15% of cases
— thyrotoxicosis
— bronchial carcinoma (Eaton–Lambert syndrome)
— disseminated lupus erythematosus
The disease itself is rare and it is very rare for it to be a manifestation of these associated conditions.

Clinical presentation

Muscular weakness is produced by repetitive or sustained contraction. It is usually most marked in the face and eyes producing ptosis and diplopia. Weakness of speech and swallowing may occur. The proximal muscles are more often affected than the distal, and the upper limb muscles more than the lower.

Prognosis

The disorder may never progress beyond ophthalmoplegia and periods of remission up to 3 years are common. Death may be rapid if the respiratory muscles are involved. Pregnancy may make the weakness either more or less severe.

Diagnosis and treatment

Edrophonium (Tensilon) 10 mg i.v. reduces the weakness of affected muscles for 3–4 minutes. Long-term therapy is achieved with longer acting anticholinesterases orally such as neostigmine or pyridostigmine (Mestinon), preferably by slowly increasing the dose until measured muscular strength is optimal. Overdose may give depolarisation block with weakness. In intractable cases thymectomy may be performed (less effective if there is a thymoma). The differential diagnosis is from other causes of ptosis (page 4), muscular dystrophies involving the face, familial hypokalaemic paralysis and the Eaton–Lambert syndrome. In this, the myasthenia is associated with a carcinoma, usually of the bronchus. It differs from classical myasthenia gravis in that the eyes are less frequently affected, that proximal limb muscle weakness is common and their strength initially *increased* by repeated movement, and that there is no response to edrophonium. Oral guanidine is specific.

Myotonia

Myotonia is the inability of muscles to relax normally after contraction.

Dystrophia myotonica

A hereditary disorder producing progressively more severe symptoms and signs with succeeding generations, i.e. 'anticipation'. It is rare.

Clinical presentation

Both males and females are affected. The 'classical' case demonstrates:

Abnormal facies—with frontal balding, ptosis, a smooth expressionless forehead, cataracts and a 'lateral' smile.
Wasting of the facial muscles, sternomastoids, shoulder girdle and quadriceps. The forearms and legs are involved and reflexes lost.
Myotonia which increases with cold, fatigue and excitement.
Testicular or ovarian atrophy.
Mental deficiency.

NB The heart may be involved and diabetes mellitus may develop.

Myotonia congenita This is an hereditary disorder, transmitted as a Mendelian dominant which affects both sexes equally, and first presents in childhood. There is no muscle wasting and no long-term effects. It is very rare. The myotonias should not be confused with two disorders of children:

Amyotonia congenita A congenital disorder producing weakness and hypotonia which is first noticed in children at the head-lifting stage. The muscle disturbance becomes less severe as the children grow older although contractures may produce scoliosis.

Progressive spinomuscular atrophy (Werdnig-Hoffmann) An hereditary disorder involving progressive degeneration of the anterior spinal horn cells starting in the first year of life and producing weakness, muscle wasting and fasciculation, and death within 6 months.

Muscular dystrophies Each family produces its own pattern of disease but some forms are more common than others. They are all rare.

Pseudo-hypertrophic (Duchenne) Recessive sex-linked disorder affecting males. The age of onset is 5–10 years with symptoms of difficulty climbing stairs, or even walking. On examination the posture is lordotic and the gait 'waddling' due to weakness of the muscles of the pelvic girdle and proximal lower limb. The calves are hypertrophied but weak. In later stages muscle contraction of the legs may produce talipes equinovarus and muscle weakness may spread to the upper limbs, though not to the face. The child dies in the early teens.

Facio-scapulo-humeral (Landouzy–Déjèrine) Transmitted as an autosomal dominant and affects both sexes equally. The onset is at puberty with progressive wasting in the upper limb-girdle and face. The disorder may abort spontaneously or progress to the muscles of the trunk and lower limbs. Individuals usually live to a normal age.

Limb-girdle (Erb) Transmitted as an autosomal recessive and affects both sexes equally. It presents at 20–40 years. It involves the muscles of the shoulders and pelvic girdles and is slowly progressive with death usually in middle age.

Other forms may affect the muscles of the face and eyes (oculo-muscular dystrophy) or the distal limb muscles (Gower's muscular dystrophy). They are very rare.

Hereditary ataxias

These are familial disorders usually transmitted as Mendelian dominants. Pathological changes of degeneration are present in one or more of the optic nerves, cerebellum, olives and long ascending tracts of the spinal cord. Each family presents its own particular variants, but tends to breed true. All are rare.

Friedreich's ataxia

Pathology

Degeneration is maximal in the dorsal and lateral (pyramidal) columns of the cord and the spino-cerebellar tracts.

Clinical presentation

Cerebellar ataxia is noted at 5–15 years affecting first the lower and then upper limbs. Pes cavus and spinal scoliosis may be present. Pyramidal tract involvement produces upper motor neurone lesions of the legs, and dorsal column involvement sensory changes and absent ankle jerks. Arrhythmias and heart failure are common due to cardiomyopathy. There may be optic atrophy. Mild dementia occurs late in the disease and patients die from cardiac disease in their forties.

Cerebellar degenerations

This group of hereditary ataxias affect primarily the cerebellum and the cerebellar connections of the brain-stem. All are rare. These disorders may present in late middle age and must be distinguished from:

— tumours of the posterior fossa
— primary degeneration secondary to bronchial carcinomas
— myxoedema

Hereditary spastic paraplegia

The pyramidal tracts are affected and the patients develop progressive spasticity. The onset occurs from childhood to middle age. The disorder, when first seen, must be distinguished from cord compression (which may require emergency decompression).

Syphilis of the nervous system

Tertiary syphilis of the central nervous system never develops in a syphilitic patient who has received early and correct treatment. All forms are now rarely seen except as chronic cases with residual symptoms and signs. Tertiary syphilis may be divided into four groups:

Meningovascular disease occurring 3–4 years after primary infection
Tabes dorsalis—10–35 years after primary infection
GPI—10–15 years after primary infection
Localised gummata

The first three produce symptoms by a combination

of primary neuronal degeneration and/or arterial lesions.

Meningovascular syphilis This affects both the cerebrum and the spine ('*meningo*': producing fibrosis of the meninges and nipping of nerves; '*vascular*': producing endarteritis and ischaemic necrosis). Headache is a common presenting symptom.

Cerebrum Syphilitic leptomeningitis produces fibrosis and thickening of the meninges with nipping and paralysis of cranial nerves. The second, third and fourth are most frequently involved.

Vascular endarteritis Produces ischaemic necrosis. Hemiplegia may result. Syphilitic endarteritis is one cause of isolated cranial nerve lesions.

Spinal meningovascular syphilis Meningeal thickening involves posterior spinal roots to produce pain and anterior roots to cause muscle wasting.

Endarteritis May produce ischaemic necrosis, and transverse myelitis and paraplegia.

Tabes dorsalis The signs result from degeneration of the dorsal columns and nerve roots.

Clinical presentation Lightning pains due to dorsal nerve root involvement characterise the disease. These are severe paroxysmal stabbing pains ('crises') which occur in the limbs, chest or abdomen. Paraesthesiae may also occur. Ataxia follows degeneration of the dorsal columns of the spinal cord. The gait is wide-based and stamping because position sense is lost.

Examination The facies is characteristic. Ptosis is present and the forehead wrinkled due to overactivity of the frontalis muscle. Argyll Robertson pupils are small, irregular pupils which do not react to light, but do react to accommodation. There may be optic atrophy. Cutaneous sensation is diminished typically over the nose (tabetic mask), sternum, ulnar border of the arm and outer borders of the legs and feet. Vibration and position sense are lost early in the disease. Deep pain sensation (pressure on testicles or Achilles tendon) may also be lost. Absence of visceral sensation results in overfilling of the bladder. The reflexes are diminished or absent in the legs. The plantar responses are flexor in pure tabes dorsalis. Romberg's sign (increased unsteadiness on closing the eyes) is present and is evidence of loss of position sense.

GPI (general paralysis of the insane) A late manifestation of systemic syphilis. Pathologically the meninges are thickened, particularly in the parietal and frontal regions. Primary cortical degeneration produces a small brain with dilated and enlarged ventricles. The dorsal columns degenerate.

Clinical presentation The pathological changes are associated with marked mental impairment. This may produce loss of memory and concentration with associated anxiety and/or depression. Later, insight is lost and the patient may become euphoric with delusions of grandeur and loss of emotional response. Epilepsy occurs in 50% of cases.

Examination

Euphoria may be present. The face is 'vacant' and memory lost. Argyll-Robertson pupils are present. The tongue demonstrates a 'trombone' tremor. Dorsal column involvement produces limb ataxia from loss of position sensation. Upper motor neurone lesions occur in the legs with increased reflexes and up-going plantar responses.

NB In tabo-paresis there is a combination of the lower limb upper motor neurone signs of GPI and the signs of dorsal root degeneration from tabes dorsalis. This produces a combination of absent knee reflexes with up-going plantar responses.

WR, TPI and VDRL tests

The Wassermann Reaction in syphilis is virtually always positive in GPI but not in tabes dorsalis (75%) or meningovascular syphilis (CSF 90%, blood 70%).

The Treponema Pallidum Immobilisation (TPI) and Venereal Disease Reference Laboratory (VDRL) tests are more specific for syphilis than the WR (which may give false positives in rheumatoid arthritis, SLE, glandular fever and chronic active hepatitis).

Management

Penicillin by injection is the drug of choice for active syphilitic infection. Improvement, stabilisation or deterioration may occur in any one case despite adequate penicillin therapy.

The Herxheimer reaction is an acute hypersensitivity reaction and results from toxins produced by spirochaetes killed on first contact with penicillin. Death has been reported and some authorities give steroids during the first days of penicillin therapy.

Disorders of spinal cord

Syringomyelia

A longitudinal cyst in the cervical cord and/or brain-stem (syringobulbia) occurs just anterior to the central canal and spreads, usually asymmetrically, to each side. It may be due to outflow obstruction of the fourth ventricle from congenital anomaly. It starts in young adults and is usually very slowly progressive over 20–30 years. It is very rare.

Damage to the cord occurs:

At the root level of the lesion

— in the decussating fibres of the lateral spinothalamic tracts (pain and temperature) since they cross anteriorly. NB Fibres of the posterior column enter posteriorly and are not involved—hence the dissociated sensory loss

— the cells in the anterior horn where the lower motor neurones start

Distant from the lesion in the upper motor neurones in the pyramidal tracts

The classical case of syringomyelia therefore presents with:

— painless injury to the hands (sensory C6–8)

— weakness and wasting in the small muscles of the hands (T1)

Examination may reveal more extensive dissociated sensory loss in the cervical segments, and upper motor neurone signs in the legs. These are usually asymmetrical. All signs and symptoms are ipsilateral to the lesion. In treatment, surgical decompression and aspiration of cysts should be considered.

Syringobulbia

With progressively more cephalad lesions, the descending root of the trigeminal nerve (pain and temperature) may be involved from first division downwards, and a Horner's syndrome from involvement of the cervical sympathetic tract. The motor nuclei of the lower cranial nerves may be involved in syringobulbia (true bulbar palsy) and there may be nystagmus from involvement of vestibular and cerebellar connections.

Subacute combined degeneration of the cord (SACD)

The neurological consequences of B_{12} deficiency include SACD, signs of peripheral neuropathy and, very rarely, dementia and optic atrophy.

'Combined degeneration' refers to the combined demyelination of both pyramidal (lateral columns) and posterior (dorsal) columns, the signs and symptoms being predominantly in the legs. It is now rare.

Clinical presentation

Sensory peripheral neuropathy with numbness and paraesthesiae in the feet are the usual presenting symptoms. Less commonly the disease presents as a spastic paraparesis. The signs are of:

— posterior column loss (vibration and position senses, with positive Rombergism)

— upper motor neurone lesion (weakness, hypertonia and hyper-reflexia, with absent abdominal reflexes and up-going toes)

— peripheral neuropathy (absence of all the jerks, reduced touch sense, and deep tenderness of the calves)

Investigation

The following are indicated:

Serum B_{12} and folate levels
Marrow histology for megaloblastic change
Pentagastrin test for achlorhydria
Schilling test for B_{12} absorption
Parietal cell antibodies

Only the last three tests are of value if the patient has previously been given vitamin B_{12} injections.

Management

Vitamin B_{12} (hydroxocobalamine 1 mg daily for one week, and then 1 mg monthly for life).

Prognosis

Neurological symptoms and signs usually improve

to some degree. However, they may remain unchanged or, rarely, continue to progress. Sensory abnormalities resolve more completely than motor, the peripheral neuropathy more than the myelopathy.

Peroneal muscular atrophy (Charcot–Marie–Tooth)

This condition is often confused with the muscle dystrophies. It is rare.

Pathology

It may be transmitted as a Mendelian dominant, or in some families is recessive and sex-linked. There is degeneration in the dorsal columns and anterior horn cells and less so in the pyramidal tracts. Characteristic interstitial neuronitis of the nerves produces typical atrophy of the muscles supplied.

Clinical presentation

Classically it presents about the age of 20 years with wasting and weakness of all the distal lower limb muscles. Later, the upper limbs may be affected. The wasting stops at mid-thigh, producing an 'inverted champagne bottle' appearance, and at the elbows. Fasciculation and sensory loss are sometimes present. The disease usually arrests spontaneously and life expectancy is normal. Contractions may produce talipes equinovarus.

Cord compression

Aetiology

Disorders of vertebrae (*extradural*) These constitute 45% of cases.
— prolapsed intervertebral disc
— collapsed vertebral body (usually secondary to carcinoma, myeloma or, rarely, osteoporosis)
— rarely, tuberculosis, abscesses, Paget's disease, reticuloses and angiomata

Meningeal disorders (*intradural*) Also constitute 45% of cases.
— neurofibroma (dumb-bell tumours)
— meningioma (usually thoracic and more common in women)

Disorders of spinal cord (*intramedullary*) 5–10% of cases.
— gliomas
— ependymomas

Clinical presentation

Patients present with a spastic paraparesis: there is upper motor neurone weakness in the legs, loss of sphincter control (an ominous sign) and loss of abdominal reflexes if the lesion is in or above the thoracic cord. The level of the sensory loss indicates the level of the neurological lesion. Remember that compared with the vertebral column, the cord is about 1 segment short in the lower cervical region, 2 segments short in the upper thoracic region, and 3–5 segments short in the lower thoracic region. The sacral segments and end of the cord lie opposite the L1 vertebra. Remember, also that the cervical spine has 7 vertebrae and the cervical spinal cord 8 segments.

It is important to consider the possibility of cord compression in all cases of spastic paresis. Cord compression is a neurosurgical emergency, particularly if of recent onset and rapid progression. Decompression must be performed as early as possible if recovery is to occur.

NB The tumours which commonly metastasise to bone arise in: bronchus, breast, prostate, thyroid, and kidney.

Investigation

X-ray of the spine.
X-ray of the chest for carcinoma of the bronchus.
Lumbar puncture for spinal block and raised protein.
Myelography to delineate the level and character of obstructing tissues—this investigation may increase the severity of transverse myelitis and should therefore be performed only after careful consideration.

Differential diagnosis

Other causes of spastic paraparesis are:

Disseminated sclerosis. Demyelination may cause isolated slow progressive paraparesis in the middle-aged
Subacute combined degeneration of the cord
Parasagittal cranial meningioma
Transverse myelitis
Anterior spinal artery thrombosis

PSYCHIATRY

Depression and anxiety are the most frequent psychiatric disorders seen in general practice and general medical out-patients. Confusional states are common in the elderly.

A working classification, adapted from Willis (*Lecture Notes on Psychiatry*, Blackwell), is shown in table 14.

Depression

There is often a familial factor and a history of 'moodiness.' There is no obvious cause for so-called 'endogenous depression'. Depression may, however, follow acute infections, e.g. influenza, glandular fever and infectious hepatitis. It may result from therapy with antihypertensive agents, particularly reserpine and methyldopa. It is sometimes the first symptom of cerebrovascular disease.

Depression, particularly in the elderly, is commonly confused with myxoedema and Parkinson's disease. Mood changes may be an obvious presenting feature and the patient may be unaware of his depression. It is surprising how many of the patients, on direct questioning, reveal a history of difficulty in sleeping, early morning wakening, weeping spells and guilt feelings. Depression is very common in chronic painful disease, and at the menopause.

Table 14 Classification of common psychiatric disorders (Willis)

Affective (mood) disorders	Anxiety, depression and manic states (common)
Organic disorders	Dementia and confusional states (relatively common, especially in the elderly)
Schizophrenia	Simple (relatively common) Hebephrenic (disorders of the content of thought and ideas) Catatonic (catatonia denotes the assumption of abnormal postures) Paranoid (persecution complexes)
Personality disorders	Obsessional personality Psychopathic personality
Addiction	Drugs and alcohol (common)
Mental subnormality	(Common)
Hysteria	(Rare)

Management In general medical practice, sympathetic support is often sufficient to allow time for spontaneous recovery, particularly after acute grief.

Drug therapy Tricyclic drugs, e.g. imipramine (Tofranil) 25–50 mg tds, may be required in addition. This is slower acting than amitriptyline (Tryptizol) (25–50 mg tds) but has fewer side-effects. Side-effects of imipramine and amitriptyline result from atropine-like effects and include dry mouth, blurred vision, postural hypotension and tachycardia, and urinary retention. Amitriptyline is also relatively contra-indicated in the presence of ischaemic heart disease since it may produce arrhythmias.

Monoamine oxidase inhibitors (MAOI) may be less effective and produce more serious side-effects. They inhibit deaminating enzymes which normally inactivate pressor amines. Hence acute hypertensive encephalopathy and cerebrovascular accidents may result from the combination of MAO inhibitors with amphetamine or ephedrine and tyramine-containing foods (Marmite, cheese, yoghurt).

In severe cases, and especially in the presence of suicidal tendencies, or if the above regime is in-effective within 3–4 months, patients should be referred to a psychiatrist. Electroconvulsive therapy (ECT) is still widely used.

Mania Patients with mania and hypomania show elevation of mood, flight of ideas and talk loudly, forcefully and rapidly. Sedation and sometimes ECT may be necessary. Periods of mania may alternate with periods of depression.

Anxiety The essential feature is an irrational degree of anxiety and worry accompanied by the somatic mani-festations of fear, for example sweating, tremor and tachycardia. Fear may amount to panic. Specific fears, such as fear of confined or open spaces, are called phobias. The somatic symptoms and signs resemble those seen in thyrotoxicosis and in both conditions there is a disturbance of the autonomic nervous system. Anxiety may be associated with depression.

Management

Mild anxiety is usually self-limiting and requires sympathetic support with or without sedation. Diazepam (Valium 5–10 mg tds) or chlordiazepoxide (Librium 10–20 mg tds) are commonly used. Anxiety which fails to respond to simple therapy which is associated with phobias should be referred to a psychiatrist.

Acute confusional states

These occur during medical or surgical illness and involve clouding of consciousness with loss of contact between the patient and his environment. There is failure of recent memory, disorientation, emotional lability. Hallucinations may occur. Confusional states occur relatively frequently in the elderly. Acute confusional states occur in:

Small cerebrovascular accidents
'All the failures,' i.e. cardiac, respiratory (often hypoxia), renal and liver
Severe acute infections including meningitis, pneumonia and malaria, particularly with high fever.
Drug overdosage, e.g. alcohol, phenobarbitone, salicylates, amitriptyline, LSD, cannabis
Hypoglycaemia and hyperglycaemia
Other endocrine disorders, i.e. thyrotoxicosis, myxoedema, Cushing's syndrome and corticosteroid therapy
Hypercalcaemia, commonly resulting from multiple secondary tumours in bone
Alcoholics may develop an acute encephalopathy possibly related to vitamin deficiency (Wernicke).

Treatment

This will depend on the diagnosis. For sedation, chlorpromazine (50–100 mg) intramuscularly can be used. Thioridazine (Melleril) 25 mg tds is a suitable tranquilliser especially in the elderly.

Dementia

Dementia means 'loss of mind'. The earliest feature is loss of memory for recent events. There is a global disruption of personality with the gradual development of abnormal behaviour, loss of intellect, mood changes often without insight, blunting of emotions, and failure to learn. Eventually there is a reduction in self-care, restless wandering, paranoia and incontinence. In patients under 60 years of age it is usually termed pre-senile dementia. Senile dementia is usually due either to neuronal degeneration, or to cerebral ischaemia and in this case the deterioration is classically stepwise. There are a number of treatable disorders which must always be excluded:

Subdural haematoma—common in the elderly, alcoholics and cirrhotics

Myxoedema ('myxoedema madness') (page 131)
Cerebral tumour—meningiomata may grow very slowly (page 95)
Chronic phenobarbitone therapy

The remaining causes are either less amenable to treatment or uncommon:

Cerebrovascular disease
Bronchial carcinoma—dementia usually results from secondary deposits
Primary cerebral atrophy is uncommon
Trauma
Vitamin B_{12} deficiency
Cerebral syphilis (page 102)
Pick's disease (*Picks* out the frontal lobe) and Alzheimer's disease (*All* the brain)
Huntington's chorea (page 95)

NB Primary dementia is a diagnosis made only by exclusion (in the absence of brain biopsy) and all 'pre-senile dementias' should be investigated.

Investigation

Chest X-ray for bronchial carcinoma
Skull X-ray for shift of pineal, calcification in tumours, erosion of posterior clinoids in the presence of raised intracranial pressure
TPI or VDRL tests for syphilis
Thyroid function studies
Serum B_{12}

It may be necessary to proceed to:

Examination of CSF
Brain scan, EEG, ultrasound
Air encephalography to demonstrate cortical thinning or dilated ventricles, and arteriography to delineate a subdural haematoma or tumour

Schizophrenia

The general physician is unlikely to have patients with this disorder referred to him in the first instance. It affects about 0·5% of the general population but the 'schizoid personality' is said to occur about four times more frequently. The essential features of the illness are due to a lack of contact with reality and involve disturbances of thought, mood and conduct. Hallucinations occur and delusions are common especially delusions of persecution (paranoia). There is evidence of a familial factor and the schizoid personality occurs more commonly in relatives of the frankly schizophrenic than in the general population. Such persons show withdrawal from life, shyness, suspicion and they may become alcoholic or commit suicide.

Management

Treatment by the phenothiazines has greatly improved the prognosis. Chlorpromazine (Largactil) is the most widely used phenothiazine. It may give rise to a Parkinsonian syndrome, rashes (including light sensitivity) and mild jaundice. It can depress the bone marrow.

Schizophrenia is best managed by experienced psychiatrists.

Connective tissue and rheumatic diseases

The connective tissue disorders have usurped syphilis as the 'great imitator' and must often be considered in differential diagnoses even though they remain uncommon diseases. SLE and PN in particular should come to mind in the clinical situations of:

— PUO, malaise, and weight loss
— multisystem disease
— renal disorders

The connective tissue diseases are non-organ specific autoimmune disorders where the lesions affect chiefly skin, glomeruli, joints, serous membranes and blood vessels. The following named diseases describe the commoner clinical pictures though any individual patient may exhibit other features from the total spectrum of the connective tissue disorders.

Systemic lupus erythematosus (SLE)

It is most common in women aged 30–50 years (90%) and is predisposed to by sunlight and infection. Hydrallazine in heavy prolonged dosage may give a similar picture as may methyldopa, procainamide and PAS, but renal involvement is rare.

Clinical presentation

The commonest early features are fever, arthralgia and general ill health, with weight loss. It can mimic rheumatoid arthritis, subacute bacterial endocarditis and may produce the nephrotic syndrome. The typical 'butterfly' rash on the face may not be present. One or more of the following systems may be involved.

Joints (90% of cases)

A migratory, usually symmetrical polyarthralgia, not unlike rheumatoid arthritis and affecting the fingers, wrists, elbows, shoulders, knees and ankles.

Skin (60%)

A 'butterfly' rash over the nose and cheeks. Follicles are blocked and telangiectases present. It may involve the ears, neck, chest and upper limbs.

Kidneys (75%)

Renal involvement is common and associated with a poor prognosis. Antigen-antibody complexes have been demonstrated by immunofluorescence in the arterioles of the glomerular tuft. The clinical presentation is usually of the nephrotic syndrome but asymptomatic proteinuria, an acute nephritic syndrome and chronic renal failure with hypertension may occur.

Lungs (30%)

Pleurisy with effusion is relatively common. Patchy consolidation and plate-like areas of collapse, and/or diffuse reticulo-nodular shadowing on chest X-ray may be seen.

Cardiovascular system (40%)

Pericarditis is sometimes the first indication of SLE. Raynaud's phenomenon (10–15%), cardiac failure of cardiomyopathy and non-bacterial endocarditis of mitral and aortic valves (Libman-Sacks) all may occur.

Nervous system (25%)

Direct involvement is uncommon and symptoms mostly result from arteritis and ischaemia. This may produce peripheral nerve lesions—single or multiple, motor or sensory. Central nervous system manifestations include confusion and hallucinations but these are more commonly secondary to the corticosteroids used in therapy. Very rarely epilepsy is the first presenting feature.

Blood

The sedimentation rate in the acute phase is greatly raised (90%) and it is this which often leads to first suspicion of the disease. Thrombocytopenia (30%) with purpura may be the first indication of SLE. Anaemia (partly haemolytic with reticulocytosis and hyperbilirubinaemia) and leucopenia may occur. There may be splenomegaly.

Lymphatic system

Generalised lymphadenopathy (45%) with or without hepatosplenomegaly (25%) may occur.

Investigation

LE cells are usually present (80%) and if so are diagnostic. The antinuclear factor (ANF) is positive in over 95% of cases. The anti-DNA antibody titre is more specific.

With renal disease, the diagnosis may be made on renal biopsy. Initially a focal nephritis may be seen. Later there is diffuse thickening of the basement membrane of the glomerulus producing the 'wire loop' appearance.

Management

Antibiotics for intercurrent infection, analgesics (salicylates) for joint pain, and blood transfusion if indicated for anaemia.

Steroids in high dosage (prednisolone 40–60 mg daily) for the acute phase. The dosage is slowly reduced depending upon symptoms and severity of involvement of vital organs. Activity is in part reflected by changes in the sedimentation rate (ESR).

Immunosuppressive therapy with azathioprine tends to be used to enable a reduction in steroid dosage if side-effects are troublesome.

Chloroquine in subacute or chronic forms has been used usually when skin disease predominates. It can cause cataracts and retinal degeneration.

Prognosis

The history is of episodic relapses and remissions lasting months to years. The two-year survival rate is 80% and the ten-year survival 50%, in the absence of renal or cerebral disease. Death usually results from renal failure or the complications of steroid therapy.

Polyarteritis nodosa (PN)

This is a very rare disease which presents in a wide variety of ways. It is commonest in young men (20–50 years). There is fibrinoid necrosis of the media of small and medium sized arteries with polymorph infiltration (eosinophils may predominate). The lumen is narrowed and may thrombose giving rise to ischaemic lesions. Healing by fibrosis leads to the formation of small aneurysms (hence the name 'nodosa').

Clinical presentation

Ill-defined malaise, fever, weight loss.

Hypertension (sometimes malignant) occurs almost invariably at some stage.

Renal disease (80% of cases) with an acute nephritic syndrome, nephrotic syndrome, or progressive renal failure.

Heart (70%) Angina, myocardial infarction, pericarditis.

Gastrointestinal tract (50%) Abdominal pain.

Lungs (40%) Asthma of late onset with diffuse transient patchy lung infiltration and eosinophilia. The differential diagnosis includes allergic aspergillosis and Loeffler's syndrome.

Nervous system Mononeuritis multiplex or polyneuritis. Occasionally subarachnoid haemorrhage.

Skin Tender subcutaneous nodules, arteritic lesions around the nail bed and splinter haemorrhages may mimic bacterial endocarditis (particularly if combined with fever).

Investigation

There is usually anaemia, leucocytosis with eosinophilia. Albuminuria, microscopic haematuria and a raised ESR are common. Diagnosis is occasionally confirmed from biopsies of tender muscles, but more reliably from renal biopsy which demonstrates changes of segmental fibrinoid necrosis of the walls of medium-sized arteries and arterioles with cellular infiltration. This causes multiple cortical infarcts.

Management

Symptomatic therapy and steroids as for SLE.

Prognosis

The overall five-year survival is 10%. The disease may progress rapidly to produce death within weeks or continue for 10 years or more. Renal failure is the most common cause of death, although in a few patients evidence of renal disease may disappear with steroid therapy and not return even after withdrawal.

Dermatomyositis

Mainly affects women of 40–50 years. At least 20% of all cases are associated with underlying malignancy (bronchus, breast, stomach, ovary) and in men presenting over the age of 50 years, over 60% have carcinoma, usually of the bronchus. An acute form occurs in children and is often fatal.

Clinical presentation

The onset may be acute or chronic. Skin and muscle changes occur in any order, or together, sometimes with 2–3 months separating their appearance. General ill health and fever are common.

Skin involvement Classically purple 'heliotrope' (a lilac-blue flower) pigmentation occurs around the eyes. The remainder of the face may be involved.
Violet, oedematous lesions over the small joints of the hands with telangiectasia.
Arteritic lesions around the nails.
There may be generalised telangiectasia, especially of face, chest and arms.

Muscle involvement Tenderness and weakness of muscles occurs, commonly of the shoulder and proximal muscles of the upper limb, and if this predominates the disease closely resembles polymyositis (page 98). Muscle wasting and fibrosis with fixed joint deformity may occur in chronic disease.

Other systems Lungs with plate-like areas of collapse and diffuse fibrosis.
Heart with cardiomyopathy and cardiac failure.

Investigation Investigation of myositis (page 99). As for SLE unless an underlying carcinoma is present.

Management Steroids are given in high doses (e.g. prednisolone 60–80 mg per day) in the acute stages but are relatively ineffective in the chronic cases.

Prognosis Depends upon the underlying neoplasm if present. The disease may progress rapidly but exacerbations and remissions are the rule and continue for 10–20 years until respiratory or cardiac failure occurs.

Polymyositis (page 98)

Scleroderma (systemic sclerosis) A disease mainly of middle-aged women. Collagen fibres initially swell and later become sclerotic. Blood vessels show initial thickening.

Clinical presentation The following systems may be involved:

General Lassitude, fever and weight loss.

Skin Raynaud's phenomenon with sclerodactyly and telangiectasia. In the early stages there is non-pitting oedema of the skin of the hands and feet, later involving the face, neck and trunk. The skin becomes smooth, waxy and tight and finally thin, atrophic and pigmented. Changes are maximal over the hands, ankles and face, producing a typical mask-like face. Subcutaneous calcification may be present. (Morphea is a localised indurated sclerodermatous lesion usually on the trunk, neck or extremities. It is benign and only rarely proceeds to systemic sclerosis.)

Lungs Overspill pneumonitis.
Diffuse interstitial fibrosis progressing to respiratory failure.

Locomotor system Polymyositis.
Polyarthralgia.

Heart Pericardial effusion, cardiomyopathy and heart failure.

Oesophagus and intestine Dysphagia.
Steatorrhoea and malabsorption.
Barium studies may reveal deformity and diminished peristalsis in the oesophagus and dilatation of the second part of the duodenum.

Kidney Progressive renal failure, with or without hypertension, is a late but often fatal development.

Management Symptomatic treatment is commonly all that is required. Antacids and sleeping upright may assist in preventing reflux pneumonitis. Physiotherapy may help stiff fingers and joints and maintain muscle activity. Steroids are sometimes required in an attempt to suppress systemic symptoms but are usually completely ineffective.

Prognosis Morphea is usually benign. Systemic sclerosis is a slow progressive disease. Death occurs from lung or cardiac complications. Severe renal involvement is uncommon but is rapidly fatal in association with severe hypertension.
NB Most patients with Raynaud's phenomenon do not have or develop systemic sclerosis.

Polymyalgia rheumatica

Clinical presentation Occurs in patients over 60 years old and more commonly in women. It presents with muscle tenderness usually in the shoulder girdle and neck, but sometimes in the pelvic region, and is worse on waking. There is little if any weakness or wasting. Joint swelling or pain may occur. The associated findings are headache, lassitude, depression and weight loss. It may be associated with temporal arteritis. The ESR may be very high (more than 70 mm/h).

Management Steroids (40–60 mg prednisolone daily) may be required initially if the symptoms are severe and unresponsive to analgesics. The response is characteristically good and the dose is reduced whilst monitoring symptoms and the ESR.

Prognosis A self-limiting benign disease which recovers within 6 to 12 months.

Temporal arteritis

(giant cell arteritis, cranial arteritis)

Clinical presentation A disease in patients usually over the age of 60 who develop severe headache, with burning and tenderness over the scalp and tenderness over the temporal arteries. Systemic manifestations are common with fever, weakness, weight loss, arthralgia and myalgia. The ophthalmic arteries may be involved and blindness of one or both eyes may result. Personality changes may occur from involvement of the cerebral vessels. The coronary arteries or other vessels may be involved.

Investigation

The ESR is markedly raised (often above 90 mm/h). Diagnosis is confirmed on temporal artery biopsy which shows patchy involvement of the arterial wall with areas of necrosis, large mononuclear cell infiltration and giant cells.

Management

Steroids in high doses (Prednisone 40–60 mg daily) are given to suppress symptoms (this usually occurs within days) and to prevent blindness. Approximately 10–15% of patients develop blindness but some may rarely recover vision to some degree if steroids are given rapidly after it occurs. Treatment is given for about 5–6 months, gradually reducing the dosage whilst checking that symptoms do not recur and observing the ESR.

Organ-specific autoimmune disease

This refers to a group of disorders characterised by the presence of antibodies to a specific organ which may fail in function. The disorders are more common in women, are familial, and may result from a genetically-determined defect of immune mechanisms. Patients with involvement of one organ have an increased incidence of involvement of one or more of the others.

The following disorders characterise this type of disease: Hashimoto's thyroiditis, Addison's (adrenal) disease, idiopathic hypoparathyroidism, premature ovarian failure, pernicious anaemia, alopecia, vitiligo (both skin-markers of organ-specific autoimmune disease), rheumatoid arthritis.

Rheumatoid arthritis

Women are more frequently affected than men (3 : 1). It is usually insidious in onset but may be an acute or a chronic relapsing disease marked by ill health and chronic joint deformity. The dominant clinical feature is a chronic synovitis. However the name 'rheumatoid disease' may be more appropriate since tissues other than the joints are frequently affected. The overall picture is of a connective tissue disease with the brunt of the disease falling upon the joints. Diphtheroid bacilli and mycoplasma have been implicated as part of the pathology but the importance or relevance of either has yet to be defined. There is often a family history.

Diagnostic criteria for rheumatoid arthritis have been laid down by the American Rheumatism Association (*Annals of Rheumatic Disease*, 1959, **18,** 49).

Clinical features

Musculoskeletal

The small joints of the hands and feet are the most commonly affected, usually symmetrically, but other large synovial joints (hips, knees, elbows) are often also involved. The onset may be gradual with progressive pain, early morning stiffness and swelling of joints. The acute onset is associated with fever and general constitutional illness. Examination may show:

— tenderness and diminished movement of involved joints with characteristic fusiform soft tissue swelling of the metacarpophalangeal and interphalangeal joints of the hands. (The metatarsophalangeal joints of the feet may also be tender on pressure.) The wrists are commonly involved. The terminal interphalangeal joints of the fingers are spared (except in psoriatic arthropathy, page 121). The chronic disease may produce fixed deformities and ulnar deviation at the metacarpophalangeal joints.

— wasting of the small muscles of the hand is common and results from a combination of disuse atrophy, vasculitis and peripheral neuropathy. Wasting may occur in the muscles around any affected joint.

— inflammation of the soft tissues surrounding inflamed joints causes swelling, tenosynovitis (Achilles tendinitis, olecranon bursitis) and even tendon rupture. Localised subcutaneous nodules occur over the dorsal aspect of the elbow in about 20% of cases.

Joints less commonly involved are the ankles which have relatively little synovial tissue, the costovertebral joints producing diminished chest expansion, temporomandibular joints, the cricoarytenoid joints (which causes hoarseness and, rarely, acute respiratory obstruction) and the cervical spine. (Laxity of the atlantoaxial joint ligaments with some erosion of the odontoid peg may result in acute or chronic cord compression and death. It is necessary to X-ray the cervical spine in all patients with rheumatoid arthritis prior to general anaesthesia.)

NB Acute septic arthritis may occur in rheumatoid joints. Acute solitary effusions should be aspirated and examined microscopically and bacteriologically.

Lung

Lung involvement is clinically uncommon. It may occur before the arthritis and usually in seropositive disease. It presents as:

— isolated unilateral pleural effusion must be differentiated from primary tuberculosis

— rheumatoid nodules, single or multiple, which may be present throughout the lung parenchyma. They are commonly subpleural

— diffuse fibronodular infiltration or fibrosing alveolitis may occur

— Caplan's syndrome is the presence of large (up to 5 cm) rheumatoid nodules in the lungs of coal miners with silicosis but also occurring in other pneumoconioses. They may calcify, cavitate or coalesce and may precede clinical arthritis. The patients are sero-positive

Vascular

Raynaud's phenomenon is common. Arteritic lesions characteristically produce minute 'splinter' necrosis in the digital pulps (this form of vascular necrosis is characteristic of arteritic lesions seen in the collagen diseases although multiple emboli in infective endocarditis may produce a similar picture). Chronic leg ulcers result from skin necrosis secondary to vasculitis—the ulcers are frequently on the lateral aspect of the tibia (*cf.* varicose ulcers).

Neurological

— peripheral neuropathy: this is usually predominantly sensory. Arteritis of the vessels supplying the nerves may be responsible. Neuropathy may also follow therapy with gold and chloroquine

— mononeuritis multiplex, particularly of digital nerves, ulnar nerves and lateral popliteal nerves

— entrapment neuropathy, e.g. carpal tunnel syndrome and the ulnar nerve at the elbow

— spinal cord lesions secondary to cervical disease

Reticulo-endothelial

The spleen is enlarged in about 15% of cases and generalised lymphadenopathy present in 10%.

Blood

Normochromic normocytic anaemia is common and its severity related to that of the disease. Iron deficiency may result from overt bleeding secondary to salicylate or phenylbutazone therapy but this is uncommon and peptic ulceration and colonic neoplasms should be excluded. Pernicious anaemia may be more common in patients with rheumatoid arthritis than in the general population. The height of the ESR reflects the activity of the disease (page 116).

Renal

Amyloidosis though common on biopsy is seldom clinically important in rheumatoid disease. Proteinuria or nephrotic syndrome may complicate treatment with penicillamine and gold.

Ocular

— scleritis presents as pericorneal injection with pain and tenderness. It may lead to uveitis and glaucoma

— scleromalacia perforans: a rheumatoid nodule in the sclera which may perforate

— keratoconjunctivitis sicca: see *Sjögren's syndrome* (page 121)

— iatrogenic: cataract and retinal degeneration with chloroquine and cataracts from steroids

Iatrogenic

From gold (proteinuria, nephrotic syndrome, skin rash, marrow suppression); aspirin (gastric erosion); phenylbutazone (gastric erosion and marrow suppression); phenacetin (nephropathy), penicillamine (nephropathy), steroids (page 134) and chloroquine (cataract, retinopathy, photosensitivity).

Radiology

The joints may be normal in early rheumatoid disease. The characteristic sequence of abnormalities is:
— soft tissue swelling and periarticular osteoporosis
— narrowing of joint space and periarticular erosions
— subluxation and osteoarthritis occur in long-standing disease
— fibrosis or bony ankylosis

Management

The object of therapy is to reduce pain and enable the patient to maintain as near normal existence as possible. A social assessment of occupation, of family help and home conditions is essential when planning therapy.

Rest diseased joints in splints especially at night to reduce pain and prevent deformity.

Physiotherapy to maintain full joint movement and strengthen weak muscles. Early attention and advice regarding posture may prevent chronic deformity and degeneration of all involved joints.

Analgesics Salicylates are the drugs of first choice and prescribed to the limits of tolerance if pain is sufficiently severe e.g. blood levels of 20–30 mg% (usually given by a dosage of approximately 4–8 g of aspirin per day). Other analgesics commonly used when aspirin is ineffective or produces toxicity include paracetamol, codeine phosphate and dihydrocodeine, mefenamic acid and indomethacin. Phenylbutazone (Butazolidine) is effective but often (30%) causes nausea, vomiting, skin rashes, and oedema due to sodium retention. More rarely it may cause haematemesis, agranulocytosis and aplastic anaemia.

Gold (intramuscular sodium aurothiomalate) 50 mg weekly up to a total of 1 gram, is of proven value but tends to be reserved for otherwise unresponsive disease in view of side-effects including skin rashes and bone marrow depression. Renal and liver damage are rare complications. Proteinuria is common but nephrotic syndrome rare.

Penicillamine is mainly of value in severe rheumatoid arthritis associated with arteritic lesions.

Systemic steroids should be considered in patients with progressive rheumatoid arthritis who have not responded to less dangerous therapy and whose life and/or occupation is threatened. They should also be considered if severe systemic involvement occurs and fails to respond to other drugs.

Systemic steroids are *very rarely needed* in the treatment of rheumatoid arthritis. In view of the serious side-effects of systemic steroid therapy, they must only be given after very careful assessment and probably only by an experienced rheumatologist. Local injection of steroids into joints (or other painful sites) may give relief, but if repeated frequently leads to further and often symptomless deterioration.

More recently immunosuppressive therapy has been used—cyclophosphamide or azathioprine may be as effective and less toxic than steroids and may allow a reduction in steroid dosage.

NB Some patients fail to respond to therapy and should be admitted to hospital for rest and further careful assessment of analgesic therapy.

Surgical management Synovectomy (especially of the knee joint), realignment and repair of tendons, joint prostheses (hip, knee, fingers) and arthrodesis may be required for severe pain or deformity.

Advice of an expert in rehabilitation may allow a severely disabled patient to continue a tolerable and even happy existence at home.

Prognosis

About 60 % of patients suffer minimal or only mild disability and are able to continue a full active life; 30–35% suffer serious disability with varying degrees of restriction of activities; 5–10% progress relentlessly to serious and almost complete disability. The following features indicate a poor prognosis:

— insidious onset
— persistent activity for over a year
— positive serology within a year
— early bony erosion and subcutaneous nodules

Rheumatoid factor

This is a circulating immunoglobulin of the IgM class which is an antibody to the patient's own (IgG). It agglutinates sensitised sheep red cells (sheep cell agglutination test: SCAT) and also latex particles which have been coated with denatured γ globulin (latex agglutination tests, e.g. F_2LP test in which the 'F_2' fraction of denatured γ globulin is used to coat the latex particles). High titres correlate with more severe arthritis with a worse prognosis, and with a higher incidence of extra-articular diseases (nodules, arteritis, leg ulcers, digital gangrene, neuropathy, Felty's syndrome and fibrosing alveolitis).

Rheumatoid factor is positive in:

50–70% of outpatients with rheumatoid arthritis
(100% in patients with nodules and Sjögren's syndrome)
25–35% of patients with collagen disease
15% of patients with juvenile rheumatoid arthritis (Still's disease)
4% of the general population, rising with age. Its presence does not necessarily indicate that the rheumatoid disease will later develop

Rheumatoid factor is usually negative in ankylosing spondylitis, Reiter's syndrome, psoriatic arthropathy and colitic arthropathy.

Diseases resembling rheumatoid arthritis

Still's disease (juvenile rheumatoid arthritis)

A childhood disease usually of acute onset with fever and skin rashes. Joint pain is not an essential feature (absent in 25% at onset) and may be monoarticular (30%) at the onset. Subcutaneous nodules are rare. One-third of patients present with a history of insidious polyarthritis as in adult rheumatoid arthritis. Tests of rheumatoid factor are usually negative (85%).

Prognosis

The majority of cases settle spontaneously with minimal or no disability. Bone growth may be retarded. In one-third the disease continues into adult life.

Sjögren's syndrome

It is commoner in women than in men (9:1). The major clinical features (sicca syndrome) result from reduced secretions from the lachrymal and salivary glands which produce dry 'gritty' eyes and corneal ulcers (keratoconjunctivitis sicca) and a dry mouth (xerostomia) with dysphagia. Recurrent respiratory infections occur from diminished bronchial secretions. About 50% are associated with rheumatoid arthritis, 30% are uncomplicated and 20% associated with other autoimmune disease (mostly non-organ specific). Rheumatoid factor is usually present, antinuclear factor frequently present (70%), and LE cells seldom present (15%). In Schirmer's test, filter paper is hooked over the lower eyelid; in normal people at least 15 mm is wet in 5 minutes and in the sicca syndrome usually far less. Fluorescein demonstrates corneal ulceration. Treatment is symptomatic with artificial tears (1% methyl cellulose) and the arthritis is treated as uncomplicated rheumatoid arthritis.

Felty's syndrome

Some patients with severe rheumatoid arthritis have enlarged lymph nodes, splenomegaly, and hypersplenism (anaemia, leukopenia and thrombocytopenia). Removal of the spleen reverses blood abnormalities but the underlying rheumatoid process is not affected.

Psoriatic arthritis

An arthritis similar to but distinct from rheumatoid arthritis may complicate psoriasis. The clinical picture resembles rheumatoid arthritis but:
— psoriasis is present
— joint involvement is usually asymmetrical and involves the terminal interphalangeal joints which may be the only affected joints
— pitting occurs in the nails
— subcutaneous nodules do not occur
— sacroileitis is more common
— tests for rheumatoid factor are negative

Ankylosing spondylitis (sacroileitis)

Clinical features

A disease of young adult males (20–40) (*cf.* rheumatoid arthritis) with a marked familial incidence. Joint involvement affects the sacroiliac joints causing low back pain with morning stiffness. The disease may involve the spine, producing pain and stiffness initially of the lumbosacral region and eventually of the thoracic and cervical spine. The hips are involved in 50% of patients. Examination reveals decreased spinal movements and loss of the normal lumbosacral curvature. 'Springing' the pelvis (i.e. pressing the iliac crests towards each other) causes sacroiliac pain.

Peripheral joints are involved relatively infrequently. The arthropathy differs from rheumatoid arthritis in that it is asymmetrical and affects large joints more than small joints.

Other features of ankylosing spondylitis are:
— general ill health
— iritis (in 25–30% of cases)
— ulcerative colitis is more common in patients with ankylosing spondylitis and vice versa
— aortic incompetence due to aortitis
— respiratory failure may result from the fixed rib cage with kyphoscoliosis, and from fibrosing alveolitis

Investigation

Tests for rheumatoid factor are usually negative. The sedimentation rate is usually but not always raised. There is a high correlation with human lymphocyte antigen (HLA) 27.

Radiology

The sacroiliac joints are irregular with sclerosis of the articular margins. Bony ankylosis occurs late. The intervertebral ligaments calcify and finally ossify to produce a 'bamboo' spine.

Differential diagnoses

Osteoarthritis of the spine
Prolapsed intervertebral disc

and rarely

Psoriatic arthritis
Reiter's disease
The sacroileitis of ulcerative colitis
Tuberculosis which may affect only one sacroiliac joint

Management

Bedrest is contraindicated because it increases stiffness and ankylosis.
Analgesics. Phenylbutazone (Butazolidine) 200–300 mg/day is particularly effective. Indomethacin may be given as an alternative.
Careful posture with spinal muscle exercises is essential to prevent chronic deformity. Sleeping on a firm bed without pillows should help prevent fixed spinal flexion.
Radiotherapy although effective in reducing pain is inadvisable except in those with intractable pain as there is an increased risk of leukaemia (0·3%).

Prognosis

Many mild cases may never present to a physician. With expert care 70–80% will maintain complete or almost complete activity. More severe cases develop moderate to severe bony ankylosis of the spine to produce fixation of mobility and rounded kyphosis of the cervical and thoracic spine. This may impair ventilation. In severe cases extreme rigidity of the spine may occur within 3–5 years. The disease may remit at any stage but recurrent episodes may occur.

Reiter's disease

A disease usually of young men presenting with urethritis, conjunctivitis and arthritis. There is usually a history of sexual intercourse but the disease may, rarely, follow bacillary dysentery.

Clinical features

Arthritis: typically acute or subacute. Usually polyarticular and asymmetrical affecting large joints of the lower limbs. Sacroileitis is common. Plantar fasciitis and Achilles tendinitis may occur.
Conjunctivitis is common in the acute disease. Iritis is associated with chronic recurrent disease, particularly when associated with sacroileitis.
Skin lesions: mouth ulcers are common. Urethritis and prostatitis are associated with superficial skin ulceration around the penile meatus. Pustular hyperkeratotic lesions of the soles of the feet and less frequently the palms of the hands (keratoderma blenorrhagica) may occur.
Tests for rheumatoid factor are usually negative.

Differential diagnosis

Gonococcal arthritis
Ankylosing spondylitis
Behçet's syndrome
Psoriatic and rheumatoid arthritis

Management

The treatment of the acute stage is symptomatic.
Rest the inflamed joints.
Analgesics. Phenylbutazone is the drug of first choice. The majority of cases settle spontaneously within 4–10 weeks, but the disease may recur. (The urethritis may respond to tetracycline 2 g/day for 10 days.)

Endocrine disease

Diabetes mellitus (page 143) and disorders of the thyroid gland (page 128) are the only common forms of endocrine disease.

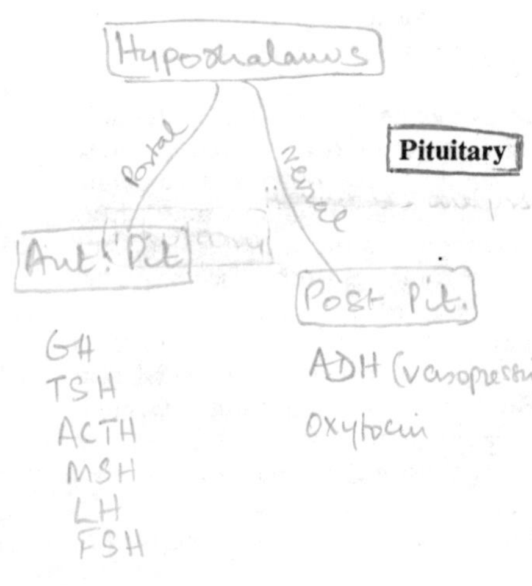

Pituitary

The anterior lobe produces six types of hormone—growth hormone (GH), follicle stimulating hormone (FSH), luteinising hormone (LH), thyroid stimulating hormone (TSH), adrenocorticotrophic hormone (ACTH), melanocyte stimulating hormone (MSH) and prolactin. The posterior lobe secretes two hormones, antidiuretic hormone (ADH) and oxytocin. The gland has a close anatomical and physiological relationship to the hypothalamus. The anatomical relationship to the optic chiasma is important and all patients with suspected pituitary tumours should have their visual fields plotted. X-ray of the pituitary fossa is essential.

The hypothalamus controls the secretion of the anterior pituitary hormones. Hypothalamic nerve fibres liberate substances which are carried in the portal blood stream to the pituitary gland and there cause release, synthesis or inhibition of pituitary hormones. At least nine factors have been suggested and two, thyrotrophin releasing hormone (TRH) and luteinising hormone releasing factor (LHRF) have been isolated and their chemical structure determined: TRH is a tripeptide and LHRF a polypeptide. The latter causes release of both LH and FSH. A growth hormone release inhibiting factor (GIF) has been shown to inhibit GH in acromegaly and diabetes mellitus. A long-acting form would be useful in treatment.

The clinical features of pituitary disease differ according to the type of the lesion and the region of the gland which is predominantly affected. Failure of secretion is more common than increased secretion. The commonest tumour is a chromophobe adenoma and this is the commonest cause of hypopituitarism. It also gives rise to increased intracranial pressure and to local pressure effects. The commonest tumour in childhood is the craniopharyngeoma which often calcifies. Classically eosinophilic tumours (rare) give giantism in the child or acromegaly in the adult and basophil hyperplasia or adenoma produce Cushing's syndrome. However, acromegaly may be associated with eosinophil, chromophobe or mixed-cell tumours.

Hypopituitarism (Simmond's disease)

The pattern of deficiency depends on the nature of the lesion and its rate of progress. In general, deficiencies of FSH and LH secretions occur early, GH and ACTH next, then TSH. Last of all ADH secretion fails if the posterior lobe is involved by surgical intervention or suprasellar disease. Deficiency of each hormone is measured by suitable blood hormone assay and the integrity of the target organs assessed by applying the appropriate physiological stimulus, e.g. ACTH or TSH.

Aetiology

Iatrogenic from hypophysectomy or irradiation—adequate replacement therapy prevents symptoms from occurring.

Chromophobe adenoma.

Post-partum pituitary necrosis in the female (Sheehan's syndrome). This is now extremely rare with improved standards of midwifery.

Other tumours (including secondary tumours), granulomas (sarcoid and tuberculosis) and head injury—all rare.

Clinical presentation

In children hypopituitarism produces pituitary infantilism (Peter Pan dwarfs). In adults the presentation depends upon (*a*) the pattern of deficiency of the various hormones and (*b*) associated pressure symptoms. The symptoms and signs can be worked out from a knowledge of the functions of the target organs involved.

Hormone deficiency

Loss of sexual function occurs, both primary with amenorrhoea and loss of libido, and secondary with loss of body hair (male patients may find shaving unnecessary).

Adrenal insufficiency (page 135) from failure of ACTH occurs but there is little change in electrolyte metabolism since aldosterone is still secreted.

Pallor and skin depigmentation of the skin occur due to failure of MSH secretion.

Symptoms of hypothyroidism (page 131) from lack of TSH appear but there is no myxoedema, e.g. the face is not coarsened.

Coma may occur from low cortisol levels, spontaneous hypoglycaemia or hypothermia.

Pressure effects

Compression of the optic chiasma produces bitemporal hemianopia and optic atrophy.

Pressure on the hypothalamus may cause somnolence and weight gain.

NB In the male, hypopituitarism is usually due to a chromophobe adenoma. In Sheehan's syndrome, there is a history of post-partum haemorrhage, failure of lactation with atrophy of breast tissue, and amenorrhoea in addition to the other effects described.

Investigation

Assessment of pituitary function involves:

— measurement of pituitary hormones (TSH, ACTH, FSH, LH, GH)

— measurement of target organ secretion (thyroid and adrenal, page 138, and sex hormones)

— dynamic tests of pituitary function (e.g. insulin hypoglycaemia, page 137)

Treatment

The pituitary is removed if there are pressure symptoms, particularly visual loss.
Replacement therapy by:
— cyclical oestrogen-progesterone therapy in women or sublingual testosterone, 4–10 mg four times a day in men
— hydrocortisone 20 mg in the morning and 10 mg at night. Fludrocortisone is not required
— thyroxine 0·1 to 0·3 mg daily
— coma is treated as in hypothermia or the Addisonian crisis (page 136)

Acromegaly

Excess growth hormone gives acromegaly in the adult (after the epiphyses have fused) and giantism in earlier life.

Giantism is almost always the result of the action of excessive secretion of GH before the epiphyses have united. Later in life pituitary failure tends to occur and giants are therefore not usually strong, aggressive or virile.

Aetiology

Excessive secretion of growth hormone from an adenoma of the pituitary often of eosinophil cells. Growth hormone causes overgrowth of soft tissues including the skin, tongue and viscera and of bones. It has an anti-insulin action.

Clinical presentation

The onset is insidious often with early changes (look at old photographs). Headache occurs early due to stretching of the dura mater. Pressure effects with bitemporal hemianopia are rarer. Excessive secretion of GH causes:

Face. Increase in size of skull, supraorbital ridges, lower jaw (separation of teeth) and the sinuses
The tongue is enlarged
Vertebral enlargement and kyphosis
Hands and feet are spade-shaped and carpal tunnel syndrome may be present
Enlarged heart, liver and thyroid
Hypertension (15%)
Diabetes mellitus (10%) and reduced glucose tolerance (30%)

The following also occur:

Acne, hirsutes, excessive sweating
Gynaecomastia and galactorrhoea (prolactin excess)
Hypogonadism, oligomenorrhoea

Investigation

Assay of growth hormone by radioimmunoassay; the levels are raised only in active disease and are not suppressed by glucose in a standard GTT.
X-ray of skull for enlargement of the sella, supraorbital ridges and lower jaw.
X-ray of hands for tufting of the terminal phalanges and increased joint spaces due to hypertrophy

of the cartilage. The heel pad is usually thickened. The glucose tolerance curve may be diabetic.
Fasting serum phosphate may be raised but is of no diagnostic value.
Chest X-ray and ECG may show left ventricular hypertrophy.

Prognosis and treatment

The disease tends to be self-limiting and rarely produces isolated hypothyroid or hypoadrenal function but may progress to hypopituitarism. However, life expectancy is halved due to cardiovascular complications. Surgery is indicated for progressive visual deterioration—regular perimetry is obligatory. Yttrium-90 implants or external irradiation are alternatives to surgical removal in active disease, but may cause further damage to the optic tracts, diabetes insipidus and aseptic bone necrosis. Cerebrospinal rhinorrhea may result from yttrium implantation.

(3) *Diabetes insipidus*

A very rare disease due to deficiency of ADH.

Aetiology

Idiopathic, often familial. The commonest form.
Tumours. Craniopharyngioma or secondary. Rare unless treated by surgery or irradiation.
Surgery or radiation to pituitary gland.
Head injury.
Granulomas, e.g. sarcoid; or infections, e.g. basal meningitis.

Clinical presentation

Polyuria and polydipsia—5–20 litres urine a day.

Investigation

The specific gravity of the urine is very low and fails to increase with water deprivation. Fluids are allowed overnight and stopped in the morning. It is dangerous to lose more than 2–3% of the body weight. In normal people plasma osmolality does not rise above 300 mosmol/kg and urine osmolality rises to 600 mosmol/kg. In diabetes insipidus the former rises and the latter does not, or remains at about plasma level. Vasopressin corrects the abnormality in ADH deficient diabetes insipidus but not in the nephrogenic type.

Differential diagnosis

Psychogenic polydipsia Thirst dominates the picture. The patient resents the water deprivation test, and surreptitious drinking is common. Renal concentrating power may be moderately reduced due to the prolonged polyuria.
Nephrogenic diabetes insipidus This is a primary renal tubular defect of water reabsorption in which there is poor response to ADH. It is an isolated hereditary disorder.
Other causes of polyuria
— diabetes mellitus
— chronic renal failure
— hypercalcaemia
— hypokalaemia

Treatment

Lysine vasopressin snuff by nasal spray.
Pitressin tannate in oil 5–10 units intramuscularly every 2–3 days.
Chlorpropamide, 100–300 mg a day, increases renal response to ADH. The patient should be warned about hypoglycaemia.
Thiazide diuretics probably act by reducing glomerular filtration rate.

Thyroid

Thyroid disease is relatively common. Enlargement of the thyroid of varying degrees is frequent, especially in women. Large non-toxic goitres are not uncommon. Both hypothyroidism and hyperthyroidism are relatively common. Thyroid cancer is rare.

Non-toxic goitre

Aetiology

The enlargement of the gland (visible and palpable) is due to an increased secretion of thyroid stimulating hormone (TSH) secondary to diminished output of thyroid hormones. The causes are:

Simple goitre Iodine deficiency especially in areas of endemic goitre. Sporadic goitre is probably due to relative iodine deficiency for that patient. Iodine requirement is increased at puberty in girls and during pregnancy. The gland tends to become nodular as age increases.
Goitrogens, e.g. iodides in large doses, antithyroid drugs such as PAS, phenylbutazone and many others, are rare as causes (except when used therapeutically, e.g. carbimazole).
Inborn errors of thyroid hormone synthesis (dyshormonogenesis). Six types of enzyme defect are known. All are rare. They are autosomal recessive and the commonest is associated with nerve deafness (Pendred's syndrome) and due to impaired organic binding of iodine.

Clinical presentation

A painless swelling of the thyroid is usually noticed by the patient or relatives. If untreated it may develop into a large nodular goitre and give pressure symptoms, especially if there is a retrosternal extension.

Differential diagnosis

Autoimmune thyroiditis (Hashimoto's disease).
Toxic goitre.
Cancer of the thyroid.
Solitary nodule—benign (rare) and carcinoma (very rare).

Investigation

Free thyroxine index or PBI—for hyper- and hypothyroidism (page 140).
Thyroid antibodies for Hashimoto's disease.
X-ray of neck and thoracic inlet if pressure symptoms are present.
Scanning of thyroid with radioiodine—hot nodules are not malignant, cold ones may be.

Prophylaxis Iodised salt, especially during pregnancy. Seafish in the diet.

Treatment Iodides in childhood.
Thyroxine 0·1 to 0·3 mg daily for long periods to suppress TSH hypersecretion (rarely used).
Surgery for pressure symptoms (rarely necessary).

Thyrotoxicosis (hyperthyroidism)

Aetiology The clinical picture results from an excess of thyroid hormones. Some regard Graves' disease in which eye signs are prominent, and toxic multinodular goitre, as different conditions but it is probable that the difference depends on the age at which the disease occurs. Rarely a single toxic nodule may produce thyrotoxicosis but this is more commonly a primary disorder of the whole thyroid gland. Long-acting thyroid stimulator (LATS) is an immunoglobulin found in at least half the patients with thyrotoxicosis. Another immunoglobulin, LATS protector (LATSP), is found in the serum of LATS-negative patients. One or other thyroid stimulating immunoglobulin is probably responsible for most cases of hyperthyroidism. There is a strong genetic factor. Self-administered thyroxine should not be forgotten as a cause of hyperthyroidism, particularly in doctors and nurses.

Clinical presentation The symptoms and signs, except the eye signs, can be deduced from a knowledge of the pharmacological action of thyroxine (T_4) and triiodothyronine (T_3).

The most helpful symptoms are preference for cold weather, excessive sweating, increased appetite and weight loss, 'nervousness', tiredness, and palpitations.

The most helpful signs are goitre, especially with a murmur over it, exophthalmos, lid retraction and lid lag, hot moist palms, tremor and excessive movements, tachycardia or atrial fibrillation.

Atypical presentations Atrial fibrillation or tachycardia in middle age or older should always suggest thyrotoxicosis.
Unexplained weight loss in apparently euthyroid patients.
Very rarely Toxic manic confusion. Proximal limb girdle myopathy. Diarrhoea. Pretibial myxoedema (always with eye signs and excess LATS) may occur in hyperthyroid or euthyroid persons.

Differential diagnosis Thyrotoxicosis is often difficult to differentiate from an anxiety state particularly when this is associated with a simple goitre.

Investigation Always carry out at least one, and preferably two, tests before starting treatment to confirm and document the diagnosis (page 140).

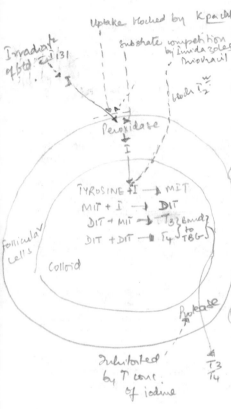

Treatment

Antithyroid drugs Carbimazole 10 mg four times a day for three weeks reducing to 5 mg three times a day or more according to the response and maintained for 12–18 months. 0·1 to 0·2 mg thyroxine a day may be given in addition to suppress TSH overactivity and prevent hypothyroidism. Review at 6 months, 1 year and 18 months. A radioiodine uptake on this regime may indicate those liable to relapse. Those in whom the gland is still autonomous have a high uptake despite TSH suppression by the prescribed thyroxine. When the drugs are stopped and if relapse occurs (up to 50%) either surgery or radioiodine is used (see below). Side-effects of carbimazole include skin rashes, loss of hair and neutropenia (sore throat is usually the first symptom).

Propranolol 40 mg four times a day may give rapid improvement if symptoms are due to sympathetic overactivity. It should not be used in asthmatics, or as the sole therapy.

Radioiodine Used in patients over 40, especially if relapse after drugs or surgery has occurred. The gland diminishes in size after treatment. The main advantage is that treatment is simple and atraumatic but there is a high incidence of late hypothyroidism as the dose is difficult to judge.

Surgery This requires an experienced surgeon and adequate pre-operative treatment with carbimazole and later potassium iodide. Surgery is advised for (*a*) failure of medical treatment, and drug sensitivity in the young; (*b*) large multinodular goitres especially with pressure symptoms as they may enlarge with medical therapy, and for cosmetic reasons; (*c*) rapid results in severely toxic patients. Complications include hypothyroidism, recurrence of hyperthyroidism, recurrent laryngeal nerve palsy (rare), hypoparathyroidism (rare).

Treatment of complications

Eye Lid retraction (sclera visible below the upper lid) usually responds to treatment of the thyrotoxicosis. Exophthalmos (sclera visible above lower lid) results from the swelling of retro-orbital tissues and does not improve and may progress. In malignant exophthalmos there is weakness of the external ocular muscles, often with diplopia, oedema of the conjunctivae and corneal damage from exposure. Treatment is difficult. Local or systemic steroids may be required with tarsorrhaphy in severe cases. Orbital decompression may be required. The condition remits slowly over years with or without treatment.

Atrial fibrillation responds poorly to digitalis until the patient is euthyroid. Cardioversion may then be used. Propranolol or other β-blocker may control severe tachycardia. Heart failure is unusual and responds to antithyroid drugs plus conventional treatment.

Thyrotoxic crisis This is rare but dangerous. Chlorpromazine, intravenous corticosteroids, oral carbimazole and potassium iodine (60 mg daily in divided doses), and propranolol may all be required. Oxygen should be given and particular attention paid to fluid balance since sweating is marked.

Hypothyroidism

This results from a low level of circulating thyroid hormone, either free thyroxine (T_4) or triiodothyronine (T_3). The term 'myxoedema' means that there is a deposition of a mucopolysaccharide beneath the skin producing a non-pitting swelling of the subcutaneous tissues.

Aetiology

Autoimmune thyroiditis. This may present as Hashimoto's disease when a goitre is present, or as 'spontaneous' or 'primary' hypothyroidism if the gland atrophies without producing a goitre. Circulating thyroid antibodies are present.

Destructive therapy for hyperthyroidism or carcinoma by operation or by radioiodine.

Primary thyroid agenesis may produce cretinism in infants.

Ingestion of goitrogens, usually an antithyroid drug (including iodine) in too large doses or for too long.

Secondary to hypopituitarism; this is rare. The thyroid gland still responds to TSH.

Inborn errors of thyroid metabolism (dyshormonogenesis).

There may be a family history of thyroid disease or of autoimmune disease, e.g. 10% have pernicious anaemia.

Clinical presentation

The onset is insidious, difficult to distinguish from depression and the condition may be far advanced before it is recognised even in doctor's families. All those who have had destructive therapy to the thyroid should be followed up at 6-monthly intervals. Many of the symptoms occur also in euthyroid individuals, e.g. tiredness, loss of hair. Those which have the greatest diagnostic value are intolerance of cold, diminished energy, physical tiredness, slow cerebration, increase in weight, hoarseness of voice, diminished sweating, dry and rough skin, dry and unruly hair, deafness, constipation, muscular pains and paraesthesiae (carpal tunnel syndrome).

The physical signs include a typical facial appearance with periorbital puffiness and pallor, coarse and cold skin, slow movements, hoarse voice, slow pulse and a slowing of the recovery phase of the ankle jerk reflexes.

Ischaemic heart disease is common. CNS involvement may produce intellectual impairment and dementia (myxoedema madness) and coma (with hypothermia).

Investigation

All suspected cases should be investigated (page 140):

Free thyroxine index (FTI) or PBI

Diminished radioiodine uptake $<20\%$ at 24–48 hours

Raised serum cholesterol
Anaemia (normochromic or macrocytic) and raised ESR
ECG shows low voltage with flattened or inverted T waves
Rise in titre of thyroid antibodies

Treatment

Thyroid extract is variable in composition and should never be used. Thyroxine is given in doses of 0·05 to 0·3 mg a day, always starting with a low dose and raising it every fourteen days. If ischaemic heart disease is present, the lowest dose should be used initially. β-blockade may help to prevent angina. Patients should be warned that treatment is for life.

Autoimmune thyroiditis

This term usually refers to disorders of the thyroid gland in which circulating thyroid antibodies are present in the plasma; in addition lymphoid and plasma cells are found in excess in the thyroid gland. The patients may be hypothyroid, euthyroid, or very rarely hyperthyroid. Hashimoto's disease refers to the condition in which autoimmune thyroiditis has produced a hard nodular goitre. Destruction of thyroid-hormone-producing tissue causes a rise in TSH which leads to thyroid enlargement. At this stage, the level of the circulating thyroid hormones, although reduced for that person, may be within the 'normal limits' and there is no evidence of hypothyroidism. However, thyroid reserve is diminished, and later the free thyroxine index fall further and symptoms of hypothyroidism occur. By then the patient has a goitre which is often hard and sometimes nodular. In some patients the development of autoimmune hypothyroidism is associated with progressive fibrosis of the gland without the production of a goitre. These patients present as cases of hypothyroidism without goitre.

Clinical presentation

Hashimoto's disease presents as a patient with a goitre who is either euthyroid or hypothyroid. The goitre must be distinguished from other types of non-toxic goitre and from carcinoma of the thyroid.

Investigation (page 140)

Thyroid antibodies may be directed against thyroglobulin or the microsomal fraction of thyroid cells. The former include the highly specific but relatively insensitive precipitin test, and the sensitive but less specific tanned red cell agglutination test. The complement fixation test against microsomal antibodies is not very specific. The gland usually takes up a normal amount of iodine, i.e. the radioiodine uptake is within normal limits but there is faulty utilisation of iodine and the iodine is discharged from the gland by potassium perchlorate in about half the cases. The FTI or PBI are in the lower range of normal or in the hypothyroid range. Biopsy will confirm the diagnosis.

Treatment Thyroxine in full doses will suppress TSH, cause the gland to diminish in size, and relieve any symptoms of hypothyroidism if present.

Thyroid cancer

All types are rare and some carry a relatively good prognosis. Ionising radiation during childhood is a predisposing factor. The main types and their clinical features are:

Papillary Commonest type. It occurs in the relatively young and may present with lymph gland enlargement (lateral aberrant thyroid). It is often TSH-dependent and regresses if thyroxine is given. The prognosis is relatively good.

Follicular Often produces functioning secondaries which are sensitive to radioiodine. It has a relatively good prognosis and is relatively common.

Anaplastic Usually presents with gland enlargement in the elderly and is highly malignant.

Medullary Rare. It secretes calcitonin and may produce ectopic corticotrophin. The prognosis is relatively good.

A thyroid nodule which appears to be single is usually not single. Even if it is, the likelihood of malignancy is low. If thyroid scanning shows a 'hot' nodule it is not malignant. A 'cold' nodule may or may not be, and is better excised.

Adrenal

Adrenal glands

The medulla secretes adrenaline and noradrenaline. The cortex produces steroid hormones of which the most important are cortisol (hydrocortisone) and aldosterone. The secretion of most of the steroids is controlled by pituitary corticotrophin (ACTH) which itself is released by the hypothalamic hormone—corticotrophin releasing factor (CRF). But the secretion of aldosterone is independent of the pituitary. The adrenals also produce androgens and oestrogens. The effects of the three main groups of adrenocorticol hormones differ. In summary they are:

Glucocorticoids (e.g. cortisol) Raise the blood sugar and antagonise insulin. They suppress the reaction to injury, infection and inflammation. They reduce the circulating eosinophil and lymphocyte counts. They cause sodium retention and potassium depletion and alkalosis, when given in large doses or over a long period.
Cortisone and synthetic analogues, e.g. prednisone, have similar actions.

Mineralocorticoids (e.g. aldosterone) Cause sodium retention and potassium depletion, with hypertension, alkalosis and oedema. The synthetic steroids, fludrocortisone and deoxycorticosterone acetate have similar actions.

Sex hormones

Produce effects depending on the dominance of male hormone, e.g. androsterone, or female hormone, e.g. oestrogens and progesterone. Hence they may be virilising or feminising. Androgens antagonise some of the metabolic effects of the glucocorticoids.

Cushing's syndrome

Aetiology

The syndrome is the result of excess corticosteroids and by far the commonest cause is *prolonged treatment with relatively large doses*. Most of the synthetic analogues of cortisone produce these side-effects but they are less liable to give rise to sodium retention. Apart from iatrogenic disease, this disorder is very rare.
The other causes are:

Basophil hyperplasia or *adenoma* of the pituitary gland, with excess production of corticotrophin (60%).
Primary tumours of the adrenals, either adenoma (20%) or carcinoma (10%).
Secondary to carcinoma elsewhere—usually an oat cell carcinoma of the bronchus causing the 'ectopic ACTH syndrome'. Other sites are the thymus, pancreas, thyroid or ovary. Pigmentation may occur in this condition due to MSH secretion.

Clinical presentation

The onset is insidious with:

Alteration in appearance with redistribution of body fat, 'mooning' of the face and truncal or 'buffalo' obesity (about 90%). The limbs are often spared but the obesity may be generalised.
Protein breakdown leads to muscle weakness, wide purple striae (50%) on the abdomen, thighs and buttocks, and easy bruising (30%).
Osteoporosis with backache and vertebral collapse (50%).
Disturbance of carbohydrate tolerance which may amount to diabetes (10%).
Electrolyte disturbance with sodium retention, potassium loss and hypokalaemic alkalosis—especially in the ectopic ACTH syndrome, where ACTH levels are very high. Renal stones may occur (20%).
Hypertension, probably related to sodium retention (60%).
Masculinisation—amenorrhoea, hirsuitism, deep voice, acne in the female (80%).
Mental disturbance—depression or mania and sometimes exaggeration of previous psychiatric abnormalities.

Investigation (page 138)

First confirm the raised cortisol level and then determine the reason.
Estimation of plasma cortisol—looking for absence of normal diurnal variation.
Radioimmunoassay of ACTH.

Increase in urinary 24-hour 17-hydroxycorticosteroids.
Dexamethasone suppression of the pituitary.
Perirenal air insufflation with or without aortography to delineate the adrenals.

Treatment

Bilateral adrenalectomy followed by replacement therapy—cortisol 20–40 mg daily and fludrocortisone 0·1 mg daily.
Removal of ACTH source if practicable (bronchial carcinoma).

***Conn's syndrome* (primary hyperaldosteronism)**

This is a very rare condition caused by a solitary benign adenoma of the zona glomerulosa producing excess of aldosterone.

Clinical presentation

Hypokalaemia and muscle weakness often in attacks. Polyuria and polydipsia secondary to the hypokalaemia.
Sodium retention often leading to hypertension but there is usually no oedema.
It may mimic hypertension from other causes especially when potassium-losing diuretics are being given.

Investigation

The serum potassium is low and usually associated with metabolic alkalosis. The serum renin is low and this differentiates it from secondary aldosteronism (which occurs in the nephrotic syndrome, cirrhosis of the liver with ascites and, rarely, in congestive cardiac failure and bronchial carcinoma).

Treatment

Surgical resection should be considered because some tumours are malignant.

Spironolactone is an antagonist to aldosterone and may be given in primary or secondary aldosteronism.

Adrenogenital syndrome

A very rare condition of infancy or childhood due to a congenital enzyme defect (usually of 21-hydroxylase) affecting cortisol synthesis. The resulting decrease in circulating cortisol stimulates overproduction of ACTH, which in turn stimulates the adrenals to produce excess of androgenic steroids. Females show virilisation early in life and are treated with cortisol. Males are less often diagnosed and may die in acute adrenal insufficiency, but if the infant survives growth is excessive and precocious puberty occurs. Treat with corticosteroids.

Adrenal insufficiency

Acute

Adrenal crisis. There is apathy, coma and epigastric pain. The blood sugar is low.
NB The Waterhouse-Friderichsen syndrome of severe acute meningococcal septicaemia associated with purpura, is usually associated with raised levels of circulating corticosteroids despite the massive bilateral adrenal haemorrhage.

Chronic Insidious onset of weakness and fatigue with gastrointestinal symptoms of anorexia, weight loss, nausea, vomiting, intermittent abdominal pain and diarrhoea. There is hypotension, often postural, and tachycardia. Hyperpigmentation occurs in exposed areas, friction areas, hand creases, and buccal mucosa.

Aetiology It may occur acutely in patients previously (within 1–1½ years) or currently being treated with corticosteroids when there is trauma, surgery or acute infection or withdrawal of steroids.

It may follow surgical removal of the adrenals for Cushing's syndrome or in the treatment of breast carcinoma unless there is adequate replacement therapy.

Chronic adrenal insufficiency (Addison's disease) is very rare and causes include: autoimmune adrenal destruction; adrenal infiltration with secondary carcinoma, Hodgkin's or leukaemic tissue; destruction in haemochromatosis, amyloidosis and infection (tuberculosis and histoplasmosis) where prevalent.

It may occur secondary to hypopituitarism (page 124) and in the adrenogenital syndrome (page 135).

Investigation (page 139) Plasma 'cortisol' levels (11-hydroxycorticosteroids) allowing for diurnal variation which diminishes in adrenal failure.

Low 17-hydroxy corticosteroid excretion (17-OHCS) in the urine.

No increase in output after tetracosactrin (Synacthen).

Serum electrolytes usually normal but in impending crisis the sodium may be low, the potassium high and the blood urea raised.

Failure of water diuresis is rectified by cortisone.

Treatment Maintenance therapy—cortisone 25–50 mg daily. Fludrocortisone 0·1 mg daily.

In acute crisis—intravenous hydrocortisone, intravenous saline and glucose are required. Underlying infection must be treated.

Phaeochromocytoma This is usually a benign tumour of the adrenal medulla. It can arise from other chromaffin tissues of the sympathetic nervous system, e.g. the para-aortic ganglia. It may be associated with neurofibromatosis, medullary thyroid carcinoma (calcitonin-producing) and parathyroid adenoma. Very rarely it is malignant.

It is a very rare cause of hypertension (less than 1 in 200) but it is important to recognise, since it is treatable. It can be familial and bilateral.

Clinical presentation The clinical features depend on the activity of the tumour and the relative amounts of adrenaline (β- and some α-effects) and noradrenaline (α-effects). Usually α-effects predominate. Some tumours secrete intermittently.

The β-effects include a rise in systolic blood pressure with an increase in heart rate, increase in the cardiac output and dilatation of muscle vessels. The α-effects include a rise in both systolic and diastolic blood pressure with reflex slowing of the heart rate and constriction of blood vessels.

A few patients have normal blood pressure between attacks of paroxysmal hypertension, but most are hypertensive all the time. In a typical attack there is pallor, palpitation, anxiety and sometimes angina, headache, sweating and nausea. The blood pressure may be very high and death may occur from myocardial infarction or a cerebrovascular accident. Hyperglycaemia may occur if adrenaline is secreted.

NB Paroxysmal bradycardia (an α-effect) may occur.

Investigation

Estimation of catechol amines (adrenaline and noradrenaline) in the blood or urine or the urinary metabolite vanillyl mandelic acid (VMA).

An intravenous pyelogram or aortogram may help to localise the tumour, but may precipitate an attack (use α- and β-blockade).

Treatment

The tumour is removed under cover of α- and β-blocking agents given 3–4 days previously to prevent the effects of the release of catechol amines during operation. Plasma volume must be monitored throughout the period of sympathetic blockade and during surgery the CVP should be monitored because changes in pulse and blood pressure are blocked.

In emergencies, α-effects may be antagonised by phentolamine (short-acting) or phenoxybenzamine (long-acting) and β-effects are antagonised by propranolol.

Carcinoid syndrome

Aetiology

This is a rare disorder and results from a malignant carcinoid tumour of the ileum which has metastasised to the liver. Carcinoid of the appendix rarely metastasises. The majority of bronchial adenomas are carcinoid but only a few metastasise and produce the syndrome.

Clinical presentation

The symptoms of the primary disorder may be present, e.g. episodic diarrhoea or recurrent haemoptysis. The carcinoid syndrome is due to the secretion of 5-hydroxytryptamine and kinin peptides. Attacks are episodic and symptoms include facial flushing, fever, acute dyspnoea from bronchospasm, nausea, vomiting and diarrhoea. Later valvular stenosis of the pulmonary and tricuspid valves may develop.

Investigation

The 24-hour urinary excretion of 5-hydroxyindole

acetic acid (5-HIAA) is estimated. Normal range: 2–10 mg in 24 hours.

Shortness of stature

The term dwarf is better avoided. The common cause is short parents. Other causes are:

Deficiency of growth hormone—sometimes familial (see *Hypopituitarism* page 124), often associated with delayed or failure of sexual development. Bone age is retarded.
Bone diseases, e.g. achondroplasia and rickets.
Malnutrition including the malabsorption syndrome.
Renal, liver or heart failure in early childhood.
Large doses of steroids in childhood.
Cretinism.

Tests of endocrine function

The tests used are determined by the suspected diagnosis and are directed towards:
— establishing this diagnosis
— determining whether it is a pituitary or a target organ disease
— elucidating the underlying pathology

Cushing's syndrome

Screening of basal function

24-hour excretion of steroid metabolites, 17-oxogenic steroids. This measures the compounds which can be converted to oxosteroids by oxidation and includes cortisol, its metabolites and some other steroid compounds. Normal ranges: 7–20 mg (male) and 5–15 mg (female). The test is not specific and values are often slightly raised in simple obesity. Up to 25% of patients with Cushing's syndrome may have normal results.
Diurnal variation in serum cortisol. This level is normally highest at 9 AM (7–25 μg/100 ml) and lowest at midnight. The midnight value is almost always raised in Cushing's syndrome. It is the loss of diurnal variation which is the important observation.
Basal cortisol secretion rate (10–20 mg/24 h).
24-hour urinary free cortisol (less than 100 μg).
Basal plasma ACTH assay There is a normal diurnal variation similar to that of cortisol.

Dynamic tests of adrenocortical-pituitary function

Metyrapone (metopirone) test 750 mg is given 4-hourly for 24 hours. It inhibits 11-β-hydroxylase in the adrenal gland which then produces 11-deoxycortisol instead of cortisol. The fall in serum cortisol stimulates ACTH and the consequent increased 24-hour urinary output of 11-deoxycortisol (measured as 17-oxogenic steroids) is a measure both of pituitary sensitivity and of adrenal response. The test differentiates between Cushing's syndrome due to bilateral adrenal hyperplasia (i.e. pituitary-dependent) where there is a rise in urinary 17-oxogenic steroids, and adrenal adenoma or carcinoma where there is no change (or a fall).

Dexamethasone suppression tests
Short screening test. 2 mg is taken between 10 PM and midnight and the 9 AM serum cortisol estimated (normal $<6{\cdot}5$ mg/100 ml).
Six-day tests. 24-hour urines for 17-oxogenic steroids are collected; 2 days control, 2 days while the patient takes 0·5 mg 6-hourly and 2 days on 2·0 mg 6-hourly.

In patients with Cushing's syndrome 17-oxogenic steroids do not fall below 5 mg on the low dose. (Many 'normal' patients do not suppress either—40%.) The high dose of dexamethasone may help to differentiate between pituitary-dependent disease (which should suppress at this dose) and patients with ectopic ACTH or adrenal tumour. The results of this test are not always reliable.

Adrenocortical insufficiency (Addison's disease)

Screening of basal function

Both 24-hour urinary 17-oxogenic steroids and some cortisols may be well in the normal range, even in strongly suspected cases. Unless results are consistently at the upper end of the normal range dynamic ('stress') tests are indicated.
A single basal plasma ACTH assay shows high levels (500 pg/ml) in primary adrenal disease and undetectable values in pituitary disease.

Dynamic tests

Synacthen (tetracosactrin) tests
Half-hour screening test. This measures the serum cortisol response after 250 μg Synactin i.m. In normal patients the initial level should be over 5 μg/100 ml, the half-hour level over 20 μg/100 ml and the difference between them not less than 7 μg/100 ml.
Five-hour test to 1 mg of depot tetracosactrin. In normal patients the serum cortisol more than doubles in the first hour.
Three-day test. This involves two baseline and three post-stimulation 24-hour urine collections for 17-oxogenic steroids. 1 mg tetracosactrin i.m. is given daily. Adrenals suppressed by prolonged steroid therapy may show a response to this prolonged stimulus when they may not to a short one.
Insulin hypoglycaemia test A blood sugar of less than 40 mg/100 ml stimulates the hypothalamic pituitary to produce ACTH and growth hormone. Soluble insulin 0·1 to 0·2 units/kg is given intravenously (with an indwelling needle for resuscitation). The lower dose is used in patients with suspected hypofunction (of pituitary and/or adrenal) and the higher dose for those with suspected hyperfunction. The serum cortisol, sugar, growth hormone and ACTH may be measured half-hourly for 2 hours. This is a fuller test of function than that below (and quicker to perform) because it includes 'stress' in the test.

Metyrapone test A reduced response occurs with suppression or hypofunction of the pituitary and/or adrenal cortex. It is necessary first to show that the adrenal can respond normally to ACTH before ascribing a reduced response to pituitary disease. The test should not be performed within 1 week of ACTH.

Thyroid function

Screening tests of basal thyroid secretion function (figure 32)

PBI This refers to the iodine precipitated with the plasma proteins and includes administered iodine (e.g. pyelography and myelography).

T_4 This gives much the same information as the PBI but administered iodine does not interfere. Thyroxine from the patient's serum is added to a standard solution of thyroid binding globulin which has radioactive thyroxine already bound to it. The displacement of this radioactive thyroxine is related to the amount of thyroxine present in the patient's serum.

T_3 (resin) uptake This is a measurement of the unoccupied binding sites on thyroid hormone binding protein (TBP). The unoccupied sites are increased when:

— there is little thyroid hormone (myxoedema)

— there is excess of TBP (pregnancy and 'the pill')

and vice versa. A known amount of radio-T_3 is added to a known volume of the patient's serum and a portion of it becomes fixed to the unoccupied sites of the patient's TBP. The portion of radio-T_3

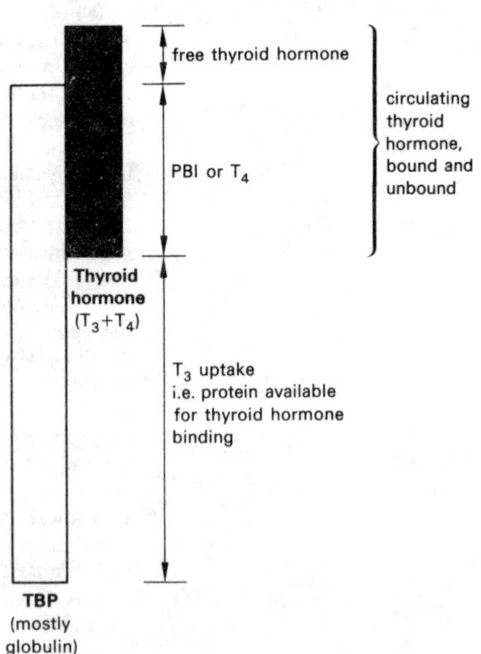

FIGURE 32 Screening tests of basal thyroid secretion function.

which remains unbound (e.g. little in hypothyroidism) is removed attached to a resin and this is counted. The resin uptake is thus small in hypothyroidism but the results are often expressed, confusingly, in terms of the quantity of radioactivity remaining in the patient's serum (i.e. high in hypothyroidism). Numerically the results are expressed as a percentage of normal (e.g. 85–115%).

FTI (free thyroxine index) This is derived mathematically from the T_4 and T_3 uptake. This automatically compensates for variations in TBP (increased in pregnancy and the pill) and variations in available binding sites on TBP (decreased with phenytoin and salicylates). It approximates to free thyroid hormone, i.e. the physiologically relevant quantity. Serum T_3 may be raised (when T_4 is normal) in hyperthyroidism.

Screening test of basal thyroid uptake

^{132}I uptake The radioactivity of the thyroid gland is measured at a standard time (e.g. 4 hours) after the patient has been given radioiodine (usually ^{132}I because of its short half-life of 2·3 hours). It is increased in thyrotoxicosis and in iodine deficiency. It is decreased in hypothyroidism and when the patient is taking certain compounds: phenothiazines, phenylbutazone, PAS and INAH, and tolbutamide (therefore note patients with tuberculosis, diabetes and arthritis, and those requiring sedation).

Basal TSH measurements

TSH is increased in hypothyroidism of thyroid origin.

Dynamic tests of thyroid/pituitary function

T_3 suppression test In the normal person, exogenous thyroid hormone (in this test, T_3 40 μg 8-hourly for 1 week) suppresses pituitary TSH and, in turn, the thyroid gland radioiodine uptake. If the thyroid/pituitary axis is autonomous (LATS, autonomous nodule, pituitary autonomy), exogenous T_3 does not suppress gland uptake. The test is usually used to determine the return of physiological (TSH) control of the thyrotoxic gland (previously under LATS stimulation) at which time antithyroid drugs can be stopped.

TSH stimulation test If hypothyroidism is due to thyroid failure (as it usually is), TSH given 5–10 units intramuscularly daily for 3 days will cause little or no increase in radioiodine gland uptake. This test may be used on patients who are on thyroxine.

TRH test There is negative feedback control of TRH (thyrotrophin releasing hormone) effect on pituitary. Raised serum levels of T_4 and T_3 thus reduce serum TSH levels, e.g. thyrotoxicosis, administered thyroxine. In the standard test, 200 μg of TRH is given intravenously and the blood is taken for TSH assay immediately before and 20 and 60 minutes afterwards. (Assessing results by thyroid hormone assay is less reliable.) In hyperthyroidism (even if mild), there is no TSH response to TRH. In hypothyroidism there is a high basal level of TSH and an exaggerated response to TRH. In hypothyroidism there is a high basal level of TSH and an exaggerated response to TRH. In hypothyroidism due to pituitary disease or hypothalamic disease there may be a reduced response. The TRH test is tending to replace the T_3 suppression test and has replaced the TSH stimulation test.

Peripheral thyroid effects

BMR, ECG, serum cholesterol and measurements of tendon reflex relaxation time are of little diagnostic value but easy to perform.

Metabolic disease

The commonest metabolic diseases are obesity and diabetes mellitus. Osteoporosis is common in the elderly.

Diabetes mellitus

The clinical picture of diabetes is due to diminished availability or effectiveness of insulin.

Primary (essential, idiopathic) diabetes

There are half a million cases diagnosed in the United Kingdom and surveys suggest another half a million undiagnosed.

Secondary diabetes

This is, in comparison, very uncommon and due to
— pancreatic destruction: carcinoma of the pancreas, pancreatitis, pancreatectomy, haemochromatosis
— insulin antagonism: steroid therapy, Cushing's syndrome, acromegaly and phaeochromocytoma
— other causes of glucose intolerance: thyrotoxicosis, pregnancy, thiazide diuretics and advanced liver disease

Clinical presentation (pages 76–78)

There are two main groups of patients.
'*Maturity onset*' diabetes which tends to occur in the overweight and elderly. They are often asymptomatic and detected by routine urine testing. They often present with the common complications of vascular insufficiency or infection.
'*Juvenile onset*' diabetes which tends to occur in the thin and young. They often present acutely with severe systemic disease—malaise, fatigue, weight loss, polyuria, polydipsia, infection and sometimes pre-coma or coma.

Diagnosis

This is made on finding:

Random blood glucose of more than 200 mg/100 ml in the presence of symptoms.
Glucose tolerance test: (*a*) 2-hour blood glucose of more than 160 mg/100 ml (suspect if more than 120 mg/100 ml); (*b*) high fasting glucose level (more than 100 mg/100 ml); (*c*) high peak of more than 170 mg/100 ml (over 200 mg/100 ml in over forty-fives) and a delayed peak.

Complications

Vascular

These account for 75% of deaths.
Large vessel disease Atheroma (page 152) is widespread and early in onset. Ischaemic heart disease produces angina and myocardial infarction (five times more common in middle aged diabetics than in the general population). Atheromatous occlusion of large vessels is forty times more common and may produce gangrene of the feet (page 244) (see *Hyperlipidaemia* page 152).

Small vessel disease Diabetic microangiopathy is associated with homogeneous thickening of the vascular basement membrane and endothelial proliferation. It produces renal failure (invariably associated with retinopathy) and gangrene of the skin of the feet with wedge-shaped infarcts—arterial pulses are usually present and the skin warm. It carries a poor prognosis for life.

Eye

20% of diabetics.
Non-proliferative (exudative) retinopathy This is characterised by haemorrhages, exudates and microaneurysms and although common has little effect on vision. Microaneurysms are bulges in capillary walls, usually appearing first on the temporal side of the macula, which leak plasma to produce hard exudates. Soft 'cotton wool' exudates are small deep retinal infarcts.
Proliferative retinopathy presents chiefly in the young-onset diabetic, usually 15–20 years after initial diagnosis. Once it occurs, blindness follows within 5 years in 50%. It is still not clear that improved diabetic control and control of hypertension improve the ocular prognosis. New vessel formation occurs mainly near the disc which later fibroses and contracts. Haemorrhage both subhyaloid and into the vitreous cause sudden blindness. Retinal detachment may also occur.
Cataracts (20% of diabetic blindness) occur at a younger age in diabetic patients.

Kidney

Renal disease accounts for 30% of diabetic deaths under the age of 40 years. Uraemia and hypertension are the common terminal events. Nephrotic syndrome occurs in under 10%; it is associated with a high mortality (within 3 years of onset).
Diffuse glomerular sclerosis This occurs in over 50% of diabetics (100% on electron microscopy). Its severity tends to correlate with the degree of renal failure. There is thickening of the basement membrane and hyaline degeneration of afferent and efferent arterioles. Similar changes may occur with arteriosclerosis and glomerulonephritis.
Nodular glomerular sclerosis (Kimmelstiel-Wilson lesion) There are focal homogenous acellular eosinophilic nodules usually at the periphery of the glomerulus consisting of excess mesangial matrix. There may be localised basement membrane thickening. This lesion is pathognomonic of diabetes; but its severity correlates poorly with the nephrotic syndrome.
Pyelonephritis (acute and chronic) This is predisposed to by glycosuria and catheterisation.
Renal papillary necrosis may occur in diabetes in the absence of analgesic abuse. It is caused by infarction of the papillae producing haematuria and renal failure.

Neuromuscular

These occur in 30% of cases.
Peripheral neuropathy This is the commonest

neurological complication. Patients present with numbness, night cramps and paraesthesiae in the feet. The neuropathy is predominantly sensory and affects the lower limbs with early loss of vibration sense and absent ankle jerks. Later there is loss of pain sensation resulting in chronic painless ulcers at pressure points (even if good arterial pulses are present).

Mononeuritis Single nerve palsies may result from occlusion of the nutrient artery to the nerve, commonly the third cranial nerve, ulnar nerve or lateral popliteal nerve. These are often transient.

Diabetic amyotrophy This usually occurs in middle-aged diabetics who develop painful, asymmetrical weakness and wasting of the quadriceps muscles. Recovery is the rule and appears to be related to good diabetic control.

Autonomic neuropathy This may produce impotence (25% in male patients), nocturnal diarrhoea, postural hypotension and occasionally urinary retention with overflow.

NB The autonomic effects of hypoglycaemia especially pallor, sweating and tachycardia may be reduced or absent in diabetics with an autonomic neuropathy and in patients on β-blockers.

Skin

Insulin-sensitivity may occur in the first month of insulin therapy with the production of tender lumps after each injection. Spontaneous recovery occurs and no change of therapy is indicated.

Lipodystrophy There is painless fat atrophy at injection sites. The patient should discontinue using these sites for injections because there is unpredictable absorption of insulin from them.

Necrobiosis lipoidica diabeticorum This is very rare but pathognomonic of diabetes and may precede it. It occurs usually over the shins and is characterised by atrophy of subcutaneous collagen. The lesions are violet rings with yellow masses at the periphery and scarring and atrophy at the centre.

Photosensitivity with chlorpropamide may occur.

Intercurrent infection

This is common in diabetic patients, particularly of the urinary tract and skin. Tuberculosis and moniliasis (vulvitis and balanitis) are more common in diabetes.

Management

Maturity-onset diabetes

Reduction of dietary carbohydrate to 120 to 150 grams daily (roughly 1200–1500 calories) with weight loss may be sufficient to reduce the blood sugar towards normal and to abolish symptoms. If not, oral hypoglycaemic agents—sulphonylureas or biguanides—should be added. In the elderly obese patient metformin (500 mg bd or tds) or phenformin (50 mg bd or tds) are often the drugs chosen since they decrease appetite (sulphonylureas may increase it) and are unlikely to produce hypoglycaemia (some sulphonylureas may).

NB Metformin and phenformin may occasionally produce megaloblastic anaemia, and phenformin predisposes to lactic acidosis.

Particular attention must be paid to the care of the feet and toenails which are frequently infected.

Insulin-dependent diabetes (page 77)

The object of therapy is to prevent hypoglycaemic and hyperglycaemic states. Good control decreases the incidence of intercurrent infection, coma, and possibly decreases neurological disability. The other complications appear not to be affected by the standard of control. Hypoglycaemia remains the major complication of insulin therapy.

The new patient is usually admitted to hospital for diet and insulin therapy and instruction in injection technique. There are many successful schemes including a 'sliding scale' (page 148) or empirical twice daily soluble insulin injection (e.g. 12–20 units bd depending on the blood sugar). When controlled and on discharge from hospital the total daily dose of insulin is reduced by 10–20% as requirements are less during activity. The dose may be given as before (soluble insulin twice daily) or a long-acting preparation such as lente insulin once in the morning before breakfast. A common combination is PZI and soluble (2/3 : 1/3) in one morning dose. Many diabetics, understandably, mix these together in one syringe and a variable proportion of soluble is converted to PZI by the excess protamine contained in this preparation. Nevertheless many achieve satisfactory control. Dietary carbohydrate intake, unless excessive, is best chosen by the individual patient according to his personal needs, and insulin therapy adjusted for the chosen diet. Patients with pancreatectomy usually need 20–30 units per day.

Diabetic coma

There are two common types:
— hypoglycaemic
— hyperglycaemic ketoacidosis

In clinical practice there is rarely any difficulty in differentiating between these two clinical situations. Should there be any difficulty the problem may be solved by estimating the blood sugar at the bedside with a Dextrostix. Unfortunately these 'stix' may be unreliable in hypoglycaemia and if still in doubt i.v. glucose can do no harm (take a blood sample first). Insulin may be fatal in hypoglycaemic coma.

Hypoglycaemia

The patients are usually known diabetics on insulin (rarely sulphonylurea therapy, insulinoma or Addison's disease). It is caused by excess antidiabetic therapy, excess exercise or decreased food intake. The rate of onset of symptoms is rapid. Most patients are aware of impending coma and may prevent it by taking sugar (2 lumps equals 20 grams). Patients present either in pre-coma with agitated, often aggressive confusion, or in coma when marked sweating is usually present.

Management Oral glucose in water or, if necessary, i.v. glucose (20–40 ml of 50%) will reverse symptoms within a minute. Glucagon 1 mg i.m. acts as rapidly. NB Hypoglycaemia must be treated rapidly since it may produce irreversible brain damage. Rarely corticosteroids may be required in addition to glucose if Addison's disease is present.

The hypoglycaemia of chlorpropamide therapy may require continued sugar administration for 24 hours (the drug's effects last up to 48 hours).

Hyperglycaemic keto-acidotic coma

This appears to be occurring less frequently perhaps due to better education of patients.

Pre-coma is of slow onset, i.e. hours or days. There is often evidence of infection (25–35%) particularly of the renal, respiratory or gastro-intestinal tracts. Septicaemia and meningitis are uncommon but important causes. The patient has usually not been eating properly and has stopped taking insulin. In 25–35% there is no obvious precipitating cause and 10–20% are new cases. The patient may be confused, vomiting, hypotensive, severely dehydrated and overbreathing. The breath may smell of ketones.

Management Venous blood should be taken for glucose, urea and electrolytes (including bicarbonate) haemoglobin and haematocrit. (Arterial acid-base studies and blood gases may demonstrate hypoxia and quantitate acidosis.)

There is usually gastric dilatation, and death can occur from aspiration pneumonia. The gastric contents should, therefore, be aspirated, preferably continuously.

Urinary catheterisation is unnecessary in mild cases where confusion is minimal, but is required in those who are in coma as it is otherwise not possible to assess urine output. A diabetic urine chart and fluid balance chart are started and urine sent to the laboratory for bacteriology.

Soluble insulin must be given immediately (100 units: half i.v. and half i.m. is one commonly used scheme) or use the slow infusion technique (page 148).

Start intravenous fluid therapy immediately. No fixed regime can be given and therapy depends upon an assessment of the degree of dehydration. (The average deficit is 6–8 litres—to be replaced in the first 24 hours in addition to the daily requirement.) The patients are water, sodium and potassium depleted and acidotic. For moderate to severe cases, in young people, 1 litre of normal saline may be given in the first half-hour containing 100 mEq of bicarbonate and repeated in the following hour.

Nearly all these patients have a low total body potassium (deficit 200–400 mEq) and about 15% have hypokalaemia on admission. Both insulin and bicarbonate will tend to exacerbate the dangers of this situation. As soon as polyuria is observed (it is usually present on admission) potassium chloride should be added at a rate of 2 g (26 mEq) per litre of intravenous fluid. Severe cases (serum bicarbonate below 5 mEq/l) may require 250 mEq of bicarbonate and 3 g (39 mEq) per litre of potassium. The potassium may be monitored by the ECG, though this is not fully reliable—if signs of hyperkalaemia are present on the ECG (page 63), potassium is withheld until plasma results are known.

The use of bicarbonate to correct acidosis is disputed. Some consider that correction results in quicker control of symptoms, whilst others underline the danger of inducing further hypokalaemia. It would seem reasonable to correct partially, e.g. half the bicarbonate deficit calculated as described (page 176), at a rate not exceeding 50 mEq/15 min.

Intercurrent infection must always be considered and treated. In the absence of obvious infection, it is advisable to perform urine microscopy and culture, chest X-ray and blood culture.

Laboratory results should be available after 30 minutes and give a baseline potassium level. The degree of acidosis may be calculated from the serum bicarbonate and used as an (approximate) guide to bicarbonate dosage. Intravenous normal (0·9%) saline with potassium as above is continued at a rate of 0·5–2 litres per hour for the first 2 hours depending upon the degree of dehydration.

A second blood sample is taken 2 hours after the initial insulin is given.

If sugar levels are unchanged, repeat soluble insulin 100 units.
If sugar levels are rising, give 200 units.
If sugar levels are falling, caution is required as too much insulin may precipitate hypoglycaemia. A rough rule is 'the 10% rule', i.e. give 10% of the blood sugar value as soluble insulin i.m.

If in doubt, i.e. the sugar is falling very rapidly, repeat blood sugar levels (Dextrostix may be useful). Insulin is rarely required at blood sugar levels below 250 mg/100 ml.

At this stage it is usually feasible to return the patient to his normal insulin dosage divided into two to four doses per day. If the patient is awake, fluid and food are given by mouth. Some physicians use the 'sliding scale' (table 15) for patients whose sugar has fallen to less than 300 mg/100 ml but who are still unconscious and not yet eating and drinking. Urinary sugars are estimated 6-hourly and insulin and fluids given according to scale, which assumes a urinary glucose threshold of 180 mg/100 ml.

Slow insulin infusion

Recently the technique of slow insulin infusion has been introduced. After a loading dose of about 8 units, soluble insulin is given at a rate of between 4 and 12 units per hour. The blood sugar falls at a rate of about 75 mg/100 ml each hour, and blood levels of under 200 mg/100 ml are reached in 3–6 hours. Intravenous saline, often with the addition of

TABLE 15 Typical 'sliding scale'

Urinary sugar	*Fluid replacement (6-hrly)*	*Insulin*
2%	1 litre N saline	32 u/i.m.
1%	1 litre dextrose/saline	16 u/i.m.
¾%	1 litre dextrose/saline	8 u/i.m.
½%	1 litre dextrose/saline	Nil
¼%	1 litre dextrose/saline	Nil

potassium chloride and occasionally sodium bicarbonate, is required as above.

Other forms of diabetic coma

Hyperosmolar non-ketotic coma

This occurs in the elderly obese diabetic, is often previously undiagnosed and may follow myocardial infarction and strokes. The onset is slow with polyuria over 2–3 weeks and progressive dehydration. Blood sugar levels are very high (often above 800 mg/100 ml), plasma osmolality is increased (often above 400 mosmol/l). Plasma bicarbonate is usually normal and there is little or no ketonuria. These patients require insulin—often in small doses over the acute episode (10–20 units may suffice)—and hypotonic (e.g. 0·5N saline) fluid replacement given slowly but usually in large quantities. The mortality is high (50%) and cerebral oedema from treatment a real risk.

Lactic acidosis

This occurs in the elderly obese diabetic and is precipitated by phenformin and alcohol. It may occur in shocked patients. The patients are acidotic. Blood sugar may be normal and there is little or no ketonuria. Blood lactic acid levels are raised and serum bicarbonate levels reduced.

The cation total (Na^+ plus K^+) may exceed the anion total (Cl^- plus HCO_3^-), the difference (of up to 25 mEq/l) being lactate. These patients require insulin in large doses, glucose, bicarbonate (up to 1000 mEq in 24 hours), and fluid replacement. The mortality is very high (80%).

NB Cerebrovascular accidents and aspirin overdosage may both produce a combination of coma plus glycosuria.

Diabetics also have strokes, take overdoses and become concussed.

Porphyria

This describes four syndromes in which there is increased intermittent excretion of porphyrins in the urine and/or faeces. The first three are hepatic porphyrias.

There are two important inherited (autosomal dominant) varieties in both of which there are acute episodes with gastrointestinal, neuropsychiatric and cardiovascular features precipitated by administration of drugs—usually barbiturates (especially intravenous general anaesthetics), sulphonamides and the contraceptive pill. The clinical features (which bear a superficial resemblance to lead poisoning) are:

— abdominal pain, vomiting or constipation
— peripheral neuropathy with weakness or paralysis
— confusion and psychosis
— tachycardia and hypertension

In both, during attacks there is increased urinary porphobilinogen (pbg) and δ-amino-laevulinic acid (ALA) and increased faecal porphyrins. Pbg is detected by Ehrlich's aldehyde reagent (water-soluble, page 35) and porphyrins recognised by fluorescence in ultraviolet light. Pbg in urine darkens on standing (oxidation).

Acute intermittent porphyria (AIP)

This is the Swedish type and the commonest in the UK. The skin is 'never' affected. In remission the urine still has excess pbg and ALA but the faeces are relatively normal. The best screening test is the urinary pbg.

Variegate porphyria (VP)

This is the South African type. The skin, photo-sensitised by porphyrins, is fragile particularly on the backs of the hands. In remission the faeces contain excess porphyrins but the urine may be normal. The best screening test is thus for faecal porphyrins. Latent forms are common.

Cutaneous hepatic porphyria (porphyria cutanea tarda)

There is an important variety which may be acquired or, less commonly, inherited. This is usually secondary to liver disease from alcoholism (hence 'symptomatic' porphyria) but perhaps only occurs in genetically predisposed subjects. There are no acute attacks and the patient is usually not sensitive to drugs (except occasionally barbiturates). The patient usually presents after an alcoholic binge. The signs are predominantly cutaneous with porphyria-induced photosensitivity leading to bullae on exposed areas. There is no family history of porphyria and the liver function tests are usually abnormal. There is no excess porphyria in the stool and no excess pbg or ALA in the urine. There is excess uroporphyrin in the urine.

Congenital erythropoietic porphyria

It is extremely rare, inherited as an autosomal dominant and characterised by extreme skin manifestations plus red-staining of the teeth and bones. There are no acute attacks. There is increased uroporphyrin and coproporphyrin.

Management of hepatic porphyrias

Avoid the usual precipitant drugs (the patient should carry a complete list) and alcohol. Shield the skin in photosensitive patients. Pregnancy can be dangerous in acute intermittent porphyria.

During attacks. Use morphine, diazepam and promazine and propranolol as necessary. Circulatory and respiratory failure may occur and artificial ventilation may be necessary. Intravenous fluids are given if vomiting is severe.

TABLE 16 The hyperlipoproteinaemias (Fredrickson/WHO classification)

Type	I	IIa	IIb	III	IV	V
Name	Hyperchylomicronaemia	Fat-induced hyperlipidaemia Familial essential hypercholesterolaemia	Mixed hyperlipidaemia	Broad β disease	Carbohydrate-induced hyperlipidaemia	
Electrophoresis	↑Chylomicrons	↑β	↑β ↑Pre-β	Broad β ↑Pre-β	↑Pre-β	↑Chylomicrons ↑Pre-β
Nephelometry	(M)L	S	SM	(S)ML	M(L)	ML
Treatment						
diet	↓Fat	↓Saturated fats ↓Cholesterol	↓Saturated fats ↓Cholesterol ↓Carbohydrate ↓Weight	↓Saturated fats ↓Cholesterol ↓Carbohydrate ↓Weight	↓Carbohydrate ↓Weight	↓Fat ↓Carbohydrate ↓Weight
drugs	Nil	Cholestyramine Clofibrate D-Thyroxine? Nicotinic acid?	Clofibrate D-Thyroxine? Nicotinic acid?	Clofibrate D-Thyroxine? Nicotinic acid?	Clofibrate Nicotinic acid?	Clofibrate Nicotinic acid?

Types IIa, IIb and IV are relatively common. I, III and V are rare.
All types except I have a raised cholesterol.
All types except II have raised triglycerides.
β particles are 50% cholesterol and 20% triglyceride.
Pre-β particles are 50% triglyceride and 20% cholesterol.
Normal ranges (fasting): cholesterol 140–280 mg/100 ml, triglyceride 70–180 mg/100 ml.

Lipid disorders (table 16)

The hyperlipoproteinaemias have been classified on the basis of electrophoretic mobility (α, β, pre-β and chylomicrons—Fredrickson, table 16), centrifugation (high, low and very low density bands—Strisower), and turbidity or nephelometry (small, medium and large size particles which correspond to β, pre-β and chlyomicrons respectively). Each subfraction produced by any of these techniques carries a variable proportion of the different fats which can be measured chemically (i.e. cholesterol and triglycerides). Endogenous triglycerides are predominantly pre-β lipoproteins and respond to clofibrate.

NB Blood samples should be taken after an overnight fast. Results may be misleading within 3 months of myocardial infarction.

'Low-fat diet' means low cholesterol, low saturated fats: poly-unsaturated fats are substituted.

Types IIa, IIb and IV (Fredrickson) are important because they are relatively common, are associated with common diseases, and are treatable.

Type IIa

Fat induced hyperlipidaemia, hyper-β-lipoproteinaemia or hypercholesterolaemia. The triglycerides are relatively normal. Commoner in women than in men.

It may be primary, or secondary to hypothyroidism, nephrotic syndrome or prolonged obstructive jaundice.

It produces corneal arcus, tendon xanthomata (Achilles tendons and extensor surfaces of hands) and tuberous xanthomata (extensor surfaces over joints). It is associated with premature coronary artery disease.

Treatment is by reduction in dietary saturated fats and cholesterol with the addition if necessary of an iron exchange resin, e.g. cholestyramine (Questran) or polidexide (Secholex), clofibrate, nicotinic acid and/or D-thyroxine (in that order).

Type IIb

Mixed hyperlipidaemia. The cholesterol and triglycerides are both raised. It is associated with coronary artery disease, hypertension and diabetes mellitus.

It produces xanthelasmata rather than tendon xanthomata and corneal arcus are frequently present. Treatment is by dietary restriction of saturated fats, cholesterol and carbohydrate with the addition of clofibrate and possibly D-thyroxine if necessary.

Type IV

Carbohydrate induced hyperlipidaemia or hyper-pre-β-lipoproteinaemia. Commoner in men than in women. This is the commonest hyperlipidaemia. The triglycerides are raised and to a lesser extent the cholesterol.

It may be primary, or secondary to diabetes mellitus and obesity. It is associated with gout, alcoholism and pancreatitis. Premature atherosclerosis with coronary artery disease and hypertension is common. It produces eruptive cutaneous xanthomata.

Treatment is by dietary restriction of carbohydrate and weight reduction with the addition of clofibrate and if necessary nicotinic acid. The diabetes mellitus may require specific therapy.

Types I, III and V

These are all rare:

Type I High chylomicron level. This presents in childhood and is due to a failure to clear fat. Patients have xanthomata and pancreatitis, but no excess of atherosclerosis. Treatment is by a very low fat diet. No drug is useful.

Type III (broad-β disease) Cholesterol and triglyceride levels are raised. Patients may have fat deposition in the palm creases. Treatment is by weight reduction with a low fat diet, low carbohydrate diet and clofibrate. Dextrothyroxine and nicotinic acid may be helpful.

Type V This is equivalent to a combination of types I and IV, i.e. raised chylomicrons and pre-β-lipoprotein. Like type IV it may be secondary to diabetes mellitus and obesity. It is associated with alcoholism and pancreatitis. The symptoms of pancreatitis respond to dietary treatment. Treatment is by low fat and carbohydrate diet and weight reduction. Clofibrate and nicotinic acid may be helpful.

Metabolic bone disease

Bone normally consists of 60% mineral and 40% organic matter (matrix). The former is mostly calcium and the latter mostly collagen.

Osteoporosis

This may be determined chemically or histologically (bone biopsy) or, less well, by X-ray. Osteoporosis as judged by these criteria increases steadily with age in the normal person. 'Osteoporosis' is a word also used to describe the clinical syndrome of a spinal disorder characterised by intermittent severe backache with crush fracture of vertebral bodies and kyphosis with loss of height. X-rays of the lumbar spine in this syndrome show loss of bone density (the bodies being nearly as transradiant as the discs) with increased trabeculation and biconcavity of the bodies with anterior wedging and kyphosis. The diagnosis in the age chiefly at risk (i.e. the elderly) is from myelomatosis and secondary carcinoma.

Aetiology

Nearly all cases are of unknown cause and generalised. Decreased bone density is more marked in women than men particularly following the menopause. The roles of calcium intake, calcium absorption, vitamin D, oestrogens, and gonadotrophins remain uncertain. A negative calcium balance due to reduced intake or absorption, or excessive excretion has been suggested, and the role of calciferol and oestrogens emphasised.

Classification

General Normal ageing—increased after the menopause

Idiopathic—any age, but excessive in degree when

compared within the age group. It is usually more dramatic, therefore, in the young
Endocrine
— Cushing's syndrome (including steroid therapy)
— thyrotoxicosis
— pregnancy and the puerperium

Local Immobilisation and paralysis
Rheumatoid arthritis

Diagnosis and treatment

If the point of diagnosis is to allow prognosis and treatment, then there is quite correctly little attention paid to the diagnosis of idiopathic osteoporosis in the elderly. The condition usually presents with fracture—vertebra or femoral neck (in both sexes) and Colles' fracture (especially in the female). The treatment of these fractures is little altered by the diagnosis of coexistent osteoporosis. The process is essentially irreversible. There is no convincing evidence yet of successful results from treatment with oestrogens, high calcium intake, dietary phosphate supplements, or small doses of vitamin D
It is important to avoid immobilisation (including the use of corsets) and treat pain symptomatically. Even correction of a Cushing's syndrome is not followed by clear evidence of healing of osteoporosis, though its progress may be arrested.

Investigation

Biochemistry Serum calcium, phosphorus and alkaline phosphatase and urinary calcium are normal.
Radiology Lateral lumbar spine and indices of cortical narrowing (e.g. metacarpal index).
Histology This is not indicated routinely but shows a diminished number of normally calcified trabeculae, the changes being most marked in the vertebrae.

Osteomalacia and rickets

This refers to the situation in which there is inadequate mineralisation of bone in situations known to produce reduced vitamin D activity (see below). There is usually a reduced serum phosphate level and (less commonly) a reduced serum calcium level. The alkaline phosphatase tends to be raised (biochemical osteomalacia or rickets). Clinically adult osteomalacia may present with:

Bone pain ('rheumatism' in the elderly) and tenderness.
Weakness most marked in the quadriceps and glutei which results in a waddling gait and difficulty in rising from a chair.
The other signs of disease causing reduced vitamin D activity, e.g. malabsorption—the osteomalacia being diagnosed in the course of investigation.

NB Tetany and fractures are relatively uncommon.

Rickets (juvenile osteomalacia) presents differently because the reduced mineralisation can affect the epiphyses, as yet unfused, and the modelling of bones, with:

Deformities in the legs (bow-legs, knock-knees).
Deformities in the chest (early sign—ricketic rosary).
Deformities in the skull (craniotabes, open fontanelles and delayed eruption of the teeth).
Hypotonia, weakness, tetany.
NB Rickets in Britain now present chiefly in pigmented immigrants due to a combination of poor sunlight and a diet poor in vitamin D.

Aetiology

Reduced intake of vitamin D.
— dietary calciferol
— cutaneous cholecalciferol (from 7-dehydrocholesterol)
— usually both (dark skin, northern climate, poor diet)
Malabsorption (page 187), especially gluten sensitive enteropathy and postgastrectomy states.
Vitamin D resistance. Uraemia (page 156) and hypophosphataemia.
Increased vitamin D inactivation with chronic anticonvulsant therapy.

Diagnosis and investigation

Clinical
Biochemistry Reduced serum phosphorus and calcium with increased alkaline phosphatase. The calcium × phosphorus product is reduced (normal over 40 and abnormal levels about 25–30). Urinary calcium is reduced and there is a tendency to mild renal tubular acidosis.
X-ray Deformities, especially rickets with slight biconcavity of the vertebral bodies in the lumbar spine with normal or even increased density.
Pseudofractures (Looser's zones). These are translucent 2 mm bands perpendicular to the surface of the bone extending from the cortex inwards, best seen in the pubic rami, the necks of the humeri and femurs and in the outer borders of the scapulae which are 'points of stress'.
Secondary hyperparathyroidism which occurs as a consequence of the low serum calcium level.
Rickets. In addition to the deformity there are cupped and irregular epiphyses which are delayed in appearance.
Histology The number of bony seams is normal.
There is excess volume of osteoid tissue.
There may be an absent calcification front.
There is usually some evidence of hyperparathyroidism.
Investigate the underlying disease, e.g. malabsorption, uraemia.

Differential diagnosis

In the elderly, rheumatism and senility.
Paget's disease (because of the raised alkaline phosphatase).
Osteoporosis which often coexists.

Treatment

Vitamin D (calciferol) The dose depends upon the aetiology. The serum calcium must always be monitored. NB Calciferol 10 micrograms equals 400 units.

— in deficiency states: 1000–4000 units per day. Maintenance requirements for health in the normal individual are probably about 500 units per day, including children.

— in vitamin D resistance—see uraemia.

— in malabsorption states: 50,000–100,000 units orally daily or smaller doses intramuscularly (e.g. 300,000 units monthly).

— in post-parathyroidectomy maintenance: up to 50,000 units daily (some patients do not require any).

Calcium 1–3 grams a day. NB About 1 gram of calcium is contained in 1½ pints of milk, three tablets Sandocal, 20 tablets calcium gluconate, and 25 tablets calcium lactate.

Treat the underlying disease e.g. malabsorption or uraemia.

Uraemic bone disease

Chronic renal failure has two direct effects on calcium metabolism (figure 33), phosphate retention and vitamin D resistance.

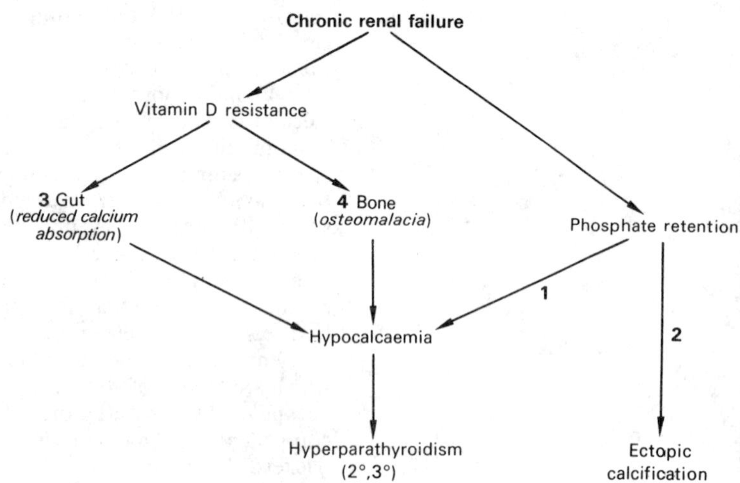

FIGURE 33 Effects of chronic renal failure on calcium metabolism.

Phosphate retention

This has two secondary effects:

1 Reciprocal depression of serum calcium level (mediated at the bone surface).

2 Rise in the calcium × phosphorus product (despite the serum calcium depression) which may lead to ectopic calcification and pseudogout.

Vitamin D resistance

This is expressed at two important sites.

3 The gut where there is reduced calcium absorption.

4 The bone to produce osteomalacia and hypocalcaemia.

The ionic hypocalcaemia produced by the

first and fourth mechanisms is a physiological stimulus to the parathyroid glands (phosphate has no direct effect on parathyroid activity) which are thus in a state of chronic hypersecretion, tending to return the serum calcium level (and phosphate level) towards normal but doing so only incompletely. This (secondary) hyperparathyroidism (page 159) may be demonstrated on bone X-rays and the serum level of parathormone is raised. The hypocalcaemia only rarely leads to tetany because of two other biochemical changes which may occur in chronic renal failure:

— acidosis reduces the protein binding of calcium and thus increases the levels of ionised calcium

— hypoproteinaemia has a similar effect

The clinical consequences of renal failure on calcium metabolism are thus:

— osteoporosis produced by hyperparathyroidism

— osteomalacia due to vitamin D resistance

— ectopic calcification

— hypocalcaemic tetany

Management

There are five chief therapeutic manoeuvres.

Calciferol (vitamin D) may be given to treat muscular weakness, bone pain and biochemical or radiological osteomalacia. The rise in serum calcium level should reduce hyperparathyroidism. The unwanted effect which needs to be monitored during therapy is increased absorption of phosphate from the gut (see above) which may lead to metastatic calcification and hypercalcaemia. It should not normally be used if the phosphate is much raised.

Oral aluminium hydroxide gel (dose 10 ml qds) reduces the absorption of phosphate from the gut and thus lowers the serum phosphate level (and the calcium × phosphorus product). Though this reduces the risk of metastatic calcification there is a risk of hypercalcaemia developing since the calcium cannot be incorporated into bone (insufficient phosphate to make the mineral).

Parathyroidectomy should reduce calcium and phosphate levels and permit vitamin D therapy without the risk of metastatic calcification but is very seldom necessary.

Chronic dialysis against a suitable calcium concentration (about 6 mg per 100 ml) in the dialysis fluid should return the calcium (and phosphate) levels towards normal.

Renal transplantation, if successful, may return renal function and calcium metabolism to normal. However, the side-effects of immunosuppressive drug therapy may influence the skeleton adversely.

NB No attempt should be made to treat the metabolic acidosis directly since the ionised calcium level will fall and may easily result in tetany. Fracture of the weakened bones may occur in the convulsion.

Vitamin D resistance

The term *vitamin D* refers to a number of related sterols. Calciferol (D_2) is a compound used therapeutically but is not important physiologically. Cholecalciferol (D_3) is the substance normally absorbed either as such in the diet (eggs and fatty fish) or converted from 7-dehydrocholesterol by ultraviolet light in the skin. This has antirachitic activity itself but is normally hydroxylated by the liver to 25-hydroxycholecalciferol (25-HCC) with some increase of potency. The kidney is responsible for a further hydroxylation to 1-25-dihydroxycholecalciferol (1-25-DHCC) which increases its potency further predominantly in increasing calcium absorption from the gut (and also to 21-25-DHCC which increases potency predominantly in effects on bone mineralisation). The production of 1-25-DHCC is increased by a low serum calcium level which thus forms a feedback mechanism for serum calcium regulation.

Vitamin D resistance thus appears to be due partly to a failure of the kidney to perform the second hydroxylation of 25-HCC. Dialysis would thus not be expected to improve calcium absorption and indeed does not (though it does improve bone mineralisation).

Paget's disease

This is characterised histologically by increased bone resorption associated with abnormal new bone formation. The early changes show large resorption cavities with increased vascularity and softened bone. The subsequent sclerotic areas are dense and disorganised (mosaic pattern). In Britain this occurs in 1% of the population at 50 years old rising to 10% by 100 years (males more than females). In only about 5–10% is the disease clinically important. It appears to have a familial incidence.

Clinical features

Bone pain and tenderness sometimes with a rise in temperature over the lesion.

Bone deformity, enlargement of the skull with headache or deformity, usually of a leg bone.

Complications:

— fracture of a long bone (immobilisation may produce hypocalcaemia and hypercalciuria)

— progressive occlusion of the foramina of the skull, e.g. deafness and basilar invagination

— about 2% develop bone sarcoma

— high output cardiac failure is rare

Investigation

Radiology Coarsening and disorganisation are characteristic and produce bones with thick trabeculae unrelated to the usual stress lines and thick cortices with an enlarged irregular outline. The sacrum and lumbar spine are most frequently affected followed by skull, pelvis, lower limbs and upper limbs. The clavicles may also be affected.

Biochemistry The alkaline phosphatase is often raised into the hundreds (King Armstrong units) and the 24-hour urinary hydroxyproline output raised from about 50 mg% in the normal up to 1 g or more. These two measurements tend to reflect the severity and extent of the disease and can be used to follow treatment. Immobilisation may produce hypercalcaemia.

Treatment

Analgesia.
Calcitonin—a polypeptide hormone from thyroid C-cells inhibits bone resorption (but bone formation continues) and may relieve pain.
Diphosphonates, fluoride and mithramycin have also been used.

Endocrine bone disease

Hyperparathyroidism

Parathyroid hormone (PTH) increases serum calcium by:
— increasing calcium absorption from the gut
— increasing mobilisation of calcium from bone
— reducing renal calcium clearance
It also increases renal phosphate clearance and this may also indirectly increase mobilisation of calcium from bone.

Primary hyperparathyroidism results from an adenoma (85%) or hyperplasia of the parathyroid glands. Very rarely a functioning carcinoma may occur. Ectopic PTH may be produced by carcinoma elsewhere, particularly of the lung and kidney. A parathyroid adenoma may be part of a polyglandular syndrome.

Secondary hyperparathyroidism is a physiological response to hypocalcaemia produced by another disease, e.g. chronic renal failure and hypovitaminosis D (dietary deficiency or malabsorption).

'*Tertiary hyperparathyroidism*' refers to the situation where chronic secondary hyperparathyroidism has resulted in an autonomous adenoma. This, as in primary hyperparathyroidism, is characterised by hypercalcaemia, though the hyperphosphataemia of renal failure may persist.

Clinical presentation

Hypercalcaemia may be found on routine screening (0·1% of the general population; higher in hospital admissions: up to 8%).
Hypercalciuria produces renal calculi, nephrocalcinosis and later renal failure (50–60%).
X-rays may reveal bone cysts, subperiosteal erosions in the phalanges and/or loss of the lamina dura of the teeth (25%).
Hypercalcaemia may produce anorexia, nausea, vomiting, thirst, polyuria, constipation, muscle fatigue and hypotonicity and calcium deposition in the conjunctiva, usually at the medial limbus of the eye (3%). Dyspepsia and peptic ulceration may occur (5%).
Psychiatric disorders (3%).

Differential diagnosis

This is from other causes of hypercalcaemia (page 161) and hypercalciuria.

Investigation

Biochemistry In primary hyperparathyroidism the serum calcium is raised and the phosphate reduced. A raised serum alkaline phosphatase indicates bone resorption. There is a high renal clearance of phosphate (measured by various indices, e.g. the Index of Phosphate Excretion) and a mild renal tubular acidosis (with a high serum chloride level). The serum calcium level is not reduced by corticosteroids (page 210). The serum PTH is raised. In the secondary hyperparathyroidism of renal failure, the serum phosphate is high and the serum calcium tends to be low (page 156).
Radiology There may be generalised osteoporosis. More specific changes include loss of the lamina dura of the teeth and small subperiosteal bone resorption cysts most marked in the middle phalanges of the hands (and feet). Osteitis fibrosa cystica is relatively rare.

Treatment

Surgical resection of the diseased parathyroid glands. It is important to visualise and probably biopsy all four parathyroid glands to determine whether they are normal or hyperplastic.

Hypoparathyroidism

Aetiology

Secondary to thyroid surgery.
Primary 'idiopathic'. This appears to be an organ-specific autoimmune disease (page 116) and is associated with an increased incidence of Addison's (hypoadrenal) disease, pernicious anaemia and malabsorption.

Clinical presentation

Tetany, convulsions, stridor and/or cramps from hypocalcaemia. Trousseau's and Chvostek's signs may be present.
Ectodermal changes: teeth, nails, skin and hair. There is an excessive incidence of cutaneous moniliasis.
Ocular changes: cataract and occasionally papilloedema.
Calcification in the basal ganglia and less commonly other soft tissues.
NB The hereditary syndrome of pseudohypoparathyroidism usually presents in childhood: the patients have a moonface, are short, mentally retarded and often have short fourth or fifth metacarpals. The biochemistry is similar to idiopathic hypoparathyroidism.
Tetany may also occur in osteomalacia, rickets, the malabsorption syndrome, alkalosis and uraemia.

Investigation

There is a low serum calcium and a high serum phosphate level with normal alkaline phosphatase. There is no common diagnostic radiological skeletal abnormality. X-ray of the skull may show calcification of the basal ganglia. If the patient is thought to have idiopathic hypoparathyroidism investigate for the associated pathologies.

Treatment *Emergency* Treat tetany with 10 ml of 10% calcium gluconate intravenously.
Intravenous magnesium chloride may also be required if there is no relief of symptoms due to hypomagnesaemia which may be associated.
Long-term therapy involves the use of calciferol and/or oral calcium supplements to raise the serum calcium towards normal (page 156).
Patients with secondary hypoparathyroidism may need only calcium.

Thyroid bone disease

Hyperthyroidism Increased bone resorption tends towards a raised serum calcium, phosphate and alkaline phosphatase. Frank hypercalcaemia, which is very rare, can develop. Osteoporosis also occurs.

Hypothyroidism There is a tendency to hypocalcaemia of little clinical significance.

Hypercalcaemia (see hyperparathyroidism, page 159) The physiologically relevant measurement is of ionised calcium but this is seldom performed. Some measure of this is obtained by determining what proportion of the serum calcium is protein-bound. There are a number of techniques for 'correcting' serum calcium levels for serum protein or albumin concentration.

Aetiology *Excess PTH* Primary and tertiary hyperparathyroidism and ectopic PTH syndromes (carcinoma).
Malignant involvement of bone Carcinoma, myeloma, reticulosis.
Excess vitamin D effect
— medication (self-administered or iatrogenic)
— increased sensitivity (sarcoidosis)
Bone diseases (all rare)
— thyrotoxicosis
— immobilised Paget's disease
— Addison's disease
— Milk-alkali syndrome

Investigation A detailed history and examination should eliminate most of the differential diagnoses listed above. Phosphate clearance studies and the hydrocortisone test (40 mg orally 8-hourly for 10 days) are not often required or diagnostically conclusive. Sarcoid, myeloma and occult carcinoma should not be overlooked. Serum PTH levels will be useful when routinely available.

Treatment *Emergency* Intravenous infusion of saline, sodium sulphate, EDTA (2 g per hour), or sodium phosphate (followed by oral phosphate).
Parenteral calcitonin (up to 4 units per kg per day).
Corticosteroids (ineffective in parathyroid disease).
Long-term Remove the cause by specific therapy.

Gout (page 26) A disease characterised by episodes of acute arthritis, at first affecting only one joint and associated with hyperuricaemia. Hyperuricaemia may occur without clinical gout.

Classification

Primary gout — An inborn error of purine metabolism which occurs in men (95%) and postmenopausal women. The hyperuricaemia is familial.

Secondary gout — This occurs at all ages in both sexes.
Ten per cent of all gout is associated with myeloproliferative disease which causes increased purine turnover and release and hence a rise in serum uric acid particularly with treatment (e.g. myeloid leukaemia, myelofibrosis, polycythaemia rubra vera). Secondary gout also occurs in multiple myeloma and in Hodgkin's disease (particularly after treatment with antimetabolite drugs when the serum uric acid and urea rise as a result of tissue destruction).
Drug-induced hyperuricaemia may follow treatment with diuretics, particularly thiazides, and salicylates and phenylbutazone in small doses.
Chronic renal failure may be associated with hyperuricaemia and rarely clinical gout, secondary to reduced renal uric acid excretion.

Clinical features

In the first acute attack, the big toe is affected in 50% of cases. The onset is usually sudden and the joint is red, hot, shiny and exquisitely tender. The patient is febrile, irritable and anorexic. Attacks tend to be recurrent and to become polyarticular. Chronic gouty arthritis remains asymmetrical and tophi appear especially on the cartilages of the ears and close to joints.

Complications

Renal disease. Uric acid stones may produce renal colic and chronic renal failure may follow hyperuricaemia.
Hypertension, obesity, coronary artery disease are more common in patients with hyperuricaemia.
Secondary pyogenic infection of gouty joints is uncommon.

Investigation

The serum uric acid is usually raised.
NB 5% of men have levels over 7 mg/100 ml but only 0·3% have clinical gout.
Leucocytosis is common and the ESR is raised.
Radiology: soft tissue swelling may be the only abnormality in acute gout. Chronic disease produces irregular punched-out bony erosions near but not usually involving the articular margins. Tophi may be seen if calcified. Osteoarthritic changes are common in gouty joints. Uric acid renal stones are radiolucent.
Aspirates of joint fluid contain negatively refractile crystals of monosodium urate seen under polarised light.

Differential diagnosis

Acute gout must be distinguished from other causes of acute arthritis, particularly septic arthritis and rheumatic fever. Pseudogout may occur in chronic renal failure.
Chronic gout, particularly if widespread, may resemble rheumatoid or osteoarthritis.
Hyperuricaemia may be secondary to chronic diuretic therapy.

Management

Acute episodes

Phenylbutazone (Butazolidine) 200 mg 6-hourly for 1 day, reducing to 200–300 mg daily. Hydrocortisone, 100 mg i.v. repeated as required, may be given instead and may relieve pain almost instantaneously without side-effects. Colchicine (0·5 mg 2-hourly until pain is relieved or vomiting and diarrhoea begin) may be given if phenylbutazone is contraindicated. Allopurinol may be started as soon as pain is relieved.

Chronic recurrent gout and hyperuricaemia

Probenecid, 0·5 g two or three times a day, acts by increasing renal clearance of uric acid and urates.

Allopurinol, 100 mg tds, is of particular value in the treatment of chronic tophaceous gout or chronic hyperuricaemia and when renal disease is present. It blocks the metabolic pathway at xanthine and hypoxanthine (by inhibiting xanthine oxidase), both of which are more soluble than uric acid and less liable to form stones.

Both drugs may precipitate an acute attack and 5–6 days cover with phenylbutazone, colchicine or prednisone may be advisable.

Pseudo-gout (articular chondrocalcinosis or calcium pyrophosphate gout)

This is rare and usually familial. It may occur in chronic renal failure. Chondrocalcinosis is frequently found by chance on X-ray and may be symptom-free. However, there may be episodic pain and effusions into large joints and it may thus mimic gout though the big toe is seldom affected. The effusions contain calcium pyrophosphate crystals which are positively refractile. The disease is associated with radiological calcification of the joint capsule and cartilage. The cartilages of the knee are characteristically outlined by calcium but calcification may occur in any cartilaginous joint. The patient may develop osteoarthritis secondary to the destruction of joint cartilage. Phenylbutazone may be needed in acute episodes.

Renal disease

The commonest disease especially in females is urinary tract infection, and in males prostatic hypertrophy and its consequences.

Proteinuria

Proteinuria results from urinary tract infection or leakage of protein from the glomeruli or tubules. Tubular proteinuria is very rare (Fanconi syndrome, heavy metal poisoning, recovery phase of acute tubular necrosis) and is usually of globulins. In glomerular proteinuria, the smaller molecules, e.g. albumin, usually pass through in greater quantities than the larger molecules, e.g. globulins. Bence-Jones proteins are very small in comparison (they are light-chain dimers) and pass through a normal glomerulus. Proteinuria of less than 150 mg/24 hours (100 ng/l) may occur from normal kidneys.

Aetiology

Acute and chronic pyelonephritis, acute and chronic glomerulonephritis, obstructive nephropathy, congestive cardiac failure, postural proteinuria, myelomatosis and the causes of nephrotic syndrome (page 165) and analgesic abuse.

Clinical presentation

Patients may have obvious urinary tract infection, symptomless proteinuria or the nephrotic syndrome.

Assessment

The history should include enquiry about previous urinary tract infection, sore throats, skin infections, renal disease, toxaemia in pregnancy, drug, occupational and family history.

Examination may be normal but there may be evidence of uraemia, nephrotic syndrome, heart failure, or hypertension.

The kidneys are large and palpable in polycystic disease. Postural proteinuria, absent after lying down, may be present in young patients (up to 30 years) on standing. Early morning specimens should be normal. About 30% of these patients have persistent proteinuria 10 years later and full investigation or long-term follow-up may be indicated.

Investigation

MSU for microscopic haematuria (page 166), urinary tract infection, urinary sugar, and Bence-Jones protein.

24-hour urine collection for protein content, creatinine clearance and differential protein clearance if nephrotic.

Blood urea and electrolytes. Serum proteins for nephrotic syndrome and protein strip for myeloma.

Blood sugar and glucose tolerance test for diabetes, if indicated.

Straight X-ray of abdomen for renal size ($13 \pm 2{\cdot}5$ cm: kidneys are normally the same length as the adjacent 2½–3 vertebrae) and stones, proceeding to IVP or infusion pyelogram (with blood ureas above 80–100 mg/100 ml) to assess structural abnormalities. IVP is dangerous in myeloma and renal failure unless the patient is kept well hydrated.

If the diagnosis remains obscure and the proteinuria persists, proceed to renal biopsy. This allows early detection of treatable disorders such as 'minimal change' glomerulonephritis, infective endocarditis, polyarteritis nodosa and pyelonephritis.

Other investigations not routinely required include:
— serum calcium, phosphate and alkaline phosphatase
— ASO titre, serum complement
— bone X-rays for 1° and 2° hyperparathyroidism and myeloma
— renal arteriography is of value in the differentiation of benign from malignant lesions
— isotope renography

Nephrotic syndrome

This may be regarded as a severe proteinuria but is usually considered separately because it is the presenting syndrome of a different range of renal disease.

The nephrotic syndrome is defined as:
— severe proteinuria (over 5 g/24 hours), with
— hypoalbuminaemia (less than 2 g/100 ml), and
— peripheral oedema

Hypercholesterolaemia is commonly present.

Aetiology

Up to 80% of cases are associated with the histological changes of glomerulonephritis (page 171). Other causes include diabetes mellitus, amyloidosis, systemic lupus erythematosus, myelomatosis, drug therapy (gold, pencillamine, mercury, troxidone). Renal vein thrombosis is associated with it.

Management

Treat the underlying cause.

In glomerulonephritis, renal histology and the selectivity of the proteinuria give a guide to the use of steroids and immunosuppression. Ninety per cent of children with 'minimal change lesions' respond initially to a short steroid course with complete remission, but half relapse. Cyclophosphamide therapy has been used in children. It is more dangerous but has a lower relapse rate. Spontaneous remission is common in adult nephrotics with 'minimal change' lesions on histology. 'Proliferative' and 'membranous' glomerulonephritic changes are usually unresponsive to steroids, cyclophosphamide or azathioprine, but exceptions have been described.

General management is aimed at:
— increasing oral protein intake to compensate for the renal loss—but urea levels must be carefully monitored
— reducing oedema with a low salt diet and diure-

ties and possibly salt-free albumin and intravenous diuretics in resistant cases
— treatment of intercurrent infection

Haematuria

Haematuria must always be considered abnormal and fully investigated.

Aetiology

Renal tract stones
Tumours of the bladder, kidneys and prostate
Renal tract infection including tuberculosis (tuberculosis characteristically produces 'sterile' pyuria)
Renal trauma and infarction
Acute glomerulonephritis
Malignant hypertension
Polyarteritis nodosa, lupus erythematosus, Henoch-Schönlein purpura, and infective endocarditis
Haemorrhagic disease, usually caused by anticoagulant drugs
Polycystic disease

Investigation

MSU for infection (including tuberculosis). Examine the deposit for casts, cells and microliths. The presence of red cells distinguishes haematuria from haemoglobinuria and also from other causes of red-coloured urine and drugs (phenolphthalein, phenindione and senna derivatives), food (beetroot and red sweets) and porphyria.
Plasma urea and electrolytes.
Straight X-ray of abdomen to assess renal size proceeding to IVP as in proteinuria.
Cystoscopy (early) and retrograde pyelography for tumours and structural abnormalities.
Renal biopsy may be required to provide histological diagnosis.
Renal arteriography may be of value in differentiating renal carcinoma (95% have an abnormal vascular supply) from benign avascular cysts.

MSU

NB Normal urine (centrifuged deposit) contains:

RBC 1×10^6 cells/24 hours (2 per high power field)
WBC 2×10^6 cells/24 hours (4 per high power field)
Casts $5–10 \times 10^3$/24 hours (1 per 20 high power field)

Hyaline casts arise from the tubules and may not be significant. Granular casts are composed of protein leaked from tubules in which RBCs and WBCs from glomerular leakage adhere. They are virtually always significant.

Acute renal failure
(acute uraemia)
(page 37)

Definition

Urine output of less than 400 ml/24 hours (the normal urine production is approximately 1 ml/min, i.e. 1·5 l/24 hours).
NB Non-oliguric renal failure can occur.

Aetiology

Pre-renal uraemia

Following severe hypotension from:
— hypovolaemia (road traffic accidents, burns,

postpartum haemorrhage, blood loss at operation, severe diarrhoea, vomiting or polyuria with salt-losing kidneys)
— myocardial infarction and shock
— septicaemic shock
— drug overdosage
If hypotension is severe and prolonged, acute tubular necrosis may follow.

Post-renal uraemia

Acute urinary tract obstruction from:
— prostatic hypertrophy
— renal and ureteric stones
— pelvic carcinoma
— retroperitoneal tumours and fibrosis

Intrinsic renal parenchymal disease (renal uraemia)

This includes acute glomerulonephritis, eclampsia, acute tubular necrosis, poisoning with heavy metals or barbiturates, papillary necrosis, malignant hypertension, polyarteritis nodosa, septicaemia and diffuse intravascular coagulation (DIC), including the haemolytic-uraemic syndrome, prolonged hypotension and severe acute hypercalcaemia.

NB Acute renal failure may complicate chronic renal parenchymal disease.

Assessment

Rapid correction of hypovolaemia with blood or plasma after haemorrhage or saline may prevent renal failure. Measurement of central venous pressure will confirm the diagnosis and monitor replacement of fluids.

Where there is no obvious cause for oliguria and uraemia it becomes necessary to:
— ensure that hypovolaemia if present is corrected
— check there is no obstruction to the urinary tract
— assess the presence of previous intrinsic renal disease (suggested by hypertension, metabolic acidosis, a normochromic normocytic anaemia and small renal shadows)

Clinical history and examination

A full history is taken with particular attention to previous renal disease, infection, stones, prostatism and abdominal operations. There may have been previous hypertension or a history of analgesic abuse.

Examination includes an assessment of the state of hydration. In hypovolaemia, postural hypotension, rapid small-volume pulse, cold extremities, reduced tissue turgor and thirst may be present. Rectal examination is obligatory to exclude prostatic disease in men and pelvic carcinoma in women—vaginal examination may be necessary.

Investigation

Urine

Oliguria following hypovolaemia and before the onset of tubular necrosis is indicated by the absence of casts, specific gravity above 1015 (sugar will increase the specific gravity) and urea concentration above 2 g/100 ml.

In intrinsic renal disease (including acute tubular necrosis) casts are present, the tubules are unable to concentrate the glomerular filtrate producing a specific gravity of 1010 and urea concentration of usually less than 600 mg/100 ml.

Blood Serum urea, creatinine and electrolytes are estimated as a baseline to measure the degree of uraemia, hyperkalaemia and acidosis. In hypovolaemia (in the absence of tubular necrosis) the ratio of urine to blood urea concentration is above 10. Estimation of Hb, Ca and P may give a clue to pre-existing renal failure.

Urine flow It is almost invariably necessary to catheterise the bladder if anuria is present in the absence of known previous intrinsic renal disease, despite the risk of introducing infection. This may be the only way to ensure that the bladder is not full (i.e. there is no obstruction distal to the bladder), of obtaining a urine sample and of accurately estimating urine flow. A persistent urine flow of 0·3–0·5 ml/min or less after correction of hypovolaemia may indicate the onset of tubular necrosis.

Radiology A plain X-ray of the urinary tract may demonstrate small kidneys (normal $13 \pm 2{\cdot}5$ cm) if pre-existent renal disease was present. It may demonstrate renal and ureteric stones. If renal outflow obstruction is suspected—usually on the basis of total anuria and/or a history of ureteric colic—isotope renography and infusion pyelography may confirm the diagnosis, and indicate that both kidneys are functioning. It may be necessary to proceed to cystoscopy with ureteric catheterisation.

Management

Hypovolaemia Replacement of circulating volume with blood or saline as indicated may be sufficient to prevent tubular necrosis. Replacement is most easily monitored with a central venous pressure catheter. After adequate hydration mannitol (50 ml of 25% mannitol intravenously) or frusemide (200 mg increasing to 1–2 g i.v.) may reverse the onset phase of acute tubular necrosis.

Acute tubular necrosis *Non-protein high carbohydrate diet* (e.g. Hycal 2000–2500 cal/24 hours) for 1–2 days.

Fluid replacement Give as water or glucose solution orally 500 ml (insensible loss) plus volume of urine output from previous 24 hours (ml for ml). Ice cubes (from 24 h allowance) or lemon slices relieve a dry mouth.

Assess the following daily

— weight to assess fluid retention—on the above regime patients should lose 0–0·5 kg per day

— clinical degree of hydration (thirst, tissue turgor, oedema and blood pressure)

— serum urea and electrolytes, and creatinine

and 24-hour urinary excretion of sodium and potassium

Electrolytes No electrolytes should be given in the first 24 hours. After that, if hydration is normal, replace the previous 24-hour urinary sodium loss. Potassium is usually raised in acute tubular necrosis and tends to rise. ECG changes of 'tenting' of the T wave may be the first indication of serious hyperkalaemia. This may be reduced by glucose/insulin or oral calcium-resonium resin (page 177).

Recovery is indicated by the onset of a variable degree of polyuria, usually after 1–2 weeks. There may be marked loss of water and electrolytes and these must be replaced, ml for ml, and mEq for mEq.

Indications for dialysis

Deteriorating clinical state with mental dullness, confusion and hiccough.

Blood urea above 300 mg/100 ml and rising. In anuria the urea rises by about 30 mg/100 ml/day. A rise of over 50 mg/100 ml/day occurs in hypercatabolic states and indicates early dialysis.

Serum potassium above 6–7 mEq/l.

Bicarbonate below 10–15 mEq/l.

Progressive weight gain of fluid retention.

The rates of change are more important than the absolute levels—the above levels are intended as guides and are not absolute (see page 171).

Chronic renal failure (chronic uraemia)

This clinical syndrome is common to the later stages of all chronic and insidious renal disease and is characterised by uraemia. The urine specific gravity eventually becomes fixed at 1010 (the specific gravity of filtered plasma) when the nephron number becomes too small effectively to alter glomerular filtrate.

Aetiology

Chronic urinary tract obstruction (commonly prostatic hypertrophy)
Chronic glomerulonephritis
Analgesic abuse (phenacetin and possibly aspirin)
Diabetic nephropathy
Hypertensive nephropathy
Polycystic disease
The collagen diseases
Hypercalcaemia and hyperuricaemia
Retroperitoneal fibrosis
Persisting acute renal failure
Chronic urinary tract infection—pyelonephritis, tuberculosis

Clinical presentation

The history is usually of lethargy, polyuria and nocturia, and general ill health. In later stages of the disease, symptoms of uraemia with anorexia, nausea, vomiting, hiccough, weight loss, bruising and epistaxis are common. There may be a history of prostatic obstruction, recurrent dysuria sometimes with episodic fever and loin pain, or a known story of acute glomerulonephritis or chronic analgesic abuse. Polycystic disease is familial (autosomal dominant).

Examination

In the early stages there may be no abnormal clinical signs but anaemia is common. Urinary tract obstruction secondary to prostatic hypertrophy must be excluded. In later stages of uraemia the patient shows varying degrees of mental confusion. A pericardial rub is characteristic and a neuropathy not uncommon. There is a characteristic 'dirty' yellow pallor of the skin, bruising is common and hyperventilation of metabolic acidosis occurs. Secondary infection is common. The kidneys are large in polycystic disease.

Rectal examination is obligatory in both sexes.

Investigation

MSU may reveal bacterial infection and granular casts.

Blood urea and electrolyte concentrations and creatinine clearance will indicate the degree of renal dysfunction and acidosis. The rise in urea may partly reflect the degree of dehydration. The serum calcium may fall secondary to renal phosphate retention or acquired vitamin D resistance (page 156).

Plain X-ray of the abdomen should define kidney size and IVP outline the renal tract to exclude obstructive lesions. Infusion pyelography may be required if the urea is above 80 mg/100 ml. Isotope renography may indicate obstruction to outflow. Proceed to cystoscopy and retrograde pyelography if necessary.

Renal biopsy is occasionally useful. Investigate for relevant systemic disease.

Management

Exclude or treat pre-renal disorders (e.g. sodium or water depletion) and post-renal obstruction.

Treat infection, both renal and intercurrent, which itself induces a hypercatabolic state and hence a rapid rise in blood urea.

Treat hypertension as in patients with essential hypertension. Control may improve or prevent deterioration in renal function. Reduction in dietary sodium may be effective alone. Be aware of altered drug handling in renal failure.

Dietary control The main purpose of protein restriction is to produce a fall in the blood urea and thus reduce the symptoms of uraemia, in particular anorexia, nausea and vomiting. The protein need not be reduced more than is necessary to relieve symptoms, usually achieved at blood urea levels of about 100–150 mg/100 ml. Normal diet contains about 85 g protein per day. In conservative management of chronic renal failure a 40 g protein diet is usually adequate. In severe uraemia the intake may be reduced to 20 g protein. A high calorie intake is essential to suppress breakdown of body protein, i.e. 2000–3000 cal per day as carbohydrate (Caloreen or Hycal). Vitamin supplements, particularly B and C, may be required.

Water and electrolyte control This is aimed at achieving as high a urine output as possible to eliminate urea and other toxic metabolites, without inducing heart failure. This may be achieved with oral fluids alone (up to 2·5–3·0 litres per 24 hours) or by the addition of frusemide 0·5–1·5 g daily, which may also increase the GFR. The 24-hour urinary sodium loss must be measured and replaced if excessive. Hypertension and fluid retention would suggest a reduction in sodium intake. Hyperkalaemia is treated by dietary restriction, followed, if necessary, by ion-exchange resins in the calcium phase (calcium resonium 45 g daily in divided doses). The acidosis is best not corrected as this results in further reduction of ionised calcium which may result in tetany and fractures.

Vitamin D supplements may be required if uraemic bone disease occurs with symptoms of osteomalacia (weakness and bone pain). Dietary phosphate restriction with or without aluminium hydroxide may reduce serum phosphate levels (page 157) and prevent ectopic calcification.

Anaemia tends to be unresponsive to iron or vitamins (except when on dialysis), but serum iron, B_{12} and folate should be checked.

Antibiotics Tetracyclines and nitrofurantoin are contraindicated in renal failure, and cephaloridine best avoided. Gentamicin and kanamycin are given in reduced doses or less frequently in renal failure and serum levels should be monitored. Ampicillin and lincomycin are relatively safe. Antibiotic therapy in renal infection is best withheld until urine culture and sensitivities are available.

Consider the suitability of intermittent chronic haemodialysis or transplantation.

Indications for dialysis

Severe renal failure (creatinine clearance less than 3–4 ml/min) is most easily managed by dialysis. It seems reasonable to dialyse every new patient with rapidly progressive uraemia of undiagnosed aetiology, to allow time for full assessment including renal biopsy, particularly in the presence of normal sized kidneys which indicate recent renal disease (infective endocarditis, polyarteritis nodosa, renal vein thrombosis. malignant hypertension, amyloid). Peritoneal dialysis tends to be used in these holding situations.

Indications for long-term dialysis (haemodialysis or, less commonly, peritoneal dialysis) and renal transplantation vary from place to place and time to time. Considerations taken into account are: age, marital status, home circumstances, 'emotional stability', the presence of lower urinary tract disease or of generalised chronic disease (e.g. diabetes mellitus, collagen diseases), availability of kidneys or dialysis time and Australia antigen status. Every reasonable case should be referred, preferably early in their chronic downhill course, for assessment by the regional dialysis centre.

Glomerulonephritis

This describes a bilateral disease of the kidneys, predominantly affecting the glomeruli. Clinically, patients present either with acute nephritis (the acute nephritic syndrome) or proteinuria (including the nephrotic syndrome) with or without varying degrees of renal failure.

Acute nephritis (acute glomerulonephritis)

Clinical presentation There is an abrupt onset of haematuria and oliguria. This is rapidly followed by oedema (classically ankle and periorbital), hypertension and varying degrees of uraemia.

Aetiology The majority occur in childhood and follow 10–15 days after a haemolytic streptococcal (group A, type 12) infection of the throat—antigen-antibody complexes have been demonstrated in the glomerular tufts. (The clinical picture of acute nephritis may also occur in other types of glomerulonephritis, Henoch-Schönlein purpura, polyarteritis nodosa, SLE and Goodpasture's syndrome.)

Investigation Streptococci may be isolated from the throat if penicillin has not already been given. A rising ASO titre may be demonstrable and serum complement reduced.

Management As for acute renal failure. Daily weighing and estimation of serum electrolytes are essential. In the large majority severe renal failure does not occur and uraemia is transitory. Penicillin should be given to eliminate the streptococci. Hypertension may be severe and require treatment in the usual way (page 243).

Prognosis Over 90% of children and 60–70% of adults recover fully. With advances in dialysis technique and management of hypertensive encephalopathy, death in the acute phase is uncommon. Insidious renal failure develops in a small number of cases.

Proteinuria/renal failure complex

Clinical presentation Patients present with proteinuria, often discovered at routine medical examination, or as the nephrotic syndrome.

Histological findings Three histological patterns are found:

Minimal change Light microscopy is normal but electron microscopy (EM) reveals fusion of the epithelial cell foot processes. 'Minimal change glomerulonephritis' is associated with selective proteinuria (e.g. ratio of IgG to transferrin). It accounts for 80% of cases of childhood nephrotic syndrome and up to one-third of adult nephrotics.
Proliferative Infiltration of the glomerular tuft with inflammatory cells with proliferation of the endo-

thelial cells. This is a heterogeneous group ranging from slight light microscopic abnormality difficult to distinguish from 'minimal change', to widespread crescent formation with necrosis of the glomerular tuft. Prognosis is as variable as the histology.

Membranous There is thickening of the glomerular wall with deposition of antigen-antibody complexes, on the epithelial side visible on electron microscopy. Electron microscopy shows thickening of the basement membrane. Membranous glomerulonephritis is very rare in childhood and accounts for one-third of adult nephrotics. It is associated with malignancy, e.g. lymphoma. Prognosis is poor and death occurs from progressive uraemia.

Management

Renal failure (page 170) and nephrotic syndrome (page 165) should be managed as above. It may be necessary to restrict protein intake even in the presence of the nephrotic syndrome because of progressive renal failure. Steroids and immunosuppressives are valuable in patients with 'minimal change lesions' (page 165) especially children.

Pyelonephritis

Acute pyelonephritis

The diagnosis is usually made on the history of dysuria, frequency, loin tenderness and fever, often with rigors and vomiting. It is rare in men in the absence of structural abnormalities. The diagnosis is confirmed by a urinary excretion of more than 100,000 organisms/ml (counts of less than 10,000/ml are usually due to contamination). Infection may be symptom-free.

E. coli is the most frequent organism (70–80% of cases). Other organisms (proteus, staphylococcus, streptococcus, klebsiella and pseudomonas) are usually associated with structural abnormality and reinfection, or previous catheterisation. Tuberculosis classically causes a 'sterile' pyuria.

Urinary white cell counts remain of uncertain value in diagnosis as the normal values are ill-defined. Non-inflammatory disorders may provoke their excretion, and the absence of white cells may still be associated with bacteriuria and clinically significant urinary tract infection.

Management

There may be an obvious predisposing cause, e.g. pregnancy, urinary obstruction or catheterisation. Diabetes mellitus must be excluded. More than two episodes in a woman, or a single episode in a man, suggests a structural abnormality of the renal tract and merits full investigation including IVP, a micturating cystogram for reflux, and possibly cystoscopy with retrograde pyelography.

The organism should be cultured for antibiotic sensitivities before treatment is started.

Co-trimoxazole (Septrin) is probably the drug

of first choice unless the patient is pregnant. Ampicillin can be used. After a 10-day course, cultures should be repeated at intervals (e.g. 6 months and 1 year). Recurrent infection which may be asymptomatic, occurs in 20–40% of cases, and usually with the same organism. The best treatment for chronic and recurrent infection remains uncertain. It seems reasonable to treat single recurrent episodes as new infections with short courses of antimicrobial drugs. Frequent attacks (symptomatic or asymptomatic) are sometimes prevented or reduced by continuous low-dose chemotherapy, usually taken at night (e.g. nitrofurantoin 100 mg or nalidixic acid 500 mg nightly).

Chronic infection (where the urinary excretion of organism remains above 100,000/ml) may require continued cyclical therapy (e.g. co-trimoxazole ii bd, ampicillin 250 mg qds and nitrofurantoin 100–200 mg daily for 10 days each continuously) but the organism must be carefully monitored throughout therapy and drugs chosen appropriately.

Surgical correction of structural abnormalities should always be considered in recurrent and chronic infection.

Chronic pyelonephritis

Clinical presentation

Patients present usually with insidious renal failure, hypertension or proteinuria.

There may or may not be clinical or bacteriological evidence of urinary tract infection. The diagnosis is made on IVP findings of small, scarred kidneys often with cortical thinning overlying calyceal 'clubbing'. If renal biopsy is performed the kidney shows patchy areas of cellular infiltration with plasma cells and lymphocytes between the tubules, which are atrophic or ballooned. There is periglomerular fibrosis. Some glomeruli are normal and others hyalinised.

Aetiology

The clinical, radiological and histological features of 'chronic pyelonephritis' are not necessarily the result of infection, acute or chronic. They may also be given by glomerulonephritis, diabetes and hypertension. Hence the term 'chronic pyelonephritis' with an implied infective aetiology is confusing. The term 'chronic interstitial nephritis' is sometimes used instead, and allows the inclusion of other conditions in which interstitial round cell infiltration is a principal reaction. These include obstructive uropathy, phenacetin poisoning, hypokalaemia, hypercalcaemia and amyloidosis.

The role of recurrent urinary tract infection remains uncertain. Many cases of 'chronic pyelonephritis' are certainly associated with a history of recurrent childhood infection and many adults with this syndrome excrete a significant number of bacteria. However, recurrent urinary infection beginning in adulthood does not seem to produce this syndrome. Moreover, the sex ratio is approximately equal unlike acute urinary tract infection.

Management

Urinary tract infection, if present, must be treated. Structural abnormalities are a feature of such cases. They are often congenital but other common conditions (e.g. prostatic hypertrophy, tumours and stones) must be considered.

Chronic renal failure is managed as described (page 170).

Hepatorenal syndrome

Acute renal failure may occur following surgery to the lower end of the bile duct for relief of long-standing obstructive jaundice. The causes remain uncertain but the renal failure might be preventable by maintaining mannitol diuresis from before and throughout surgery.

Haemolytic uraemic syndrome (diffuse intravascular coagulation)

A disease of children of unknown aetiology often following viral infections of the gastrointestinal or respiratory tracts. Renal failure is caused by intravascular blood-clotting in small renal arterioles. Fibrin degradation products are detectable in the blood and haemolysis and thrombocytopenia also occur. Anticoagulation with heparin is the treatment of choice. A similar, often fatal, disease occurs in adults (thrombotic thrombocytopenic purpura).

Fluids and electrolytes

60% of total body weight is water.
30% of total body weight is 'bicarbonate space'.
15% of total body weight is 'sodium space'.

These values are empirically useful in correcting deficiencies and approximate to 'spaces' determined isotopically.

Minimum daily replacement values in the normal adult:

2·5–3·0 litres water per day
80 mEq sodium (0·5 litres normal saline)
80 mEq potassium (6 g potassium chloride)

These are minimum requirements and most patients with normal kidneys are able to maintain sodium and potassium balance with higher intakes. The above schedule forms the basis of postoperative fluid replacement.

Sodium deficiency

In Britain this usually results from:
— chronic renal failure with renal sodium loss
— following relief of urinary obstruction (post-prostatectomy)
— vomiting and diarrhoea (usually pyloric stenosis)
— diuretic therapy for cardiac failure
Sodium replacement is required in all except the last.

Clinical presentation

It should be suspected following prostatectomy. Mental confusion, thirst and dry tongue are common, and tissue turgor is reduced. Oliguria is not universally present, particularly when sodium deficit follows the polyuria of chronic renal failure. In severe salt depletion hypotension and shock occur.

Investigation

Weight is usually reduced. Blood pressure tends to fall and there is a marked postural drop. Blood urea, haemoglobin and packed cell volume tend to rise. (The central venous pressure, if measured, is reduced.) Serum sodium and chloride tend to be low.

Management

If the patient is properly hydrated calculate sodium deficit (total deficit is the measured serum sodium below normal ×15% body weight in kg) and replace as Slow-sodium tabs (10 mEq/tablet) orally, or intravenously (3% saline contains 500 mEq/l; 5% contains 850 mEq/l). (It is usually nauseating orally.) In the elderly and ill it is valuable to monitor saline infusion with a central venous pressure line to prevent overtransfusion. With continuous salt loss, daily weighing gives an approximate estimate of salt loss but these are more accurately estimated by collection of urine (and faeces or vomit if necessary). Potassium loss is not necessarily associated with body sodium loss from chronic renal disease, but is invariable in losses from the gastrointestinal tract.

NB The serum sodium concentration does not necessarily give an accurate indication of total body sodium since it tends to move with water.

Metabolic acidosis

This commonly occurs in:
— cardiac arrest
— diabetic ketoacidosis
— salicylate poisoning
— renal failure

Management

Calculate bicarbonate deficit (total deficit is the measured serum bicarbonate below normal standard bicarbonate ×30% body weight in kg) and replace as 8·4% sodium bicarbonate solution (contains 1 mEq/ml). This should be rapid (give 50–100 mEq) following cardiac arrest as cardiac arrhythmias are difficult to revert in the presence of acidosis. The value of correcting acidosis in diabetic ketosis, renal failure and salicylate poisoning remains doubtful and total rapid correction is seldom indicated.

Hypokalaemia

Aetiology

This arises from:
— diuretic therapy
— vomiting and pyloric stenosis
— diarrhoea
— recovery from diabetic ketoacidosis and renal tubular necrosis
— gastrointestinal fistulae
— Cushing's disease

The clinical symptoms are of weakness and lethargy. The ECG shows flat T and prominent U waves.

Management

Treat the underlying cause.
Give oral potassium supplements as Slow-K (8 mEq/tablet).

In diabetic ketoacidosis potassium is given intravenously: 2 g (26 mEq) per litre of intravenous fluid are usually sufficient to maintain balance through the osmotic diuresis in young patients with healthy kidneys. In the elderly or in the presence of renal disease careful monitoring by ECG and serial serum levels are necessary.

NB The serum potassium concentration does not necessarily give an accurate indication of total body potassium, being mainly an intracellular ion.

Hyperkalaemia

Aetiology

This is the result of:

— renal failure

— excess potassium intake, e.g. Slow-K with potassium retaining diuretics (spironolactone, amiloride, triamterene)

— acidosis

— Addison's disease—very rare

Management

Stop oral or intravenous intake.

Ion exchange resins and dialysis (see page 170).

In emergency states: i.v. calcium 10 ml 10% calcium gluconate (this may be fatal in digitalised patients) or insulin in dextrose, e.g. 100 ml of 50% dextrose with 20 units soluble insulin (1 unit to 2·5 g dextrose) followed if necessary by 20% dextrose containing 1 unit soluble insulin per 2 g dextrose (i.e. 100 units per litre) given at the rate of 2 ml/kg over 1 hour.

The following values may be found useful:

Sodium (*mEq = mmol*)			*Na^+ mmol*
Sodium chloride	:	1 g has	17·1
Sodium bicarbonate	:	1 g has	11·9
Sodium lactate	:	1 g has	8·9

BNF Preparations

Normal saline (sodium chloride injection) 0·9%	1 l has	150
Dextrose/saline (1/5 N saline)	1 l has	30
Sodium bicarbonate injection 1·4%	1 l has	167
8·4%	1 l has	1000
Sodium lactate (M/6) injection 1·84%	1 l has	167
Sandocal tablets	1 has	6·0
Slow-sodium tablets	1 has	10·0
Phosphate-Sandoz tablets	1 has	20·9

Potassium (*mEq = mmol*)			*K^+ mmol*
Potassium chloride	:	1 g has	13·4
Potassium citrate	:	1 g has	9·2
Potassium bicarbonate	:	1 g has	10·0

BNF Preparations

Potassium chloride slow tablets (Slow K, Leo K)	1 has	8·1
Potassium chloride effervescent tablets (Sando-K)	1 has	12 K^+ (8 Cl^-)
Potassium citrate mixture	10 ml have	27·6
Effervescent potassium tablets	1 has	6·5
Sandocal tablets	1 has	4·5

N.B. A millimole is the molecular weight of an ion in milligrams

Liver disease

The commonest disease is acute viral hepatitis. Drug jaundice and bilary tract obstruction are fairly common.

Hepatitis
(pages 33–37)

This refers to inflammation of the liver with little or no fibrosis and little or no nodular regeneration. There may be minor distortion of lobular architecture. If there is extensive fibrosis with nodular regeneration (and hence distortion of architecture) the condition is called cirrhosis. These diagnoses are made histologically and there may or may not be clinical evidence of previous hepatic disease.

Acute inflammation with necrosis of liver cells results from:

— infection, most commonly acute infectious and serum hepatitis, but also with the viruses of yellow fever and glandular fever, and associated with septicaemia and leptospirosis. Amoebic hepatitis is common on a world basis and usually presents as a hepatic abscess or amoeboma.

— chemical poisons and drugs are less frequent causes of acute hepatitis. Toxic chemicals include carbon tetrachloride and ethylene glycol. Toxic drugs include halothane, gold, PAS, isoniazid and rifampicin, phenylbutazone, phenacetin, paracetamol, and the monoamine oxidase inhibitors.

If the patient recovers this is usually complete, but progressive necrosis may affect almost the entire liver (acute massive necrosis) causing hepatic coma and death.

Acute viral hepatitis

By clinical criteria acute viral hepatitis can be divided into two groups:

— infectious hepatitis (IH, short incubation hepatitis, virus A hepatitis)

— serum hepatitis (SH, long incubation hepatitis, virus B hepatitis)

'Australia antigen' consists of morphologically identifiable particles visible under the electron microscope. This 'antigen' is present during acute episodes of serum hepatitis and (usually) disappears as the hepatitis resolves. It does not occur in infectious hepatitis. It may or may not contain the 'virus' of serum hepatitis—this remains unknown. This antigen is also called hepatitis associated antigen (HAA) and is present in the blood of 0·1% of healthy people in Britain. All blood for transfusion is screened usually by immunoelectrophoresis.

Infectious hepatitis

The aetiology of this disease is almost certainly viral. The disease is endemic but small epidemics may occur in schools or institutions. Spread is usually via the faecal-oral route. The young (5–14 years) are chiefly involved.

Clinical presentation After a variable incubation period of 2–6 weeks there is a gradual onset of an influenza-like illness with fever, malaise, anorexia, nausea, vomiting and upper abdominal discomfort associated with tender enlargement of the liver and, less commonly, the spleen. There may be a distaste for cigarettes. After 3–4 days the urine becomes characteristically dark and the stools pale—evidence of cholestasis. Symptoms usually become less severe as jaundice appears although pruritus may develop. Jaundice and symptoms tend to improve after 1–2 weeks and recovery is usually complete although mild symptoms may continue for up to 3–4 months in a few patients. Recurrent hepatitis is extremely rare and immunity probably lifelong.

Differential diagnosis
Obstructive jaundice, either in the early cholestatic phase or in the rare cases where cholestatic jaundice persists after other clinical and biochemical evidence of liver cell damage have settled. It is dangerous to diagnose infective hepatitis in patients over 40 years old—a safeguard against misdiagnosing major bile duct obstruction.
Drug jaundice (page 185).
Glandular fever.
Acute alcoholic hepatitis may present with enlargement and tenderness of the liver and sometimes obstructive jaundice. There are usually other signs of alcoholism.

Management If hospitalised the patient should be isolated. The true period of infectivity is unknown but is probably about 1–2 weeks after the appearance of jaundice. Symptomatic treatment only is required in the active disease state. Most physicians would maintain bed rest until jaundice has disappeared and only moderate exertion whilst the serum transaminase levels remain elevated. No food restriction is necessary but alcohol should be avoided for at least 1 year. Liver function tests (page 35) usually return completely to normal in 1–3 months.

Recovery is the rule in virtually every case. Occasionally jaundice may be prolonged by intrahepatic cholestasis and corticosteroids are sometimes used to reduce the jaundice rapidly particularly if it is associated with pruritus. In a small number of patients (5–10%) a mild relapse occurs sometimes after the jaundice has disappeared. Acute massive necrosis is an extremely rare complication but invariably fatal.

Prophylaxis Immune γ-globulin (500–750 mg in adults) protects contacts of infectious hepatitis. It is given to travellers entering endemic areas but the period of effectiveness remains uncertain—probably about 3–4 months.

Serum hepatitis

This is spread by infected blood or serum. It is most frequently seen in heroin addicts who use contaminated syringes, and patients and staff in renal dialysis units. Most blood transfusion units now screen all donor blood for the presence of Australia antigen. Recent work has shown that the disease can also be transmitted by ingestion, although this must be very uncommon.

Clinical presentation After a long incubation period of 6 weeks to 6 months, there is a gradual onset of lethargy, anorexia, abdominal discomfort, jaundice, and hepatomegaly.

Management and prognosis While in hospital patients should be isolated, barrier nursed, and all excreta disinfected. Blood samples should be taken wearing gloves, transported in plastic bags and the laboratory informed of the suspected diagnosis.

In uncomplicated cases treatment is symptomatic as for infectious hepatitis. Complications include acute necrosis and liver failure which are more common following serum hepatitis than following infectious hepatitis.

Chronic hepatitis

Though the classification is based on pathology, there are fairly clear clinical correlations. Both forms are characterised by inflammatory infiltration around the portal tracts and may have features of superimposed acute hepatitis.

Chronic persistent hepatitis

The lobular architecture is preserved and there is little or no necrosis or fibrosis. It may follow acute viral hepatitis and carries an excellent prognosis without treatment. The patients may only have fatigue and hepatomegaly.

Chronic aggressive hepatitis (chronic active hepatitis: CAH)

Similar and overlapping syndromes include lupoid hepatitis (in the presence of LE cells) and juvenile cirrhosis. In addition to the periportal inflammatory infiltrate, there is piecemeal cellular necrosis along the interlobular septa and some fibrosis with the formation of intralobular septa and the formation of rosettes of cells. The architecture is only moderately disturbed but there is no nodular regeneration. Progression to cirrhosis is usual.

Clinical presentation It occurs chiefly in young women with the insidious onset of anorexia, abdominal pain and increasing jaundice. It may follow acute hepatitis. It tends to run a relapsing course culminating in cirrhosis. In 50% of patients, other systems are involved, e.g. fever, arthralgia, skin rashes, ulcerative colitis, lymphadenopathy, haemolytic anaemia and thrombocytopenia. Australia antigen and LE cells are associated with a proportion of cases (10–25%) and smooth muscle antibodies are present in 60%. See liver function tests (page 35).

Management Steroids and/or azathioprine improve

the symptoms, signs and liver function tests, and may improve the outcome. Steroids are more effective than azathioprine but have more side-effects, and may worsen the prognosis if ascites is present.

Cirrhosis

Cirrhosis is a pathological diagnosis and therefore implies liver biopsy in all suspected cases. It is characterised by widespread fibrosis with nodular regeneration. Its presence implies previous or continuing hepatic cell damage. See liver function tests (page 35); these are normal in inactive disease.

Classification

Micronodular (portal cirrhosis) is characterised by regular thick fibrotic bands joining the portal tracts to hepatic veins, and with small regenerative nodules. The liver is initially large with a smooth edge but subsequently shrinks with progressive fibrosis. It is often alcoholic in origin and is then associated with fatty infiltration.

Macronodular (post-necrotic cirrhosis) is less common and is characterised by coarse, irregular bands of fibrosis and loss of normal architecture and large regenerative nodules. It is believed usually to follow viral hepatitis with widespread necrosis. The liver is enlarged and very irregular due to the large nodules.

Biliary cirrhosis is less common and is characterised by fibrosis around distended intrahepatic bile ducts. It may follow chronic cholangitis and biliary obstruction (secondary), or be idiopathic (primary). In *primary biliary cirrhosis*, there is evidence of persistent cholestasis though the extra-hepatic bile ducts are patent. It occurs predominantly in middle-aged women who may be symptom-free. Xanthomata, pruritus and skin pigmentation are characteristic. The intrahepatic cholestasis results in pale stools, dark urine and steatorrhoea. The liver is enlarged. The diagnosis is confirmed by the presence of mitochondrial antibodies in the serum detected by immunofluorescence. This distinguishes it from biliary cirrhosis secondary to chronic obstruction. Chlorpromazine may produce a similar picture. Management is symptomatic for pruritus, and for the complications of steatorrhoea and hepatocellular failure. Death from hepatocellular failure with or without bleeding varices or intercurrent infection occurs in about 5–10 years.

Cardiac cirrhosis may occur in chronic cardiac failure. Centrilobular congestion leads to necrosis and fibrosis, but nodular regeneration is not marked.

Other rare causes (*q.v.*) of cirrhosis include chronic aggressive hepatitis, haemochromatosis and hepatolenticular degeneration.

NB *Schistosomiasis* causes periportal fibrosis and is not a form of cirrhosis. Liver involvement is more common (50%) in *S. mansoni* (bowel) infections than in *S. haemotobium* (bladder) due to the portal rather than systemic drainage of the primary infected area in the former. The schistosomes cause a granulomatous fibrosis in the portal tracts and enlargement of the liver. In severe cases the liver shrinks and extensive fibrosis develops leading to portal hypertension. There is little or no hepatocellular failure since the disease is presinusoidal. Late spread may occur to the lungs (cor pulmonale) and to the spinal cord (paraplegia).

Clinical presentation and management

This includes features of hepatocellular failure, portal hypertension, or both.

Hepatocellular failure (chronic)

Marked jaundice is uncommon. The oestrogen effects of gynaecomastia, spider naevi, liver palms and testicular atrophy may be present. In alcoholics, Dupuytren's contracture is common and other features of alcoholism may be present (wasting, polyneuropathy, Korsakoff's psychosis, dementia, delirium tremens and Wernicke's encephalopathy). Pigmentation, clubbing, cyanosis and peripheral oedema may occur. Portasystemic encephalopathy (hepatic coma and pre-coma) may be absent or may completely dominate the clinical picture. It may be precipitated acutely by:

— excess protein in the diet
— excess protein in the bowel, e.g. after gastro-intestinal haemorrhage
— acute alcoholic intoxication
— intercurrent infection, particularly Gram-negative septicaemia
— morphine and other alkaloids, paraldehyde and short-acting barbiturates
— minor or major surgical procedures including paracentesis
— electrolyte imbalance (potassium and/or sodium depletion)

Pre-coma is characterised by irritable confusion, drowsiness, flapping tremor, foetor and other signs of hepatocellular failure. Exaggerated reflexes and upgoing plantar responses may be present. Constructional apraxia may be demonstrated by inability to draw or copy a star. In the EEG, delta waves (3–4 c/s) are characteristic. Both the EEG and apraxia may be used to follow the course of the disease.

Specific management includes:

Sedation Despite the recognised hepatic complication, chlorpromazine is frequently used. Diazepam is also suitable.

Stop dietary protein.

Remove protein and blood (if present) from the bowel with magnesium sulphate enemas and purgation.

Decrease urea splitting bowel organisms with neomycin (1 g qds) and lactulose (50 ml tds) which also has a purgative action.

General management includes:

Maintenance of fluid balance Sodium restriction

may be required despite hyponatraemia which may be dilutional. Hypokalaemia should be treated with standard potassium preparations. Diuretics (thiazides, frusemide and/or spironolactone) may be given for ascites.

Calories are given as dextrose (up to 300 g daily) orally or intravenously. Treat intercurrent infections. Give parenteral vitamins B (particularly thiamine: B_1) and K.

If transfusion is required use fresh blood for preference to avoid further coagulation failure.

NB A reduced level of consciousness in hepatocellular failure (especially alcoholics) may be due to concussion, subdural haematoma or epilepsy. Previously healthy patients without cirrhosis who develop acute hepatocellular failure are managed similarly.

Portal hypertension

In cirrhosis, this is suggested by a patient with anorexia, vomiting, upper abdominal pain, splenomegaly and ascites. The liver may be large or small. Collateral circulation may be evident at the umbilicus (where a venous hum may be heard). Haematemesis is the commonest presenting symptom. Some evidence of hepatocellular failure and/or alcoholism may be present. Tests of liver cell function are usually slightly abnormal though not always so, and there may be hypersplenism. The bromsulphthalein excretion test may be abnormal when the standard liver function tests are not.

Management of bleeding varices The aim is to:

— replace blood lost (with blood or dextran).

— stop bleeding initially with vasopressin to lower portal pressure (20 units in 100 ml dextrose in 20 minutes intravenously repeated 2-hourly if necessary). This produces colic and diarrhoea and it is dangerous in ischaemic heart disease. Vitamin K_1 (phytomenadione) is given parenterally. If bleeding fails to stop, a Sengstaken tube may be used though it is very distressing and often ineffective. Surgery (ligation or transection) may be indicated if bleeding still continues. Portacaval anastomosis may be performed as an emergency procedure: contraindications after the first bleed are serum bilirubin (more than 2 mg/100 ml), serum albumin (less than 3 g/100 ml), age (above 45 years), and portasystemic encephalopathy during the bleed (this being accepted as a sufficient protein load). Avoid factors which may precipitate hepatocellular failure and treat if necessary (see above).

Portacaval anastomosis may be performed as an elective procedure after the first bleed and after investigation to:

— demonstrate oesophageal varices (barium swallow)

— determine the site of obstruction with splenic venography and pressure studies

— assess liver cell function with a high protein diet (120 g/day). If encephalopathy is demonstrated clinically or by EEG, surgery is contraindicated

NB Cirrhosis accounts for 80% of the portal hypertension seen in Britain. The other postsinusoidal causes (which have poor hepatic function) are exceedingly rare and result from cardiac failure, constrictive pericarditis and hepatic vein thrombosis (Budd-Chiari syndrome). Presinusoidal obstruction causes portal hypertension with normal hepatic function in schistosomiasis (granulomatous portal tract fibrosis), and in obstruction to the portal vein by tumours or following venous thrombosis with umbilical sepsis.

If cirrhosis develops in a young person (under 30 years) chronic aggressive hepatitis and hepatolenticular degeneration (Wilson's disease) must be considered.

Rare cirrhoses

Haemochromatosis (bronzed diabetes)

An autosomal dominant error of metabolism resulting in excess iron absorption and deposition chiefly in the liver, pancreas and heart, but also in endocrine glands. Alcohol seems to predispose to the development of symptoms and signs.

Clinical presentation

It occurs almost entirely in men over the age of 30 years who present with:
— diabetes mellitus (over 50%)
— skin pigmentation (due to melanin rather than iron)
— hepatomegaly (large, regular, firm); portal hypertension and hepatocellular failure are not common
— progressive polyarthropathy (50%)
— cardiac failure or arrhythmias (30%)
— testicular atrophy and loss of libido

Diagnosis

The serum iron (normally 125 μg/100 ml) is raised so that the serum iron-binding capacity (which remains normal: 350 μg/100 ml) is nearly saturated. The patient is not anaemic or polycythaemic.

Biopsy of most tissues (skin, marrow, testes) shows excess iron deposits but diagnosis is usually made on liver biopsy which shows iron staining of the liver cells with perilobular fibrosis.

Treatment

Deplete the body of the excess iron (up to 50 g) by weekly venesection of 500 ml (which contains 250 mg iron). This is continued until a normal serum iron is established and/or the patient becomes anaemic (in about 2 years). Maintenance venesection will be required (about 500 ml every 3 months depending upon the serum iron).

Treat appropriately the diabetes, hypogonadism, heart failure and arrhythmias, hepatic cell failure and portal hypertension.

NB Primary hepatic carcinoma occurs in up to 20% of cases whether treated or not.

Overload of the tissues with iron either following repeated blood transfusions (about 100 pints) or rarely after excessive iron ingestion results in *haemosiderosis*. In this the iron is in the reticulo-endothelial cells and the patients do not develop the serious sequelae. The patients are usually pigmented.

Hepatolenticular degeneration (Wilson's disease) (page 94)

An autosomal recessive disorder of copper metabolism characterised by a low serum caeruloplasmin level (and hence low serum copper) and by overabsorption of dietary copper. The urinary copper is high. Symptoms appear during adolescence or early adult life.

Clinical presentation

Copper which is bound only loosely to albumin (in the absence of the globulin caeruloplasmin) is deposited in:
— liver producing cirrhosis
— basal ganglia producing chorea-athetosis
— cerebrum producing dementia and emotional lability
— eyes producing Kayser-Fleischer rings (a brown 'fuzz' around the cornea)
— renal tubules producing the effects of heavy metal poisoning (aminoaciduria, phosphaturia, glycosuria and hypercalciuria)
The cerebral type is commoner than the hepatic type.

Management

Low dietary copper intake.
D-penicillamine (1–2 g daily for 6 months to 2 years followed by maintenance treatment) to increase urinary copper excretion.

The prognosis for improvement is good. Siblings should be examined.

Drug jaundice

Drugs are responsible for up to 10% of all hospital jaundice.

Hypersensitivity reactions

These are the commonest cause of drug jaundice. They are not dose-dependent.

Cholestasis

Clinically and biochemically this is an obstructive jaundice. Histologically there are bile plugs in the canaliculi and there may be an inflammatory infiltrate including eosinophils in the portal tracts.

The classical example is chlorpromazine jaundice which occurs 3–6 weeks after starting the drug. The prognosis is excellent if the drug is discontinued (and never given again).

Other drugs producing cholestasis are: other phenothiazines, erythromycin estolate (but not the stearate), phenylbutazone, sulphonylureas, sulphonamides, PAS and rifampicin, and nitrofurantoin. Occasionally there may be a more generalised reaction with fever, rash, lymphadenopathy and eosinophilia.

Acute hepatitis-like syndrome

Occasionally with acute necrosis. This is much less common but much more serious (mortality up to

20%). Clinically and histologically this is very like acute viral hepatitis. It is Australia antigen-negative. It occurs 2–3 weeks after starting the drug, and is caused by monoamine oxidase inhibitors, methyl dopa (which more commonly gives haemolytic jaundice), halothane (after multiple exposure), oxyphenisatin (an obsolete evacuant) and the anti-tuberculosis drugs, ethionamide and pyrazinamide.

Direct hepatotoxicity

In some cases this is dose-dependent though individual susceptibility is extremely variable.
The mechanisms are:
— cholestasis (without inflammatory infiltrate or necrosis). Chiefly due to C-17 substituted testosterone derivatives, i.e. anabolic and androgenic steroids, including methyl testosterone and most contraceptive pills.
— necrosis due to organic solvents, e.g. carbon tetrachloride, paracetamol in suicidal overdose, and antimitotic drugs, e.g. methotrexate, 6-mercaptopurine, azathioprine.

Haemolytic jaundice

This is a rare complication of therapy. It may occur with methyl dopa (which more commonly gives a positive Coombs' reaction without jaundice), phenacetin, and the 8-aminoquinolines (e.g. primaquine) in patients with glucose-6-phosphate dehydrogenase deficiency.

Gastroenterology

Symptoms arising from the gastrointestinal tract are extremely common. Most are due to disturbances of motility and/or are psychogenic. The commonest organic diseases are peptic ulcer, hiatus hernia, appendicitis, diverticulitis, haemorrhoids, acute infections and malabsorptions. Carcinoma of the colon is common. Carcinoma of the stomach is less common and carcinoma of the oesophagus relatively rare.

Steatorrhoea and malabsorption

Malabsorption signifies impaired ability to absorb one or more of the normally absorbed dietary constituents, including protein, carbohydrates, fats, minerals and vitamins.

Steatorrhoea signifies malabsorption of fat, and is defined as a faecal fat excretion of more than 6 g in 24 hours on a normal fat intake (50–100 g).

Apart from the occasions when the cause of steatorrhoea is obvious (such as obstructive jaundice) the diagnostic problem revolves around the differentiation between gluten-induced enteropathy and other causes of steatorrhoea.

Diarrhoea is not necessarily a presenting system and malabsorption may present with one or more of its complications (e.g. anaemia, weight loss, osteomalacia).

Primary idiopathic steatorrhoea

(gluten-induced enteropathy, coeliac syndrome or disease.)

Aetiology

There is mucosal sensitivity to wheat and possibly rye gluten (though not barley or oats). This may be due to the direct toxic effect of the polypeptide gliadin perhaps as a result of an immune disorder (a local deficiency of IgA or an antigen–antibody reaction at the mucosa).

NB A high proportion of patients with dermatitis herpetiformis have gluten-sensitive enteropathy.

Clinical presentation

There is usually a history of intermittent or chronic increased bowel frequency, classically with pale, bulky, offensive frothy greasy stools which flush only with difficulty. There may be a history of intermittent abdominal colic, flatus and abdominal distension. Depending on the severity and duration of the disease, there may be weakness and weight loss. If the malabsorption started in childhood, the patient may be short compared with his unaffected siblings, or parents. Children may present as 'failure to thrive'.

Since the malabsorption involves not only fat and

the fat-soluble vitamins but also minerals and water-soluble vitamins, the following deficiencies may occur:

Vitamin B_{12} and folic acid	to produce megaloblastic anaemia	or both
Iron (rare)	to produce iron deficiency anaemia	
Vitamin D	resulting in osteomalacia with bone tenderness and muscle weakness. Tetany may occur. Children may develop rickets	
Vitamin B group	glossitis and angular stomatitis	
Vitamin K	deficient prothrombin formation to produce bruising and epistaxis	
Associated impairment of amino acid absorption	may produce hypoproteinaemia and oedema	
Potassium	may produce weakness and apathy	

Examination

In addition to the features mentioned above there may be:
— evidence of weight loss
— pigmented, scaly and bruised skin
— distended abdomen with increased bowel sounds

NB Clubbing may occur. Signs of subacute combined degeneration of the cord are very rare.

Other causes of malabsorption

Bile salt deficiency

Patients present with obstructive jaundice usually secondary to carcinoma of the head of the pancreas or to gallstones (which may sometimes be seen on plain abdominal X-ray).

Pancreatic enzyme deficiency

Usually due to chronic pancreatitis or carcinoma affecting the pancreatic ducts (also rarely, fibrocystic disease, pancreatic calculi and benign pancreatic cystadenoma). The differentiation of these two diseases may be very difficult at presentation. Tests for malabsorption, glucose tolerance, serum bilirubin and barium meal are of little help. Tests of pancreatic secretion (secretin/pancreozymin/cholecystokinin stimulation) are said to give low volumes in carcinoma and low enzyme levels in chronic pancreatitis. Calcification of the pancreas on straight abdominal X-ray favours chronic pancreatitis and increasing experience of selenomethionine pancreatic isotope scanning may prove to be helpful (a normal test virtually excludes pancreatic disease). Similarly, duodenal fibroscopy with cannulation of the pancreatic duct and carcinoembryonic antigen (CEA) studies are likely to be increasingly useful.

Symptoms of pancreatic malabsorption are improved by a low fat diet (40 g/day), replacing minerals and vitamins, and giving pancreatic supplements (e.g. Nutrizym, Cotazym B, Pancrex V Forte).

Other intestinal disease

Postsurgical Incomplete food mixing may follow gastrectomy or gastroenterostomy and there may be a diminished area for absorption following small bowel resection.

Abnormal intestinal organisms The normal bacterial count in jejunal juice is less than 10^3–10^5 organisms/ml. The organisms (*E. coli* and bacteroides) breakdown dietary tryptophan to produce indoxylsulphate (indican) which is excreted in the urine. Overgrowth can be detected by a urinary indican excretion of more than 80 mg/24 hours. The aetiological role of the cultured organisms is difficult to prove but the steatorrhoea may respond to antibiotic therapy (tetracycline). There may be a close association between bacterial overgrowth and stasis from 'blind loops', diverticula and strictures.

Crohn's disease (page 193)

Rare causes

The following are very uncommon but well-recognised:

Zollinger-Ellison syndromes (page 196)

Disaccharidase deficiency Malabsorption of lactose, maltose and sucrose may occur in isolation due to primary enzyme deficiency, or as part of a general malabsorption picture. The most important is isolated lactase deficiency which presents, usually in children, with milk intolerance and malabsorption. Management consists of withdrawal of milk and milk products from the diet.

Other intrinsic disease of the intestinal wall due to tuberculosis, Hodgkin's disease, lymphosarcoma, diffuse systemic sclerosis, amyloidosis, and Whipple's disease (intestinal lipodystrophy).

Tropical sprue is a disorder which produces steatorrhoea and occurs almost exclusively in Europeans in the tropics, especially in India and the Far East. The aetiology is unknown. The most common associated deficiency is folic acid. The disease frequently remits spontaneously on return from the tropics. In some cases which do not remit a course of parenteral folic acid or oral tetracycline may be curative.

Very rarely, malabsorption is associated with diabetes, atheroma of the mesenteric arteries, cardiac failure and giardiasis.

Investigation of malabsorption

In a patient with a characteristic history, the investigation with the greatest likelihood of achieving a diagnosis is jejunal biopsy.

However, tests of absorption may quantitate the degree of malabsorption and help with the differential diagnosis between pancreatic and intestinal steatorrhoea.

NB Pancreatic malabsorption (page 188) is much less common and tends to affect the absorption only of fat and proteins and to leave the absorption of sugars, minerals, and water-soluble vitamins relatively unaffected. Intestinal malabsorption tends to give a total malabsorption.

Blood tests

Anaemia is common and may be 'iron deficient', megalobastic or dimorphic.
Blood folic acid, B_{12} and iron levels may be low.
Serum albumin may be low and the prothrombin time prolonged.
Serum calcium, phosphate and magnesium may be low and the serum alkaline phosphatase increased (osteomalacia pattern).

Tests of absorption

Faecal fat excretion The diagnosis of steatorrhoea is made by measuring faecal fat excretion over 3–5 days on a normal diet (50–100 g of fat in 24 hours). The upper limit of normal is 6 g/24 hours.
Xylose excretion More than 20% (5 g) of an oral load of 25 g is normally excreted in the urine in the 5 hours after ingestion. Less than this is excreted in intestinal malabsorption and also if there is renal dysfunction (and if the urine collection is incomplete). The 2-hour blood xylose level is normally greater than 30 mg/100 ml. The test is normal in pancreatic steatorrhoea.
NB Xylose was originally used because it was thought not to be metabolised (it is a little). It is absorbed mainly in the jejunum.
Glucose tolerance test In intestinal malabsorption, the curve is usually flat. In chronic pancreatitis and pancreatic carcinoma the curve may be diabetic.
Schilling test Megaloblastic anaemia may be caused by vitamin B_{12} deficiency in malabsorption syndromes if the terminal ileum is involved (e.g. Crohn's disease). In this case the absorption of radio-cobalt-labelled B_{12} is not improved by the addition of intrinsic factor (unlike pernicious anaemia).

Radiology

A small intestinal meal usually shows flocculation and segmentation of barium—evidence of excess mucus secretion. Of more significance are widening of the small intestinal calibre and increased distance between adjacent loops of bowel indicating thickening of the intestinal wall. Diverticula, fistulae or Crohn's disease may be seen.

The bones may show evidence of osteomalacia and/or osteoporosis.

Jejunal biopsy

In gluten-induced enteropathy, dissecting microscopic examination usually reveals flattening of the mucosae, with partial or total villous atrophy. The appearance does not necessarily correlate with the degree of malabsorption or the response to gluten withdrawal.

Management of gluten-induced enteropathy

Gluten-free diet In adults the response may take several months. Repeat biopsy is performed and the diagnosis is confirmed by a return of the appearances towards normal.
NB There may be a predisposition to malignancy—lym-

phomas and gut carcinoma (particularly oesophagus) —in gluten-induced enteropathy and there is some evidence that gluten-free diets may reduce the incidence of these. Hence the diet is continued for life.

Replace vitamins and minerals as indicated, and, if necessary, parenterally.

Laparotomy If a definitive diagnosis is not established, a laparotomy with biopsy may be indicated, to exclude other rare causes of malabsorption, especially if associated with abdominal pain (see below).

Ulcerative colitis

Clinical presentation

The disease usually presents in the 20–40 year old group but may occur at any age. First presentation over 65 years is uncommon but carries a greater mortality. Intermittent diarrhoea with mucus and blood in the stool, associated with fever and remissions to near normal are the most frequent symptoms. Three patterns may be distinguished:

— the disease may occasionally present as a single short mild episode of diarrhoea which appears to settle rapidly but may at any time relapse.

— usually the history is of months or years of general ill health with continuous or intermittent diarrhoea. In these cases the disease is usually restricted to the rectum and descending colon. General symptoms may be mild or severe. Secondary complications are frequent.

— approximately one-fifth of cases present with a severe acute episode of bloody diarrhoea with constitutional symptoms of fever and toxaemia and abdominal distension from toxic megacolon which may proceed to perforation of the intestine.

Diagnosis

This is suggested by the clinical picture and may be confirmed, except in the very ill, by sigmoidoscopy with biopsy and barium examination. The differential diagnosis includes:

— carcinoma of the colon which may present with bloody diarrhoea

— the acute case may resemble bacillary dysentery and the chronic case amoebic colitis (these should be excluded by stool examination)

— Crohn's disease of the colon appears to be increasingly recognised and may resemble ulcerative colitis

— very rarely acute ischaemic colitis may occur and affect the rectosigmoid junction (but not the rectum)

Sigmoidoscopic appearances

These may be conveniently divided into three groups:

Inactive: a granular mucosa with loss of normal vascular pattern.

Active: with pus and blood.

Very active: pus and blood with contact bleeding at the rim of the sigmoidoscope and visible ulceration.

NB The rectal mucosa is virtually always abnormal in ulcerative colitis, i.e. it is a distal disease with a variable extension proximally up the large bowel.

Radiology

Barium enema shows loss of normal haustral pattern with shortening of the large intestine. The bowel takes on the appearance of a smooth tube ('hosepipe appearance'). Undermined ulcers and pseudopolypi may be seen. Thickening of the oedematous colonic wall produces widening of the presacral space seen on lateral views of the sigmoid colon. Stricture formation or carcinoma produces fixed areas of narrowing.

Plain abdominal films will show acute dilatation when present. Barium enema examination in such circumstances may produce perforation.

Complications

General

Fever, anaemia, weight loss, iatrogenic steroid disease.

Colonic

Loss of protein with hypoalbuminaemia and oedema, loss of electrolytes (sodium and potassium) producing lethargy and contributing to intestinal dilatation. Pseudopolyps are common and possibly predispose to colonic carcinoma.

Carcinoma of the colon is more frequent if the entire colon is involved (total colitis), if the history is prolonged (10% in 10 years), if the first attack was severe, and if the first attack occurred at a young age.

Acute toxic dilatation of the colon with bleeding and perforation still has a high mortality.

Non-colonic

Skin rashes. Erythema nodosum (2%), pyoedema gangrenosum, leg ulcers (2%).

Arthritis (15%). This usually involves the joints of the hands and feet. Sacroileitis and ankylosing spondylitis are commoner in patients with ulcerative colitis.

Liver disease. Nearly all patients probably have some degree of liver involvement including fatty infiltration, chronic aggressive hepatitis, pericholangitis, sclerosing cholangitis, ascending cholangitis and carcinoma of the bile duct. These may result from a combination of malnutrition, portal pyaemia, and multiple blood transfusions. Secondary amyloidosis is uncommon but may follow prolonged chronic colitis.

Ocular. Iritis and episcleritis occur in about 5% of cases.

Venous thrombosis of the legs (5%).

Stomatitis (15%).

Management

High protein diet (150 g per day) with supplements of vitamins and potassium. Iron is given in the presence of anaemia and blood transfusion may be necessary to maintain the haemoglobin at 10–11 g%, particularly in acute cases. Intravenous feeding is sometimes necessary.

Codeine phosphate (15–30 mg tds) or *diphenoxylate* (Lomotil) is sometimes given for symptomatic control of diarrhoea if mild. Sulphasalazine (0·5 g bd to 1 g qds) may be sufficient to control symptoms in mild cases and in remission. Prednisolone phosphate retention enemas are added if symptoms persist and the rectum is involved. A course of prednisolone (40–60 mg daily) is required for more severe disease but maintenance oral steroids are not usually indicated. Some believe ACTH to be more effective in acute toxic colitis.

Surgery is indicated if severe haemorrhage or perforation has occurred and in acute toxaemia with dilatation of the colon which fails to respond within 4–5 days to high dose steroids.

Surgery is usually performed in the presence of severe secondary complications if perianal sepsis or fistulae are present, and in long-term (10 years) total colitis either for treatment of chronic ill health or in view of the risk of carcinoma.

Total colectomy with ileostomy is the elective operation performed in most centres. In the absence of rectal involvement an ileorectal anastomosis may be performed in order to retain 'normal' anatomy and avoid ileostomy—this operation has not gained general popularity as bowel frequency tends to persist, as may ill health, and the risk of cancer developing in the rectum remains.

Prognosis

About 70% of all cases remit with medical treatment in the first attack, 15% improve, and 15% come to surgery or die. Young patients do better than old patients, and subtotal colitis is less severe than total colitis in terms of both general health and the risk of colonic carcinoma. Surgery is therefore indicated early in patients who are older and have total colitis. The mortality from total colectomy when performed as a 'cold' procedure is 2–4% (in severely ill acute cases including toxic dilatation the mortality may be as high as 30–40%). However 20% of these patients require further surgery usually to refashion the stoma or less commonly to divide obstructing adhesions. Impotence and loss of micturition control are serious complications of surgery.

Crohn's disease (regional ileitis)

A rare granulomatous inflammatory disorder of the intestine, of unknown aetiology usually starting in the teens and early twenties. The terminal ileum is most frequently diseased but any part of the tract may be involved. The colon may be involved in up to 10–20% of cases. The process affects short lengths of the intestine leaving normal bowel between, i.e. 'skip lesions'. The wall is thickened and the lumen narrowed. Mucosal ulceration and regional lymphadenopathy are present. The characteristic microscopic lesion is a non-caseating granuloma not unlike those found in sarcoid. It is a progressive chronic disease.

Clinical presentation

It usually presents (80–90%) as intermittent abdominal pain with diarrhoea and abdominal distension in a young thin person. There may be associated fever (30%), anaemia and weight loss in part secondary to malabsorption (50%), and rarely, fresh blood or melaena stools (10%), fistulae and perianal sepsis (15–20%). Intermittent intestinal obstruction may occur. Clubbing is fairly common (up to 50%). Occasionally uveitis (5%), arthritis (5%), and skin rashes (erythema nodosum and pyoedema) occur. Renal stones occur in 5–10%.

Less commonly it presents as an 'acute abdomen' with signs of acute appendicitis with or without a palpable mass in the right iliac fossa. Many of these patients have no further trouble. The appendix should not be removed as fistulae may result.

Radiology

The terminal ileum is most commonly involved and may produce incompetence of the ileocaecal valve. Mucosal ulceration may be deep and 'spikes' of barium may enter deep into the bowel wall. Lesions may be multiple with normal bowel between ('skip lesions'). Coarse cobblestone appearance of the mucosa appears early. Later in the disease fibrosis produces narrowing of the intestine ('string sign') with some proximal dilatation.

Diagnosis

This is usually made on the basis of the clinical picture and radiological findings. Characteristic Crohn's granulomata may occasionally be seen in jejunal biopsy specimens or in biopsy specimens taken at laparotomy for abdominal pain.

Crohn's disease of the large bowel may resemble ulcerative colitis. The diagnosis of Crohn's disease is favoured by little blood loss, a normal rectal mucosa, and the presence of perianal sepsis.

A mass in the right iliac fossa must be differentiated from a caecal carcinoma and an appendix abscess. Amoebic abscesses and ileocaecal tuberculosis are uncommon in Britain.

Prognosis and management

Approximately 25% remit spontaneously. This is most frequent in the group presenting as acute appendicitis. The appendix should not be removed as this may lead to fistula formation.

Long-term management for chronic recurrent disease requires:

— bed rest during acute exacerbations.

— high protein diet with vitamin and electrolyte supplements as required. Low roughage diet may decrease the risk of intestinal obstruction.

— steroids are sometimes effective in suppressing acute intestinal symptoms but less so than in ulcerative colitis. Low-dose steroids (prednisone 10 mg daily) may improve health and decrease the frequency of recurrence in individual cases. Steroids may also be necessary for systemic complications. Immunosuppression (azathioprine) has been used successfully in a small number of cases over a short period of time. It appears to allow a reduction in steroid dosage with apparently little detrimental effect on well-being.

Surgery is retained for the relief of acute emergencies (obstruction), abscesses and fistulae. Surgery eventually becomes necessary in a high proportion of cases (70–80%) the longer the disease is present, but this number may decrease as experience with steroids and immunosuppressives increases. Resection of diseased intestine and bypass operations may become necessary for severe chronic ill health, but these are not curative and fistula formation may result and recurrence is the rule. Intestinal obstruction is best managed conservatively in the first instance with gastric aspiration and intravenous feeding to allow time for the acute inflammation to resolve.

Gastric and duodenal ulceration

Clinical presentation

It may be impossible, on the basis of history and examination alone, to differentiate between duodenal ulceration, benign ulceration of the stomach and carcinoma of the stomach, but carcinoma is much rarer.

Duodenal ulceration is the most common and classically presents with a history of periodic epigastric pain, occurring 2–3 hours after meals, often waking the patient at 1–3 AM, relieved by food and alkalis.

Gastric ulcer pain may be epigastric or occur anywhere in the anterior upper abdomen. Anorexia, vomiting and weight loss are more frequent and severe in carcinomatous ulcers of the stomach than in benign peptic ulceration.

Examination

The patient characteristically points to the epigastrium with a forefinger when asked where the pain is and this is the point of maximum tenderness. The presence of an epigastric mass suggests a carcinoma. A gastric splash indicates pyloric obstruction due to benign duodenal stricture or to carcinoma of the pyloric antrum.

Complications

Bleeding (page 197).
Perforation (usually duodenal ulcer).
Pyloric stenosis. This presents with recurrent vomiting of food ingested up to 24 hours previously with immediate relief. Visible gastric peristalsis may be seen. Conservative management with gastric aspiration and intravenous fluids may sometimes allow time for a benign active ulcer to heal and relieve the obstruction. Surgery is usually required either on the first or subsequent admission. These patients may vomit profusely and become dehydrated and alkalotic. Fluid and electrolyte replacement is obligatory and particularly so prior to surgery.

Investigation

Barium meal. Duodenal ulcers are 'always' benign. Gastric carcinomas are commoner on the greater curve and in the antrum but lesser curve ulcers may nevertheless be malignant. The size of the ulcer is no guide to whether a carcinoma is present. Carcinomas may have a rolled edge and a translucent 'halo' around them.

Gastroscopy, fibreoscopy with photography or gastrocamera studies will distinguish benign from malignant ulcers in the large majority of cases. Biopsy and exfoliative cytology can give histological confirmation.

Management

Benign peptic ulcers tend to heal on bed rest and stopping smoking. Anticholinergic drugs, antacids and diet often ameliorate symptoms but do not hasten healing.

Duodenal ulcer

Treatment is only indicated when symptoms are present. Antacids and frequent small meals may relieve symptoms. Carbenoxolone (as Duogastrone) may relieve symptoms and favour healing but the evidence is much less convincing than for benign gastric ulcers.

Gastric ulcer

Management is directed towards ulcer healing and differentiating benign from malignant ulcers. Treatment comprises bed rest, stopping smoking and carbenoxolone sodium (Biogastrone) or deglycerinised liquorice (Caved-S: which causes less retention of sodium and less depletion of potassium). Symptoms should settle and a repeat barium meal after 3–4 weeks should show a decrease in the size of the ulcer. If neither has occurred, the presence of a carcinoma becomes more likely and exploratory laparotomy may be indicated particularly if biopsy and photography have been inconclusive.

Indications for surgery

Duodenal ulcer

Acute indications include:
— perforation
— pyloric obstruction
— persistent haemorrhage

Failed medical treatment. Surgery in chronic duodenal ulceration depends upon assessment of the degree of disability produced by the symptoms. Factors to be considered are the severity and frequency of pain, and time off work. There is an increasing tendency to perform vagotomy with pyloroplasty or vagotomy and gastroenterostomy instead of partial gastrectomy in an attempt to reduce the incidence of side-effects of malabsorption and 'dumping.'

Gastric ulcer

Acute indication: persistent haemorrhage (page 198).
Non-acute indications:
— carcinoma
— failed medical treatment either if there is a possibility of carcinoma or for persistent symptoms

Zollinger-Ellison syndrome

This rare disorder is characterised by multiple recurrent duodenal and jejunal ulceration associated with gross gastric acid hypersecretion and the presence of a gastrin secreting adenoma (which may be malignant), usually in the pancreas but sometimes in the stomach wall. Diarrhoea sometimes with steatorrhoea may be a feature. The volume of gastric secretion is enormous (7–10 litres/24 hours) and acid secretion persistently raised (and raised little further by pentagastrin).

The presence of an adenoma may be associated with adenomata of other endocrine glands, i.e. adrenals, parathyroids and anterior pituitary (pluriglandular syndrome).

Treatment is usually by total gastrectomy rather than by attempts to find and remove the tumour which is usually benign.

Gastrointestinal haemorrhage

Aetiology

Acute

Duodenal ulcers	35%	
Gastric ulcers		
acute erosion	40%	(salicylates and phenylbutazone)
chronic ulcer	20%	
Oesophageal varices	5%	(up to 50% in France and parts of U.S.A.)

Chronic

NB Bleeding from hiatus hernia and gastric carcinoma is usually insidious (but not always). Severe blood loss may result from haemorrhoids, diverticulosis, colonic tumours, ulcerative colitis, ischaemic colitis and bacillary dysentery.

Management

Initial treatment

Treat shock if present with transfusion of blood and monitor progress by pulse and blood pressure recording. If facilities and time allow, a central venous pressure monitor may be inserted as a guide to further transfusion and rebleeding. A central venous pressure of +3 to +6 cm of saline should be maintained. Oxygen should be given.

NB Always attempt to have 4 pints of blood available for further transfusion.

If blood is supplied citrated (in bottles) give 10 ml 10% calcium gluconate for every 4 bottles.

Sedate the patient if anxious. Diazepam probably causes less hypotension than morphine and heroin.

Inform the surgeons.

Vasopressin may stop haemorrhage from varices (page 183).

Vitamin K should be given if bleeding has occurred from varices. The blood urea may rise to 100–150 mg/100 ml due to absorption of protein from the gut. The serum creatinine is not increased unless renal disease is also present. Hepatic coma may be precipitated by protein in the gut.

If bleeding appears to have stopped (steady pulse and blood pressure) assess progress with repeat haemoglobin and/or haematocrit. Transfusion is usually required if the haemoglobin is less than 9–10 g/100 ml particularly in older patients.

Investigation (for site and cause of bleeding)

As soon as the patient's condition allows, a barium swallow and meal should be performed, which may show the site of bleeding. This may be of considerable value if surgery becomes necessary. Fibreoscopy is often useful in determining the site of bleeding.

If bleeding continues or recurs surgery may be necessary (see below). If bleeding has stopped the patient should be given oral iron and a normal diet. Carbenoxolone sodium or Caved-S aids healing of gastric ulcers. Patient should be advised not to smoke.

Indications for surgery (in haemorrhage from peptic ulcer)

Although there are no definite indications, surgery is usually indicated if bleeding does not stop spontaneously or the patient rebleeds in hospital (the central venous pressure may be the first indication of this, but slower continuous bleeds are indicated by a persistently low haemoglobin). The overall mortality is worse in older patients (10% in the over sixties) than in the young (2% in the under sixties). Bleeds from gastric ulcers (mortality up to 20% in the over sixties) carry twice the mortality of bleeds from duodenal ulcers. Also the operative risk for gastric ulcer surgery is less than for duodenal ulcers.

Hence the tendency is to operate early in older patients, particularly if bleeding from a gastric ulcer. Supplies of compatible blood may be a controlling factor.

Hiatus hernia

In the common type both stomach and oesophagus are present in the thorax. It occurs in midlife, in the fat and flabby, and during pregnancy.

It is often found if looked for by the radiologist but is symptomless unless there is a reflux oesophagitis (which is usually associated with hyperchlorhydria and hence with duodenal ulcer).

Symptoms

These are heartburn with acid regurgitation on bending and pain, worse on lying down and in bed. Food may 'stick'. Bleeding may give positive occult blood tests and anaemia.

Treatment

Sit up in bed with high pillows and a raised foot of the bed to stop slipping down.
Lose weight and remove corsets.
Antacids and avoid foods which give symptoms.
Treat anaemia with iron.
Avoid surgery unless symptoms become intractable and dominate the patient's life.

Diverticular disease

Diverticula occur anywhere in the alimentary tract but chiefly in the colon—diverticulosis. They are due to a weakening of the colonic wall and increased intracolonic pressure. They affect chiefly the descending and sigmoid colon. It is a disorder of mid and late age (5% of the population over 50 years in Britain), more common in women than men and usually discovered incidentally during barium enema performed to exclude colonic carcinoma.

Clinical features

Diverticulosis by definition produces no symptoms. Inflamed diverticula produce diverticulitis with:
— pain, discomfort and tenderness in the left iliac fossa (there may be a mass)—'appendicitis of the left side'
— change in bowel habit with constipation and/or diarrhoea sometimes alternating
— rectal bleeding which may be acute and sometimes massive and the first symptom
— subacute obstruction
— frequency of micturition and cystitis, and occasionally vesico-colic fistula
— perforation with peritonitis or fistulae

Management

Acute diverticulitis may be extremely painful and require rest in bed, analgesia, local warmth and antibiotics (ampicillin or co-trimoxazole). Occasionally surgery is required, particularly colostomy and resection for obstruction or if carcinoma is suspected.

Dietary fibre

Diverticulosis is rare in communities which take a fibre-rich diet. Such peoples also have far less carcinoma of the colon and appendicitis. A diet high in dietary fibre results in bulkier stools and rapid intestinal transit times. The soft stool prevents straining which may help to prevent diverticulosis. In the established disease added dietary fibre (two teaspoonsful to two tablespoonsful daily) reduces symptoms in most patients. Fibre-rich diets also decrease serum cholesterol and increase faecal excretion of bile salts and their relative absence from Western diets has been suggested as a possible contributory factor in coronary artery atheroma and gallstones.

Respiratory disease

The commonest diseases are infections of the upper respiratory tract, e.g. the common cold. The commonest diseases of the lower respiratory tract are bronchitis (acute and chronic) asthma and carcinoma of the bronchus.

Chronic bronchitis

Definition

Daily cough with sputum for 3 months a year for at least 2 consecutive years.

This is a clinical definition. Radiological, pathological and biochemical features are judged by this standard. The definition is chiefly of use epidemiologically: patients whose respiratory disease does not satisfy this definition may nevertheless have bronchitis. It causes about 30,000 deaths per annum in the United Kingdom.

'Emphysema' is a histological diagnosis and is therefore usually made with precision only post mortem. It is defined as enlargement of the air spaces distal to the respiratory (smallest) bronchioles.

Aetiological factors

Cigarette smoking. The increased mortality risk from bronchitis has an approximately straight-line relationship with numbers of cigarettes smoked per day (increased risk $= \frac{1}{2} \times$ cigarettes smoked per day).
Atmospheric pollution.
There is a relationship to lower social class and to being British.

Clinical presentation

Initially, the patient has productive morning cough and an increased frequency of lower respiratory tract infections producing purulent sputum. The organisms responsible are usually *Haemophilus influenzae* and *Streptococcus pneumoniae*. Over the years there is slowly progressive dyspnoea with wheezing, exacerbated in the acute infective episodes. There is clinical emphysema with hyperinflation of the lungs. Respiratory failure (page 204) or cardiac failure (cor pulmonale) may develop.

Investigation

Chest X-ray This may be normal. Abnormalities correlate with the presence of emphysema and are due to:
— overinflation with a low, flat, poorly moving diaphragm and a large retrosternal window on lateral X-ray
— vascular changes with loss of peripheral vascular markings but enlarged hilar vessels. The heart is narrow until cor pulmonale develops
— bullae if present

The chest X-ray is an important investigation because it excludes other disease (carcinoma, tuberculosis, pneumonia, pneumothorax).

Ventilatory function tests Spirometry shows a greater reduction in FEV_1 than in VC (and the ratio FEV%, is thus also reduced). PEFR is reduced.

Arterial blood gas estimations These may be normal. In later stages the P_{O_2} falls and the P_{CO_2} rises, particularly with exacerbations.

ECG This records the presence and progression of cor pulmonale (right atrial and ventricular hypertrophy).

Sputum for bacterial culture and sensitivity. This is useful in acute infective episodes in case infections other than *H. influenzae* or *S. pneumoniae* are present.

Haemoglobin estimation may show polycythaemia.

Management

Stop smoking (and move to a 'clean air' district).

Treat acute exacerbations. Ampicillin (0·5–1·0 g qds) or co-trimoxazole (Septrin, Bactrim, 2 tab bd) are suitable. Change of therapy is directed by the clinical condition. Bacterial sensitivities are useful if clinical improvement has not occurred.

Bronchodilators. Salbutamol (Ventolin) and terbutaline (Bricanyl) are suitable and are given by metered aerosol or in tablet form.

Treat heart failure with digitalis and diuretics.

Physiotherapy—with emphasis on coughing and relaxation.

NB Steroids are usually not indicated but in severe refractory cases they may be given a short trial while ventilatory function is monitored (page 44).

Bronchiectasis

Bronchiectasis means dilatation of the airways. It only becomes of clinical significance when infection occurs within these airways. It is now rare especially in the young.

Aetiology

Following acute childhood respiratory infection, particularly measles and whooping cough.

Fibrocystic disease (mucoviscidosis).

Bronchial obstruction predisposes to bronchiectasis (e.g. carcinoma and peanuts).

Tuberculosis has become less common as a cause.

Congenital (rare), e.g. Kartagener's syndrome.

Chronic cough, often postural.

Clinical features

Sputum often copious, especially with acute infections. Halitosis.

Febrile episodes.

Haemoptysis: may be the only symptom ('dry bronchiectasis').

Dyspnoea, coarse basal crepitations and wheeze.

Cyanosis and clubbing.

Loss of weight in advanced cases.

Management

Treatment is unnecessary in the absence of symptoms. Daily postural drainage will help to empty dilated airways and decrease the frequency of further infections. Antibiotics, as for chronic bronchitis, are given for acute infections and exacerbation. Surgery is virtually never indicated because the disease is seldom limited to one or two lung segments. Patients tend to develop respiratory failure.

Cystic fibrosis (mucoviscidosis)

A hereditary recessive disorder which occurs equally in males and females and usually presents in early childhood with repeated lower respiratory tract infections. These are secondary to bronchial obstruction from the viscid secretions of the bronchial mucosa. Secondary bronchiectasis or lung abscesses may result. Associated pancreatic malabsorption is common (80%) with weight loss and steatorrhoea from inspissation of pancreatic secretions. A high sodium concentration in the sweat (above 70 mEq/l) is characteristic, and exceptionally can lead to circulatory collapse from uncontrolled salt depletion during heatwaves.

Asthma

The diagnosis is made on a history of episodic wheeze and dyspnoea. There are two main clinical groups:

Extrinsic asthma It begins in childhood and there is usually a family history of other allergies (hayfever and eczema) and a family history of asthma.
Intrinsic asthma (late-onset asthma) It begins in adult life and there is usually no allergic or family history and no demonstrable skin sensitivities. It is associated with marked inspissation of sputum and attacks are less responsive to therapy than extrinsic asthma. Eosinophilia may be marked.

The margins between these two groups are not distinct. The differential diagnosis of late-onset asthma includes chronic bronchitis, and, far less likely, polyarteritis nodosa, extrinsic alveolitis (farmer's lung, bird-fancier's lung may present as 'asthma'), carcinoid syndrome, aspergillosis and Loeffler's syndrome.

Clinical features

Acute attacks

These may be fairly abrupt in onset and brief in duration (hours), or longer (a week or two), remittent and less severe. Longer severe attacks are called status asthmaticus (see below). In an attack the patient feels tightness in the chest and expiratory difficulty. There may be a cough which is initially dry but becomes productive later, particularly if there is infection. The patient usually sits up with an over-inflated chest, an audible expiratory wheeze and a fixed shoulder girdle using the accessory muscles of respiration. The respiratory rate may be little altered but the pulse is invariably rapid. Acute attacks are precipitated by specific allergens (e.g. pollens or house dust mite), exertion, excitement, a cold environment or a respiratory infection and some β-blockers.

Chronic asthma

Mild asthmatics (particularly with extrinsic asthma)

usually have normal respiratory function between attacks, but those with long-standing severe asthma tend to develop emphysema and some degree of dyspnoea between acute attacks.

Investigation

Investigation includes chest X-ray (for regional collapse, pneumonia, pneumothorax), haematology (eosinophilia and ESR), and spirometry (FEV_1 or PEFR, preferably at several times in a day on several days) and the response to bronchodilators. Skin hypersensitivity tests can help the patient to recognise and avoid environmental precipitants.

Management

The patient should be asked about precipitant factors including the relationship of attacks to upper respiratory tract infection, season (grass pollen and fungal spores), cold, exercise, food, house dust (contains the mite dermatophagoides), smoke, emotion and drugs (e.g. aspirin, propranolol).

Most patients and almost all extrinsic asthmatics respond to simple therapy and may be controlled by:
— removing known allergies, e.g. feather pillows and cats
— disodium cromoglycate (Intal), 2–3 Spincaps daily
— salbutamol orally 2–4 mg tds, or by inhalation
— hyposensitisation is of value in only a small number of patients who demonstrate specific allergies

Steroid therapy

In view of the serious side-effects, systemic steroids must be avoided whenever possible in the long-term maintenance of asthma. Few extrinsic asthmatics need steroids but many intrinsic asthmatics cannot be controlled without, although some may require as little as 1–2 mg prednisolone per day. Systemic steroids should only be considered after trying routine maintenance therapy with:
— disodium cromoglycate (Intal), one capsule inhaled 2–4 times daily
— salbutamol (orally or by inhalation)
— metered-dose inhaled steroids (e.g. Becotide)

The majority of acute episodes are successfully treated outside hospital and many cases admitted to hospital improve on bed rest alone.

Status asthmaticus

Status asthmaticus is defined as an asthma attack of over 24 hours' duration. This is not a clinically useful definition since of those who die in an acute asthma attack, half are dead within 24 hours. Moreover death is frequently sudden and sometimes unexpected as the patient may not appear severely ill.

Clinical presentation

Dyspnoea. Inability to speak is one criterion of severity. It also implies inability to drink (and therefore dehydration). Hypoxaemia is usually then present, and wheeze frequently absent due to poor ventilation.

Confusion and drowsiness are evidence of a perilous

situation whatever the cause (abnormal blood gases, sedation or fatigue).

Cyanosis is also an ominous sign and tends to occur at a lower Po_2 than in the chronic bronchitic (because the bronchitic tends to have polycythaemia).

Tachycardia and arterial hypotension tend to reflect the severity of the attack.

NB The useful clinical signs of drowsiness and cyanosis are those of a very severe attack and vigorous treatment is essential before they are apparent.

Investigation

A chest X-ray is mandatory to exclude a pneumothorax. Blood gases provide the most useful guide to the severity of the attack. Tests of ventilatory function (FEV and PEFR) are useful in following recovery but not at the height of the attack.

Management

All asthma attacks which do not respond to treatment with standard bronchodilators (theophylline preparations and β-stimulator drugs such as salbutamol) within a few hours should be regarded as severe. They usually merit admission to hospital. Sedation may depress respiration farther and is contraindicated.

Continuous oxygen should invariably be given and is relatively safe; 28% is usually adequate. The patient may tolerate 'uncontrolled oxygen' techniques better, e.g. nasal cannula.

Bronchodilators

— aminophylline 500 mg in 10 ml by very slow i.v. injection or infusion

— β-stimulators (e.g. salbutamol) by metered aerosol or patient-triggered ventilator. Isoprenaline and adrenaline are seldom used

Corticosteroids Hydrocortisone is given early and in large doses intravenously, e.g. 500 mg stat and 250–500 mg 4-hourly. The patient is transferred to oral prednisolone (e.g. 10 mg tds) when he has improved (24–48 hours) and this is subsequently withdrawn gradually.

Intravenous fluids are required both to make up the initial dehydration and for as long as oral fluids are not taken. Fluid charts and alterations in the patient's weight are useful guides. Central venous pressure monitoring may be helpful.

Antibiotics are given for underlying infection.

Mechanical ventilation may be necessary. Persistent or increasing elevation of arterial Pco_2, especially with accompanying exhaustion (usually becoming important by 48 hours) suggests the need for artificial ventilation by an experienced anaesthetist. Bronchial lavage with saline or 1% sodium bicarbonate can be performed after intubation but not all physicians think it valuable.

Respiratory failure

Respiratory failure is defined as an inability to maintain normal arterial blood gases, i.e. $Pco_2 = 36$–44 mmHg, $Po_2 = 80$–100 mmHg.

NB The mean Po_2 is about 90 mmHg (not 100).

Normally values are about 10 mmHg lower in the elderly.

Rarely, the Po_2 may fall while the Pco_2 remains normal. This may occur with alveolar parenchymal lung disease: infiltrations, fibrosing alveolitis and 'pure' emphysema. Much more commonly, both arterial gas levels are abnormal. This occurs with ventilatory failure.

Acute

Patients with normal lungs, with upper airways obstruction (e.g. croup) or mechanical failure (e.g. fluid in the chest, drug overdosage).
Patients with abnormal lungs (e.g. asthma, chronic bronchitis).

Chronic

Usually in patients with abnormal lungs, especially chronic bronchitis. These patients are particularly likely to develop acute failure.

Acute on chronic respiratory failure

Usually chronic bronchitis.

Clinical presentation

Peripheral vasodilatation with headache, engorged veins in the fundi, warm hands and a bounding pulse.
Varying degrees of agitated confusion, drowsiness and coma.
Increasing cyanosis.
Signs of right heart failure.
Flapping tremor of the outstretched hands and papilloedema are late signs.
NB Unfortunately the physical signs are a poor guide to the presence of respiratory failure and to its degree. It is therefore necessary to measure blood gases in all patients in whom the diagnosis is suspected.

Management

This consists of the measures used for chronic bronchitis as given above, with the addition of controlled oxygen therapy. The danger to life in this situation is hypoxia but paradoxically relief of hypoxia may make the situation worse.
Oxygen is given at 24% or 28% by Ventimask (or other controlled technique) if the arterial Po_2 is low. Oxygen is not required unless the Po_2 is less than 50 mmHg (and some authorities would withhold oxygen unless it were less than 40 mmHg). It is given continuously until the acute situation (including infection and heart failure) has recovered. The Pco_2 is monitored either by mixed venous rebreathing method or from the arterial blood.
Intravenous analeptics (e.g. nikethamide 2–6 ml as a bolus) may be used in the semi-comatose patient to provoke coughing.
Intravenous aminophylline (10 ml) slowly may be valuable.
NB Sedatives are absolutely contraindicated.

Indications for mechanical ventilation

If the Pco_2 falls or rises only slightly (e.g. by 10 mmHg) conservative therapy should be continued and reassessed periodically. If the Pco_2 rises this indicates that the patient's ventilation is inadequate and is the prime indication for mechanical positive pressure ventilation. The final decision to ventilate a patient is determined mainly on the basis of his respiratory function before the acute illness.

Pneumonia

Bronchopneumonia

It may occur in previously normal lungs or be superimposed on underlying bronchitis or other respiratory disease, e.g. bronchiectasis or carcinoma. It is preceded by bronchial infection and is commonest in children (measles and whooping cough) and the elderly (chronic bronchitis and hypostatic pneumonia in debilitated patients in bed). In normal adults it may follow respiratory viral infections.

Clinical presentation

The history is initially often of acute bronchitis. Fever and malaise develop with a cough producing infected (yellow or green) sputum. On examination coarse crepitations may be present in one or more areas of the chest. There may be areas of consolidation with dullness to percussion, increased vocal resonance and bronchial breathing.

Investigation

Diagnosis is confirmed on chest X-ray. Sputum should be cultured before starting antibiotics, but these should *not* be withheld until sensitivities are available.

Management

Haemophilus influenzae and *Streptococcus pneumoniae* are the most common organisms but other bacteria (e.g. klebsiella and staphylococcus) may be responsible. Initial therapy involves the use of:

— oxygen—about 40% (e.g. MC mask) in the absence of respiratory failure and 28% in its presence
— antibiotics—usually ampicillin or cotrimoxazole in the first instance
— physiotherapy

Important predisposing causes should be considered including diabetes mellitus and carcinoma of the bronchus. Complications include lung abscess, pleural effusion and empyema.

Lobar pneumonia

This has become uncommon since the advent of penicillin.

Clinical presentation

The onset is sudden with cough, rusty sputum, marked fever and rigors. There are signs of consolidation if a large area of lung is involved. Chest X-ray shows consolidation in lobar distribution. There may be cerebral abscess.

Management

The organism most frequently cultured is *S. pneumoniae* (pneumococcus) and this responds to i.m. crystalline penicillin (1–2 million units 6-hourly) which is the drug of first choice.

NB Lobar consolidation suggests an underlying bronchial obstruction, e.g. neoplasm, foreign body.

Recurrent bacterial pneumonia

In the absence of chronic bronchitis, recurrent pneumonia arouses the suspicion of:

— bronchial carcinoma preventing drainage of infected areas of the lung

— bronchiectasis (including fibrocystic disease)

— achalasia of the cardia, 25% of which present as chest disease, pharyngeal pouch and neuromuscular disease of the oesophagus, e.g. bulbar palsy

— hypo- or a-gammaglobulinaemia

Other bacterial pneumonias

Klebsiella pneumoniae (Friedlander's)

This is rare and often opportunistic in patients with leukaemia, lymphomas or on steroids. The history is of sudden prostration, fever, rigors and cough with blood-stained viscous sputum. The chest X-ray shows patchy areas of consolidation, often involving the upper lobe. The mortality is high (40%) and subsequent respiratory disability common.

The bacillus is not penicillin or ampicillin sensitive. It responds to streptomycin, chloramphenicol and, with some strains, tetracyclines. Lung abscess, emphysema and bronchiectasis are common complications.

Staphylococcal pneumonia

This produces widespread infection with abscess formation. It occurs in patients with underlying disease which prevents normal response to infection, e.g. chronic leukaemia, Hodgkins's disease, cystic fibrosis, and patients on steroid therapy. It may complicate influenzal pneumonia and this makes it relatively common during epidemics of influenza. The organism may not be penicillin sensitive and cloxacillin and fusidic acid are the drugs of choice. Lung abscess, empyema and subsequent bronchiectasis are relatively common complications.

Viral pneumonia

The most common virus producing pneumonia in children in this country and the U.S.A. is the respiratory syncytial virus (so called as it is a respiratory virus which produces syncytial formation when grown in tissue culture). The agent is not responsive to antibiotics and it may be indistinguishable from acute bacterial bronchitis or bronchiolitis in children and infants. The presence of an associated skin rash supports the likelihood of RSV infection.

Acute virus pneumonia in adults is very rare and occurs during epidemics of influenza A (Asian 'flu). The picture is of rapid and progressive dyspnoea. Death may occur within hours from acute haemorrhagic disease of the lungs. The most common cause of pneumonia during epidemics of influenza results from secondary bacterial infection, the most serious being staphylococcal pneumonia. The viruses of measles, chickenpox, and herpes zoster may directly affect the lung. The diagnosis is confirmed by a rise in specific antibody titre.

Mycoplasma pneumonia

This is also known as Eaton-agent pneumonia and is caused by *Mycoplasma pneumoniae*, the only mycoplasma definitely pathogenic to man. The clinical picture resembles bacterial pneumonia although cough and sputum are absent in one-third of cases.

Respiratory symptoms and signs and X-ray changes (patchy consolidation with small effusions) are usually preceded by several days of 'flu-like symptoms. Malaise and fatigue may persist long after the acute illness is over. The diagnosis is confirmed by a rise of specific antibody titre, the presence of cold agglutinins and antibodies to streptococcus MG in the serum and/or isolation of the organism. Tetracycline (0·5–1·0 g qds) is the antibiotic of choice. Psittacosis and ornithosis (Bedsoniae) may cause a similar picture and also respond to tetracycline.

Carcinoma of the bronchus

Incidence

This causes about 35,000 deaths per year in the United Kingdom, half of them under 65 years of age. Sixty per cent are squamous cell and 30% oat-cell (anaplastic). They are five times commoner in men than women. About 10% are adenocarcinoma. Alveolar cell carcinoma is very rare.

Aetiological factors

Cigarette smoking. The increased mortality risk of carcinoma of the bronchus has an approximately straight-line relationship with numbers of cigarettes smoked per day (increased risk of death = cigarettes smoked per day, numerically). Stopping smoking decreases the risk by about one-half in 5 years, and to only twice that of non-smokers in 15 years.

Other atmospheric pollution (coal smoke and diesel fumes) may prove to be aetiologically relevant, but quantitatively small compared with cigarettes.

Exposure to chromium, arsenic, radioactive materials or asbestos (which in addition produces interstitial fibrosis and mesotheliomata) is associated with a higher incidence of bronchial carcinoma.

Clinical presentation

The patient is usually, or has been until the onset of his symptoms, a cigarette smoker. Cough or the accentuation of an existing cough is the commonest early symptom, and haemoptysis the next. Dyspnoea, central chest ache or pleuritic pain, or slowly resolving chest infection are common early manifestations. The patient may present with metastatic deposits involving brain, bone, liver, skin, kidney, adrenal glands or other site, or symptoms from local extension (superior vena cava obstruction, Horner's syndrome, Pancoast syndrome, hoarseness, cervical lymph glands, dysphagia, cardiac arrhythmia or effusion). Occasionally patients are 'picked up' on routine chest X-ray.

The presence of systemic and non-specific symptoms usually (but not always) implies late or possibly inoperable disease, i.e. anorexia, weight loss and fatigue.

Blood and marrow — Anaemia (often normochromic, normocytic or haemolytic). Polycythaemia is uncommon.

Neuromuscular — Dementia (due to cerebral secondaries or rarely cortical atrophy), cerebellar syndrome, mixed sensorimotor peripheral neuropathy, proximal myopathy, polymyositis (page 98) and a myasthenic syndrome (page 100).

Skin, connective tissue, bone — Clubbing, hypertrophic pulmonary osteoarthropathy, dermatomyositis and acanthosis nigricans.

Endocrine — Syndromes due to ectopic hormone production, the pituitary-like ones (ACTH, ADH, prolactin) usually from oat-cell tumours, and parathyroid hormone from squamous cell tumours. Hypercalcaemia may be due to bone secondaries.

Cardiovascular — Atrial fibrillation (local extension) and migratory thrombophlebitis. Pericarditis.

Diagnosis

Chest X-ray:

— the tumour may be visible often as a unilaterally enlarged hilum or peripheral circular opacity occasionally cavitated

— collapse/consolidation due to bronchial obstruction by the tumour

— effusion, raised hemidiaphragm of phrenic paralysis, and bone erosion suggest local extension

Tomography may show the tumour better and demonstrate bronchial narrowing.

Exfoliative cytology may be diagnostic.

Bronchoscopy with biopsy are performed if possible. This may provide a histological diagnosis. The site of the tumour is a guide to operability (not less than 2 cm from the carina).

Treatment

Surgery offers the only 'cure'—15–20% of all cases are resectable and only 30% of these survive 5 years. Surgery is contraindicated by metastasis, local spread and inadequate respiratory function.

Radiotherapy is valuable for relief of distressing symptoms (effusions, haemoptysis, mediastinal compression, and relief of pain produced by bony secondaries). Cancer chemotherapy may also relieve symptoms, especially of mediastinal obstruction and effusions.

Bronchial adenoma

This rare tumour is usually benign but locally invasive. Ninety per cent are histologically 'carcinoid' tumours but only a few cases present with the carcinoid syndrome (page 137). They usually present with cough and haemoptysis. The tumour may either occur (*a*) anywhere within the thoracic cavity and appear as a well circumscribed peripheral mass on chest X-ray, or (*b*) in the major bronchi and appear as a pedunculated intrabronchial mass seen bronchoscopically. The tumours are removed in view of the risk of neoplastic change.

Sarcoidosis

This is a disease of unknown aetiology. It appears to be a systemic granulomatous reaction to various stimuli which may involve any tissue. It most commonly affects the lungs, mediastinal lymph nodes and skin.

Clinical presentation

Pulmonary sarcoid

Most commonly it presents as an acute syndrome in young people (20–40 years) with fever, malaise and lassitude, erythema nodosum (sarcoid is the most common cause in this country), polyarthralgia, usually of the ankles and knees, and mediastinal hilar lymphadenopathy. Dyspnoea is not usually a feature of this acute form which is self-limiting (2 months to 2 years).

Less commonly and more seriously it may present as a chronic insidious disease with respiratory symptoms of cough and progressive dyspnoea. There may be malaise and fever. Progressive pulmonary fibrosis may develop.

Non-pulmonary sarcoid

Apart from erythema nodosum this is relatively uncommon and causes:

Skin. Erythema nodosum in the acute syndrome; infiltration of scars; lupus pernio.

Hypercalcaemia: occurs in about 10% of patients with sarcoidosis and may be the presenting abnormality (page 161). Hypercalciuria is even more common (up to 50%). This is probably due to an excessive sensitivity to vitamin D and responds to steroids.

Eyes. Uveitis and keratoconjunctivitis sicca. Blindness may result.

Parotitis.

Hepatosplenomegaly.

Generalised lymphadenopathy.

Bone and joints, producing cystic lesions most commonly in the phalanges.

Nervous system, causing isolated cranial nerve lesions and peripheral neuropathy.

Endocrines, producing diabetes insipidus from pituitary involvement.

Investigation

Chest X-ray usually shows bilateral hilar gland enlargement, or less commonly parenchymal mottling or diffuse fibrosis.

The Mantoux test is usually negative (70%): a positive test is thus not uncommon but a strongly positive test very unusual.

Kveim test (subcutaneous innoculation with 0·1 ml splenic homogenate from a previous case of sarcoid). The skin becomes indurated and biopsy of the papule at 4–6 weeks shows characteristic sarcoid granulo-

mata. False negative reactions occur in up to 25%, possibly due to poor antigen.
Hypercalcaemia may be present and if so this returns to normal with steroids.
Biopsy—blind scalene node biopsy, or biopsy of mediastinal glands at mediastinoscopy may confirm the diagnosis. Liver biopsy may be diagnostically valuable if the liver is enlarged. Bronchial biopsy at bronchoscopy is positive in about 30% of cases.
Polyclonal increase in γ-globulins is non-specific but common.

Management

The differential diagnosis of bilateral hilar lymph node enlargement is from Hodgkin's disease (and other reticulosis), and any deviation of the patient's syndrome from the usual pattern makes a definite diagnosis imperative either by Kveim test or biopsy. Treatment, other than simple analgesics, is usually unnecessary.

Indications for corticosteroids in sarcoidosis (e.g. prednisolone 20 mg daily reducing after 1 month to the minimum dose necessary to suppress activity for 6–12 weeks include):
— progressive lung disease, hopefully to prevent fibrosis. The indication is progressive pulmonary shadowing or increasing breathlessness. The effect of therapy is monitored by symptoms, chest X-rays and lung function tests including blood gas analysis for $P\text{O}_2$
— hypercalcaemia
— when vital organs are threatened, e.g. eyes, nervous system, kidneys and heart

Prognosis of pulmonary sarcoid

The chest X-ray remains abnormal in about half of all cases (table 17). Clinical disability due to the disease is much less common and is related to:
— age—the younger, the better
— presence of erythema nodosum where over 95% recover by 1 year
— extent of extrapulmonary involvement. Bone or chronic skin lesions indicate chronicity and the worst prognosis
— extent of intrathoracic involvement
— the acuteness of the attack

NB In systemic sarcoidosis, the activity and clinical course of the disease in any one tissue (e.g. skin,

TABLE 17 Prognosis of pulmonary sarcoid

	Recovery	
Chest X-ray appearance	*X-ray*	*Clinical*
Hilar lymphadenopathy alone	75%	90%
Hilar lymphadenopathy with fine pulmonary reticular-nodular shadowing	50%	60%
Coarse reticular-nodular shadowing or fibrosis	30%	30%

eyes) is a guide to the activity in any tissue less easily observed (e.g. lungs).

Tuberculosis

Infection with the acid alcohol fast bacillus (AAFB) of *Mycobacterium tuberculosis* affects predominantly the lungs, lymph nodes and gut. Some features of the disease vary with the patient's sensitivity to tuberculin.

Primary tuberculosis

This is the syndrome produced by infection with AAFB in non-sensitive patients, i.e. in those who have not previously been infected. There is a mild inflammatory response at the site of infection (subpleural in the mid-zones of the lungs, in the pharynx, or in the terminal ileum), followed by spread to the regional lymph nodes (hilar, cervical and mesenteric respectively). One to two weeks following infection, with the onset of tuberculin sensitivity, the tissue reaction changes at both the focus and in the nodes, to the characteristic caseating granuloma. The combination of a focus with regional lymph node involvement is called the 'primary complex'. Patients are usually symptomless. The complex heals with fibrosis and, frequently, calcifies without therapy. The enlarged lymph node may, however, be obvious in the neck or cause obstruction to a bronchus with consequent collapse-consolidation. Blood dissemination of the AAFB may occur rarely from the primary complex to cause widespread miliary disease especially in infants.

Secondary tuberculosis (post-primary)

This is the syndrome produced by infection with AAFB in the previously infected and therefore tuberculin-sensitive patient. Reactivation (or reinfection) is thus followed by an immediate brisk granulomatous response which tends to localise the disease and regional lymph node involvement is uncommon. As with primary tuberculosis, the lesion may

— heal with fibrosis (and calcification)

— rupture into a bronchus giving tuberculous bronchopneumonia

— spread via the blood to produce miliary tuberculosis of liver, spleen, lungs, choroid, bones and/or meninges.

Presenting features Symptoms occur relatively late and in established disease. The earliest are non-specific such as malaise, fatigue, anorexia and weight loss. Of more specific symptoms, the most common is cough often with mucoid sputum. Other symptoms include repeated small haemoptysis, pleural pain, slight fever or occasionally exertional dyspnoea. Frequently the diagnosis is made presymptomatically on routine chest radiography. Erythema nodosum (page 252) does occur in pulmonary tuberculosis but is more commonly the presenting symptom of sarcoidosis (page 210). Signs also occur late in the disease and are not very specific, e.g. crepitations (usually apical) and later signs of consolidation, pleural effusion or cavitation.

Diagnosis

Diagnosis depends, in part, on clinical suspicion which should be particularly high in high-risk groups, for instance:

— the hostel-dwelling 'down-and-out', and the alcoholic

— Pakistani, Indian and Irish immigrant (glandular tuberculosis is common in Indians and Pakistanis)

— diabetics

— patients on immunosuppressive therapy (steroids or cytotoxic drugs)

— occupations at risk—doctors and nurses

Ideally the diagnosis is made by repeated examination for AAFB in sputum and gastric washings on direct smear, by culture on Lowenstein-Jensen medium, and by guinea pig innoculation. Six to twelve specimens (or more) may be required. Sometimes the diagnosis can only be made radiologically and activity is suggested by:

— changing 'soft' shadows

— progression of apical lesions

— cavitation

Tuberculin sensitivity (Mantoux, Heaf, or Tine testing) may be helpful particularly in the young. A repeated negative test after 6 weeks is strongly against a diagnosis of tubercle.

It may be necessary to treat on clinical grounds alone and response to PAS and INAH in 2 weeks is taken as proof of diagnosis.

NB AAFB on smear may not be pathogenic mycobacteria, particularly in urine specimens.

Management

Isolate and rest patients who are sputum-positive (this is standard practice in Britain but the Madras trials suggest that neither may be necessary).

Investigate family and social contacts for infection (or via the local medical officer of health) by chest X-ray and tuberculin sensitivity (Mantoux or Heaf) immediately and 6 weeks later, then:

— if both tests are negative, give BCG, check for conversion and follow up 3-monthly for 2 years

— if the initial test is negative and the 6-week test positive this indicates recent infection. These patients are treated with two antituberculous drugs (PAS and INAH) for 18 months to 2 years unless primary resistance is discovered in the contact

— if the initial tuberculin test is positive, give INAH for 1 year to children under 7 years not previously innoculated with BCG, and follow up all other patients 3-monthly for 2 years and then annually for 3 years

Start therapy if AAFB are detected in sputum. If the clinical suspicion of tuberculosis is high but the sputum smear is negative, collect sputa or gastric washings for culture and guinea pig innoculation and start triple therapy with the first-line drugs:

Rifampicin 450–600 mg daily (or PAS 12 g/day)
INAH 300 mg/day
Streptomycin 1 g/day

Therapy should be started with 3 weeks in hospital to assess the patient's tolerance to the drugs. Continue triple therapy until sensitivities are reported (6–8 weeks). If the organism is sensitive to PAS (or rifampicin) and INAH, stop streptomycin and continue PAS (or rifampicin) and INAH for 1½–2 years with 3–6 monthly follow-up, radiographic and clinical. The patient's sputum is tested regularly to detect relapse (failure to take drugs is the most common reason).

Major drug complications

PAS	Nausea, vomiting and skin rash
Rifampicin	Liver disease (not severe)
INAH	Peripheral neuropathy and encephalopathy—these are extremely rare and respond to pyridoxine, often given prophylactically.
Streptomycin	Vertigo and nerve deafness. In the elderly and in the presence of raised blood urea, the dose is reduced to 0·75 g or 0·5 g daily to maintain blood levels of 1–2 μg/ml

Second-line drugs and major complications

Ethambutol	Visual field defects
Ethionamide	Nausea and vomiting; hepatotoxic
Pyrazinamide	Hepatotoxic (severe)
Cycloserine	Neurotoxicity with confusion and depression

NB Five per cent of patients in this country are resistant to one or more of the primary drugs.

Sputum conversion, if the organism is sensitive, occurs in:

50% of patients at 1 month
80% of patients at 3 months
95% of patients at 6 months

after therapy is begun.

Corticosteroids

May be used in miliary tuberculosis; severely ill tuberculous patients at the onset of chemotherapy; tuberculous meningitis, hopefully to prevent fibrosis. The value of steroids other than when life is immediately threatened, remains uncertain and they probably do not effect long-term morbidity.

Occupational lung diseases

These may be due to mineral dusts, organic dusts, irritant gases or, rarely, bacteria.

Pneumoconiosis (the dust diseases)

These are:
— coal pneumoconiosis
— silicosis in rock drilling and crushing but also occurs in coalminers
— asbestosis in insulation workers; this can produce fibrosis, carcinoma, and pleural mesothelioma
— benign (no fibrosis). These are radiographic diagnoses made in the light of the patient's known occupational hazards, the shadows are due to the

metals themselves e.g. siderosis (iron) and stannosis (tin). All are rare

Clinical features

In the early stages there are no symptoms but X-ray changes occur; later there is dyspnoea on exertion, cough, sputum and attacks of bronchitis. Pulmonary massive fibrosis may occur and Caplan's syndrome occurs in association with rheumatoid arthritis. The patients may eventually develop cor pulmonale.

Asthma

Immediate: type I (reaginic) usually atopic subjects handling objects with organic dust, e.g. feathers, furs and wool.

Late: type III (see below) precipitin-mediated. This results in the dyspnoea rather than true 'asthma' of extrinsic allergic alveolitis.

Irritant gases

May give acute pulmonary oedema.

Extrinsic allergic alveolitis

Inhalation of organic dusts may give a diffuse allergic (type III precipitin-mediated) reaction in the alveoli and bronchioles.

Aetiology

Exposure to mouldy hay (*Micropolyspora faeni*) causes farmer's lung, to mouldy sugar cane causes bagassosis, to mushroom dust causes mushroom picker's lung, to bird droppings (containing avian serum proteins) causes bird breeder's lung, to contaminated malting barley (*Aspergillus clavatus*) causes malt worker's lung and to pituitary snuff (containing foreign serum protein) causes pituitary snuff taker's lung. Precipitating antibodies against the offending antigen can be found.

Clinical features

Acute (i.e. 4–6 hours after exposure) Dyspnoea, dry cough, malaise, fever and limb pains occur, and examination shows fine inspiratory crepitations with little wheeze. The symptoms subside in 2–3 days.
Chronic After repeated acute attacks fibrosis occurs with finger clubbing, persistent inspiratory crepitations, respiratory failure and cor pulmonale.

Investigation

Chest X-ray shows a diffuse haze initially and later micronodular shadowing develops progressing to honeycombing and cor pulmonale. Ventilatory function tests initially show an obstructive picture during the acute attacks but as the chronic disease develops a restrictive pattern is produced.

Pulmonary embolism

Emboli usually arise in the veins of the pelvis or legs and rarely from the right atrium. They occur more frequently:
— following (after about 10 days) surgery or trauma, especially to the pelvis and legs (including Caesarian section)
— following venous stasis during prolonged bed rest, particularly in the obese, in heart failure and following myocardial infarction

— in pregnancy and in patients on the 'pill' (especially the high oestrogen pills)
— possibly more common in people of blood group A

About 50% of those who die from pulmonary embolism have had premonitory signs and symptoms of small emboli or venous thrombosis in the preceding week. A deep vein thrombosis should be regarded as a potential pulmonary embolus and must be suspected, diagnosed and treated early.

Diagnosis of deep vein thrombosis is made on one or more of the following findings:

Tenderness between the heads of the gastrocnemius where the thrombosed vein may be palpable.
Stiffness of the calf muscles (increased turgor).
Delayed cooling of the involved limb on exposure.
There may be tenderness at the saphenous opening.
Oedema, cyanosis and engorged superficial veins are late signs. Homan's sign is neither specific nor sensitive.

Diagnosis is confirmed by increased ^{125}I fibrinogen uptake over the blood clot, ultrasound, or venography. Thromboses which extend above the knee are more likely to produce clinically recognisable pulmonary emboli.

Clinical presentation

This depends upon the size of the embolus:

Small

Transient faints and dyspnoea, with slight pyrexia.

Medium

Usually result in infarction and produce, in addition, haemoptysis, pleurisy and occasionally a pleural effusion.

Large

(Affecting over 60% of the pulmonary bed.) Acute cor pulmonale with sudden dyspnoea and shock. There is a small-volume rapid pulse, with hypotension, cyanosis, peripheral vasoconstriction and a raised jugular venous pressure. There may be a gallop rhythm.

Investigation

Chest X-ray to demonstrate:
—pulmonary oligaemia of the affected segment (usually present but difficult to diagnose except in retrospect)
— the corresponding pulmonary artery is sometimes dilated at the hilum
— small areas of horizontal linear collapse, usually at the bases, with a raised diaphragm
— a small pleural effusion

With larger emboli, the heart enlarges acutely and the superior vena cava distends.

ECG changes usually occur only with larger emboli but are then common. The characteristic changes are (see also page 62):
— tachycardia
— right ventricular 'strain' pattern-inverted T waves in leads V_{1-4}

— acute, often transient, right bundle branch block pattern

— S_1, Q_3, T_3 pattern

— transient arrhythmias, e.g. atrial fibrillation

Arterial blood gases With larger emboli, a fall in Po_2 is common.

Lung scan is a useful non-traumatic investigation in doubtful cases and may show underperfusion of one or more parts of the lung which are radiologically normal.

Pulmonary angiography is the most precise but also most traumatic investigation.

Treatment

Prophylaxis pre- and post-operatively and in patients confined to bed or with predisposing disorders (e.g. cardiac failure) with regular leg exercises. Low-dose subcutaneous heparin may reduce the incidence of deep venous thrombosis following major surgery.

For established deep vein thrombosis or pulmonary embolism, anticoagulate with heparin and warfarin—for 6 weeks in the first instance depending upon whether a non-recurring cause for the deep vein thrombosis (e.g. surgery) was present or not.

In massive pulmonary embolism, cardiac massage and correction of acidosis plus urgent intravenous heparin may improve survival. With large emboli, oxygen in high concentration and thrombolytic therapy with urokinase or streptokinase may be valuable. Morphine may be necessary. The operative removal of large emboli with bypass surgery may be lifesaving and may reduce the risk of long-term pulmonary hypertension if the patient survives.

Pneumothorax

Aetiology

Spontaneous. This is the most common type and usually occurs in normal thin young men following rupture of a small subpleural bulla. The history is of the sudden onset of one-sided pleuritic pain and/or dyspnoea. Dyspnoea rapidly increases in tension pneumothorax and the patient becomes cyanosed. The classical signs are of diminished movement on the affected side with deviation of the trachea to the other side. There is hyperresonance to percussion and reduced pulmonary sounds (breath sounds, tactile fremitus and vocal resonance). All pneumothoraces are best diagnosed by seeing a lung edge on X-ray (which may also show underlying disease). Conditions predisposing to pneumothorax include:

Ruptured emphysematous bulla.

Tuberculosis—often with a small effusion.

Bronchial asthma.

Other extremely rare causes include staphylococcal pneumonia, carcinoma, and occupational lung disease.

Management (of spontaneous pneumothorax)

Often no therapy is required if the pneumothorax is small. Spontaneous recovery occurs in 3–4 weeks. Indications for aspiration of air are:

— tension pneumothorax (an acute emergency)
— severe dyspnoea
— collapse of more than 50% of the total lung field on chest X-ray

Insert an intercostal tube with a water seal. When the lung is re-expanded X-ray the chest. Clip off the tube for 24 hours, then re-X-ray the chest. If the lung is still expanded the tube may be removed.

Rarely, a continuing air leak persists from the lung into the pleural space (bronchopleural fistula). Pleurodesis with defibrinated blood, camphor in oil or surgical pleurectomy may be required.

Haemoptysis

Aetiology

Bronchial carcinoma (or rarely other vascular tumours)
Tuberculosis (active or healed). NB Aspergilloma
Pulmonary embolism with infarction
Bronchiectatic cavities or chronic bronchitis
Mitral stenosis
Foreign body
Infection (pneumococcal pneumonia, *Mycoplasma pneumoniae*, lung abscess and *Klebsiella pneumoniae*)
The presence of chronic bronchitis, a common cause of slight haemoptysis, does not exclude any of the above.

Investigation

The usual clinical problem is to exclude carcinoma and tuberculosis. A full history and clinical examination will usually identify pulmonary infarction, foreign body, bronchiectasis, mitral stenosis and pulmonary oedema.
Chest X-ray.
Sputum for culture, including tuberculosis and malignant cells.
Bronchoscopy with biopsy—this is essential in all patients suspected of early bronchial carcinoma which is amenable to surgery only if diagnosed early.
Isotope lung scans for suspected pulmonary embolism.
Bronchography for suspected bronchiectasis may be diagnostic.

NB About 40% of patients with haemoptysis have no demonstrable cause. Patients who have had a single small haemoptysis, no other symptoms, and a normal chest X-ray, probably do not require further investigation, but a follow-up appointment with a chest X-ray is advisable after 1–2 months. Patients who have more than one small haemoptysis should be regarded as having carcinoma or tuberculosis until proved otherwise.

'Hysterical' dyspnoea

Breathlessness in the absence of abnormal clinical signs and increased by emotion (e.g. clinical examination and ward rounds) should never be described as psychogenic until the following diagnoses have been excluded:

— early pulmonary congestion of left ventricular failure
— 'silent' multiple pulmonary emboli (lung scan may be diagnostic)
— lymphangitis carcinomatosa
— interstitial fibrotic pulmonary infiltrations
— metabolic acidosis (e.g. uraemia, diabetic ketosis)
The chest X-ray may appear normal in all of these at the time of presentation.

The hyperventilation syndrome may be the presenting symptom of psychiatric disease and the patient should be asked about symptoms of depression and enquiries made about his pre-morbid personality. The breathlessness is usually episodic and not directly related in degree to exertion (often even occurring at rest). There are associated symptoms of hypocapnia (tingling in the fingers, dizziness, headache, heaviness in the chest, cramp). Frank tetany may occur with carpopedal spasm. Spirometry usually gives a disorganised trace but the FEV is usually normal when obtained.

Fibrosing alveolitis (diffuse interstitial pulmonary fibrosis)

Clinical features

The disease begins in middle age and presents with progressive dyspnoea and dry cough usually without wheeze or sputum. The typical signs are clubbing, cyanosis and crepitations in the mid and lower lung fields.

Investigation

The arterial $P\text{O}_2$ is reduced and hyperventilation may cause a reduction in $P\text{CO}_2$. Spirometry (page 44) demonstrates a restrictive pattern, i.e. a grossly reduced FVC with rapid initial exhalation of this small volume, thus giving a normal or high FEV%.

Chest X-ray shows diffuse bilateral basal nodular/reticular shadowing which extends upwards as the disease progresses. The differential diagnosis of the chest X-ray includes occupational dust lung diseases, sarcoidosis, scleroderma, lymphangitis carcinomatosa, collagen diseases, miliary tuberculosis and histiocytosis X. Clinically the problem is less difficult.

Management

The disease is progressive and, though steroids are usually given, there is little evidence that the course of the disease is altered. The patient eventually dies with severe hypoxia.

Cardiovascular disease

The commonest diseases are atherosclerosis and hypertension, which are associated with ischaemic heart disease and heart failure. Chronic rheumatic heart disease is still fairly common though becoming less so. Congenital heart disease is relatively rare but important because many forms can be treated surgically.

Ischaemic heart disease (IHD)

The disease is usually inferred from a history of cardiac pain (angina of effort) or of myocardial infarction. Less commonly it may present as an arrhythmia or a defect of conduction.

Myocardial ischaemia in the United Kingdom is normally due to atherosclerosis but cardiac pain can also be produced by:

— aortic valve disease (page 228)
— paroxysmal tachycardias
— polyarteritis nodosa, severe anaemia, coronary embolism and cardiomyopathy are all rare causes

Factors associated with coronary atherosclerosis

Sex: men more than women
Age: steady increase with age
Occupation: stress; lack of exercise
Diet
Medical condition: diabetes mellitus, hypertension, hyperlipidaemia, obesity, gout
Cigarette smoking. The excess risk of death is 2–3 times that of non-smokers. However ischaemic heart disease is so common compared with bronchitis and lung cancer that about 50% of all excess deaths attributable to cigarette smoking are due to ischaemic heart disease
Heredity

Angina

Diagnosis

This is a clinical diagnosis. There should be the characteristic four-feature history—site, character, radiation and precipitation/relief (NB effort, food, emotion and cold). There are no specific characteristic physical signs but evidence of the associated factors (see above) should be sought. 'Crescendo angina' refers to angina of increasing severity and frequency with decreasing effort: it may be a pre-infarction syndrome.

Investigations are used to confirm or deny a doubtful or difficult clinical diagnosis. Resting ECG is a safe investigation and an exercise (or an atrial-paced) ECG adds little to the risks though the significance of the changes may be difficult to evaluate. Apex cardiography, ballistocardiography and right heart catheter pressure studies are used at some specialist centres, but their use and significance is disputed. Coronary arteriography has a morbidity and mortality which varies from centre to centre. It may supply unequivocal evidence of arterial narrowing and define its site so that revascularisation procedures may be undertaken.

Management

The patient needs considerable reassurance about symptoms and their implications. He should stop smoking, lose weight and take regular non-strenuous exercise. The diet should be relatively low in cholesterol and saturated fats. Specific hyperlipidaemic syndromes should be treated (page 152).

Sublingual glyceryl trinitrate (0·5 mg) remains the mainstay of therapy. The major side-effect is headache and as many tablets as necessary may be taken. It should be taken for pain and prophylactically before known precipitating events. If attacks are frequent, long-term therapy with β-blocking agents (e.g. propranolol or oxprenolol 40 mg tds) may be valuable.

Anaemia should be investigated and treated.

There is some evidence that clofibrate reduces mortality and reinfarction in patients with angina but this is disputed and its value remains uncertain. (It undoubtedly reduces cholesterol and β-lipoprotein levels.)

Anticoagulants may relieve symptoms of 'crescendo angina'. There is no good evidence that anticoagulants improve prognosis in angina.

NB Hypertension should be treated as the mortality from strokes and renal failure is thereby reduced. The incidence of myocardial infarction is not affected.

Myocardial infarction
(page 50)

The predisposing and precipitating factors are those of atherosclerosis. Infarction may also occur during hypotension (including surgery). The immediate mortality (within 4 weeks) is 30–40% chiefly in the first 48 hours. There is sudden death in 25% mainly from arrhythmias. After recovery from the acute attack, 90% survive 1 year, 70% survive 5 years, and 40% survive 10 years.

Bed rest

The optimum duration of bed rest remains undetermined. There is an increasing tendency to mobilise uncomplicated cases early (after a week) to prevent venous thrombosis and progressive physical weakness. It seems sensible to keep patients in bed for longer if complications are present or fever prolonged. (*Clinical features*, page 50.)

Pain relief and sedation

Morphine and diamorphine are the drugs of choice. Both may produce hypotension. Morphine causes vomiting and diamorphine is preferred for this reason. The dose required is the minimum which will relieve pain (i.e. start with diamorphine 5 mg). Diazepam (5 mg tds) is a suitable sedative.

Oxygen therapy High concentration oxygen is given (except in chronic respiratory failure, page 204). Diuretics may also decrease hypoxia which is usually associated with pulmonary oedema in cardiac failure.

Shock (10% of hospital admissions) and cardiac failure The patient is hypotensive, pale, cold sweaty and cyanosed. Oxygen, digitalis and diuretics are given. Arrhythmias should be treated. A central venous pressure line will guide possible transfusion if hypovolaemia is present. Metaraminol and noradrenaline may raise the blood pressure but tissue perfusion is not improved. The overall mortality is over 70%.

Anticoagulants *Short-term* (until mobile) Anticoagulants are commonly used to reduce the incidence of deep venous and mural thrombosis, but there is no good evidence that mortality is reduced. It seems reasonable to give anticoagulants in cases complicated by cardiac failure, arrhythmias, obesity and after severe infarcts when prolonged bed rest will be necessary.

Long-term The MRC trial showed a marginal benefit in reducing mortality and reinfarction over 2 years, but only in men under the age of 55. Most of the advantage occurred in the first 6 months and many physicians would give anticoagulants for this period of time in young men. This decision is strongly influenced by the accuracy of anticoagulant control available since poor control has a considerable morbidity and mortality.

Arrhythmias Ninety per cent of patients develop arrhythmias.

Sinus tachycardia This may be a sign of early cardiac failure, and digitalisation (possibly with β-blockade) may be necessary. Otherwise, sedate with diazepam.

Supraventricular extrasystoles If infrequent (less than 1 in 10), sedate with diazepam. If frequent, consider digitalisation and β-blockade.

Supraventricular tachycardia (SVT) Firstly try procedures such as carotid massage (unilateral), the Valsalva manoeuvre and swallowing lumps of ice. β-blockade (e.g. practolol), possibly with the addition of digoxin, is frequently effective, and may be used orally if a rapid response is not required. DC cardioversion is used when rapid results are required (e.g. acute heart failure), and following the other procedures mentioned (though preferably not if the patient has been digitalised). If all else has failed, 'over-pacing' can be attempted with a pacing catheter.

Atrial flutter and atrial fibrillation Consider DC cardioversion (with intravenous diazepam sedation) with or without β-blockade. Some physicians prefer digitalisation, but cardioversion then becomes relatively contraindicated because of the risk of ventricular fibrillation.

NB Supraventricular arrhythmias may be caused by digitalis toxicity (serum levels are helpful) particularly if there is hypokalaemia. In this situation, stop the digitalis, give potassium if indicated, and follow with parenteral β-blocker (e.g. practolol, up to 10 mg slowly i.v.). Continue with oral β-blocker.

Sinus or nodal bradycardia This may be due to heavy sedation particularly with morphine or diamorphine. If the rate is less than 50/min, give atropine 0·6 mg i.v. and repeat twice if necessary. If unsuccessful, consider isoprenaline (5 mg in 500 ml of 5% dextrose at 5 drops/min initially) or cardiac pacing. Ventricular extrasystoles may be due to the bradycardia and should not themselves be treated unless they persist after the bradycardia has been corrected.

Heart block First degree: no immediate therapy is required but the patient must be closely monitored.

Second degree (Wenckebach): monitor and consider atropine or isoprenaline (see above). Many physicians would insert a pacing catheter for 'on-demand' pacing. Complete heart block (CHB): atropine and isoprenaline may be helpful while awaiting insertion of a pacing catheter. NB CHB is commoner in inferior myocardial infarctions because the AV nodal artery is a branch of the right coronary artery; CHB complicating anterior infarction is an ominous situation since it implies a very large muscle infarction.

Permanent pacing should be considered in patients who have had Stokes-Adams attacks and those with extensive damage to the bundle.

Ventricular tachycardia or ventricular ectopic beats if they are multifocal, close to the T waves, in pairs or short runs or more frequent than 4 per minute, give lignocaine 50 mg bolus i.v. and repeat up to twice at 5-minute intervals if necessary. If successful continue with a slow lignocaine infusion at 1–2 mg/min. (NB 2 grams lignocaine per 24 hours is about 1½ mg/min.) Boluses of lignocaine can be added to this periodically if full control is not obtained.

After 48 hours control by this regime, procaine amide (500 mg tds) or a β-blocker may be substituted and continued for 6 weeks.

If this is not successful in correcting the tachycardia, give about 50 mEq sodium bicarbonate every 15 minutes and use DC cardioversion under diazepam sedation.

Ventricular fibrillation External cardiac massage with artificial ventilation followed by DC cardioversion and intravenous sodium bicarbonate 50–100 mEq. Follow with a lignocaine drip.

Asystole Blows on the chest may be sufficient stimulus to provoke repeated systole, but if an arterial pulse is not definitely detected, external cardiac massage and artificial ventilation are essential. External pacing may be successful but a transvenous pacing catheter should be inserted as soon as possible.

Asystole may recur. Permanent pacing may be necessary.

NB After successful treatment of cardiac arrest, unless the patient is fully conscious, give dexamethasone 4 mg qds i.v. to reduce cerebral oedema.

Cardiac aneurysm

This is more common than is usually supposed. The features, which may be intermittent, are severe heart failure with gallop rhythm and considerable cardiac enlargement, and abnormal cardiac pulsation (e.g. an impulse at the sternal border). Its presence may be suggested by persistent ST elevation in convalescence.

X-ray screening may show abnormal pulsation (or lack of pulsation) with an abnormal cardiac contour. Cineventriculography may confirm these findings and operation is then indicated in suitable cases. The operative mortality is relatively low.

Discharge from hospital

Under optimal conditions, 3 weeks' rest and medical supervision (not necessarily in an acute ward) will cover the time during which later serious complications (ruptured septum, rupture of papillary muscles) occur. However, discharge at 9–14 days is not associated with increased mortality. The patient should be encouraged to increase activity gradually over about 2 months with regular walks after 1 month (1 mile per day if this is within their exercise tolerance), returning to work after 3 months. Weight must be reduced if necessary and patients should stop smoking. Arduous occupations, or stressful situations, should, if possible, be modified or avoided.

Rheumatic fever

An acute febrile systemic disorder affecting mainly the heart and joints following a streptococcal infection (group A, β-haemolytic), occurring usually between the ages of 5 and 15 years.

Symptoms

Double asterisks denote major criteria, single asterisks minor criteria. The diagnosis is made if there are one major and two minor or two major and one minor.

The disease usually presents with flitting **polyarthropathy or **carditis, the former being more common in adults and the latter in children. Both may be present at the same time but carditis is uncommon over the age of 20. The involved joints may be exquisitely *tender. There may be a history of streptococcal infection of the throat or skin 10–20 days previously. Rarely, children may present with **chorea.

Examination

General

The dominant features are *fever and arthropathy of large joints (small joints may be affected in the elderly) which are exquisitely tender. Erythema nodosum and erythema **marginatum are more common in children. Symmetrical subcutaneous **nodules lying over bony prominences and extensor surfaces occur virtually only in children and their presence probably correlates with severe carditis.

Signs of carditis

Myocarditis: tachycardia, cardiomegaly, heart failure.
Endocarditis: any valve may be involved and cause transient murmurs. A transient mitral diastolic murmur (Carey-Coombs) is the most common. Mitral systolic and aortic murmurs also occur.
Pericarditis: friction rub or small effusion.

Investigation

The *ESR is raised. *ASO titre may be raised or rising (more than 200 units/ml) and *haemolytic streptococci may be isolated from the throat. The *WBC is raised and a hypochromic normocytic anaemia, unresponsive to iron therapy, may develop. The ECG may show *first degree heart block. Almost any rhythm disorder may occur. Chest X-ray may demonstrate progressive cardiac enlargement.

Management

Bed rest.
Immobilise inflamed joints.
Acetylsalicylic acid. The oral dose is 6–12 g/day to achieve blood levels of 30–35 mg/100 ml. Side-effects of nausea, tinnitus and blurring of vision may limit the dosage. The symptomatic response to salicylates is characteristic. Steroids are frequently used with salicylates but there is no evidence that either improves the prognosis.
Penicillin G is given during the acute stages and oral penicillin (125–250 mg bd) continued in those with cardiac involvement for at least 5 years and preferably until 20 years of age to prevent recurrence. Erythromycin is used for patients sensitive to penicillin.
NB Sodium salicylate is best avoided because of the sodium load and because it is a less effective analgesic.

Chronic rheumatic heart disease

Mitral stenosis (MS)

Occurs in 60% of patients following acute rheumatic fever and is four times as common as MI and twice as common as MS and MI combined. Thirty per cent of patients with MS give no history of rheumatic fever. It is four times more common in women than men. It may occur 2 to 20 years after the acute episode of rheumatic fever.

Symptoms

Dyspnoea on exertion and paroxysmal nocturnal dyspnoea of pulmonary oedema
Palpitations or emboli from atrial fibrillation
Haemoptysis (bronchial vein rupture, bronchitis, left ventricular failure, pulmonary embolism)
Recurrent bronchitis
Fatigue and cold extremities from a low cardiac output. Angina may occur rarely

Signs Mitral facies (malar flush).
Arterial pulse: there is a small volume pulse (obstruction to flow at the mitral valve).
Apex: the apex beat is tapping (a palpable first sound). There is a left parasternal heave of right ventricular hypertrophy. There may be a diastolic thrill in severe disease.

Auscultation The mitral first sound is loud because the mitral valve is held wide open by high atrial pressure until ventricular systole slams it shut.
Length of the murmur is proportional to the degree of stenosis. The murmur starts when blood starts to flow through the mitral valve, i.e. when atrial pressure exceeds ventricular pressure. The tighter the stenosis, the higher the atrial pressure and the longer the murmur. In mild cases, exercise tachycardia may bring out the murmur and the patient should lie on his left side.
The presence of an opening snap and loud first sound denotes a pliable valve. If the valve is already rigid this cannot occur. Presystolic accentuation is due to the increased flow through the valve produced by atrial systole and it is, therefore, absent in atrial fibrillation (AF).
NB Some of the signs and symptoms of MS can be given by the Austin Flint murmur associated with AI and by a left atrial myxoma. Both are very rare.

Assessment The *degree of stenosis* is assessed from the severity of the dyspnoea, the duration of the murmur and evidence of the degree of left atrial enlargement on chest X-ray and ECG. The tighter the stenosis the closer is the opening snap to the second sound.
The *mobility of valve* is denoted by the presence of an opening snap and a loud mitral first sound (and absence of valve calcification on the chest X-ray).
Pulmonary hypertension Fatigue, symptoms of right heart failure and a reduction in dyspnoea indicate raised pulmonary vascular resistance. The development of pulmonary hypertension is indicated by right ventricular hypertrophy, a dominant 'a' wave in the jugular venous pressure (unless in atrial fibrillation), a loud pulmonary second sound and pulmonary incompetence.
Presence of other lesions e.g. MI must be noted and assessed particularly if symptoms indicate surgical intervention. AF suggests a greater degree of myocardial disease, which is always present to some degree.
ECG Atrial fibrillation may be present or, if not, the P mitrale of left atrial hypertrophy. Right ventricular hypertrophy may be present
Chest X-ray Left atrial enlargement. Upper lobe venous congestion with septal lines (Kerley B) just above the costophrenic angles may be present with enlargement of the pulmonary arteries. The mitral valve may be calcified. Haemosiderosis in the lung fields is rare.

Echocardiogram This non-invasive technique can help with the diagnosis and evaluation of mitral stenosis.

Complications

Pulmonary oedema (acute)
Right heart failure
Atrial fibrillation (40%)
Systemic embolism (10%)
Subacute infective endocarditis

Management

Prophylactic parenteral penicillin given half an hour before dental treatment, cystoscopy etc. This should be a bactericidal drug other than penicillin if the patient is already on this (e.g. cephaloridine, vancomycin).

No other treatment is indicated in the absence of respiratory symptoms, evidence of enlargement of the left atrium, pulmonary hypertension (normal 25/8 mmHg) or systemic embolism.

Anticoagulation is indicated when atrial fibrillation develops or following systemic embolism. The risk of embolism is increased by a large left atrium or atrial appendage, recent onset of fibrillation or paroxysmal fibrillation, and a low cardiac output.

Valvotomy is usually indicated in the presence of any of these. The operative risk is small (2–5%). Re-stenosis tends to occur (about 2% per year) and requires re-valvotomy, Mitral incompetence may result from closed valvotomy.

Mitral stenosis in pregnancy. Fluid retention in pregnancy may produce a 30% increase in blood volume during the last trimester and may precipitate heart failure in the presence of underlying MS. Valvotomy may be performed *at any time* during pregnancy if indicated by the above criteria. If possible this is best deferred until the last trimester to ensure viability of the fetus. However the cardiac output falls in the last 2 months of pregnancy and most patients who can manage at that time, can go to term.

Mitral incompetence (MI)

This follows fibrosis and shortening of the papillary muscles, chordae tendineae and valve cusps. About 50% are associated with mitral stenosis. It is no more common in women (compare MS).

Aetiology

Rheumatic carditis
Ischaemic papillary muscle dysfunction, particularly after inferior myocardial infarction
Severe left ventricular hypertrophy with dilatation of the mitral ring
Rarely, cardiomyopathy, congenital malformation (Marfan's syndrome), infective endocarditis and rupture of the chordae tendineae

Symptoms

Progressive dyspnoea develops as a result of pulmonary congestion and this is followed by right heart failure. Angina, systemic embolism and haemoptysis are uncommon compared with mitral stenosis. Fatigue and palpitation are common.

Signs Left ventricular hypertrophy and systolic thrill. Auscultation. There is an apical pansystolic murmur, radiating to the left axilla, sometimes with a thrill. The mitral first sound is soft. There may be a third sound (of rapid ventricular filling). A short mid-diastolic flow murmur in severe MI does not necessarily indicate valve stenosis.

NB A late systolic murmur may occur with prolapse of the posterior cusp following myocardial infarction (late because the valve only starts to leak when the ventricular pressure is at its highest).

ECG: left ventricular hypertrophy. P mitrale of left atrial hypertrophy. Atrial fibrillation is less common than in MS.

Chest X-ray: the left atrium and ventricle are enlarged, the former sometimes being enormous.

Complications As with MS, except that infective endocarditis is more common and embolism less common.

Assessment: dominance of lesions in combined MS/MI MS is more likely to be the dominant lesion if the pulse volume is small (in the absence of failure) and if there is no left ventricular hypertrophy. The final decision is made by catheterisation.

Management Prophylactic antibiotics for dental treatment.

Valve replacement is indicated if symptoms are severe and uncontrolled by medical therapy or pulmonary hypertension develops. The operative mortality is 10–20%. Patients with mitral incompetence deteriorate much faster than those with mitral stenosis.

Indications for anticoagulation are systemic embolism and prosthetic valves. Some authorities recommend anticoagulation for all patients with atrial fibrillation.

Aortic stenosis (AS)

Aetiology (of valvular stenosis) Under 60 years: rheumatic or congenital

60–75 years: calcified congenital bicuspid valve, more common in men

Over 75 years: degenerative calcification, more common in women

NB Supravalvar stenosis (associated with 'fish-face' and infantile hypercalcaemia) and subvalvar stenosis (usually due to cardiomyopathy) are both very rare.

Symptoms There may be no symptoms. They usually occur late. The symptoms are angina, syncope (which may be due to the low cardiac output) and dyspnoea. Sudden death is relatively common and symptoms of left ventricular failure may occur.

Signs Slow rising, slow falling, regular pulse ('plateau').

Small pulse pressure (e.g. blood pressure 105/90).

Left ventricular hypertrophy (sustained and heaving apex beat).

An aortic thrill in systole radiating to the carotid arteries favours organic stenosis.
Auscultation. An aortic systolic ejection murmur maximal in the right second intercostal space radiating to neck with a quiet delayed aortic second sound. An ejection click may be present.
NB Non-valvar aortic stenosis: both supravalvar and subvalvar have neither an ejection click nor a post-stenotic dilatation (see *Cardiomyopathy*, page 241).
ECG: left ventricular hypertrophy and sometimes left atrial hypertrophy. Severe stenosis in adults is unlikely if left ventricular hypertrophy is not present.
Chest X-ray: left ventricular enlargement may not be present even in the presence of a prominent apex beat, but when present, its degree is a measure of the severity of the stenosis. The aorta is small and may be dilated distal to the valve (poststenotic dilatation). The aortic valve may be calcified.

Complications

Left ventricular failure
Infective endocarditis (10% of cases)

Management

Observe if symptom-free.
Digitalis and diuretics for heart failure.
Valve replacement (Starr or homograft) is indicated for symptomatic deterioration including syncope, a rapidly enlarging heart and 'strain' on ECG, as soon as failure has occurred or as a result of catheter findings. Catheter studies and angiography are performed to determine the presence of associated disease of the mitral valve and patency of the coronary ostia and the systolic gradient across the valve (surgery considered if more than 50 mmHg).

Aortic incompetence (AI)

Aetiology

Rheumatic carditis and infective endocarditis are the most common causes. Syphilis is a rare cause. Even less common causes include seronegative rheumatoid syndromes (ankylosing spondylitis, Reiter's syndrome, colitis and psoriatic arthropathy), congenital lesions (e.g. Marfan's syndrome, coarctation of the aorta, bicuspid valves) and traumatic rupture.

Atherosclerosis and severe hypertension are of disputed importance.

Symptoms

There are usually none until left ventricular failure with dyspnoea occurs. Angina may be severe and even present at rest, especially in syphilitic aortic incompetence, but is not common.

Signs

The pulse has a 'sharp rise and fall' ('waterhammer' or 'collapsing') and there is a high pulse pressure. The carotid pulsation in the neck may be marked. The left ventricle is hypertrophied and the apex displaced laterally.

There is an immediate blowing diastolic murmur at the left sternal edge maximal in the left third and fourth intercostal spaces, heard best with the patient leaning forwards with the breath held in expiration. The second sound is quiet.

There may be a diastolic murmur at the apex (Austin Flint) which sounds like mitral stenosis. (It is usually organic.)
ECG: left ventricular hypertrophy.
Chest X-ray shows cardiac enlargement.

Prognosis Death occurs 2–3 years after the onset of left ventricular failure.

Management Digoxin and diuretics for heart failure.
Treat underlying endocarditis or syphilis.
Valve replacement should be considered for symptomatic deterioration.

Differential diagnosis of rheumatic from syphilitic aortic incompetence *Rheumatic* 20–40 years old. Angina is rare. There may be associated valve stenosis.
Syphilitic 40–60 years old. Angina occurs in 50% of cases. Calcification of the ascending aorta may be present. The WR is positive in the blood in 70% of cases and CNS signs are present. There is no valve stenosis.

Dominance of lesions in combined rheumatic AS/AI Aortic incompetence is dominant if the pulse volume is high and the pulse pressure collapsing. The left ventricle is hypertrophied and displaced. Aortic stenosis is dominant if the pulse is of small volume (plateau pulse) and the pulse pressure low. The ventricular apex, though hypertrophied, is not necessarily displaced.

Tricuspid incompetence *Rheumatic* Invariably associated with disease of mitral and/or aortic valves (rare).
Functional in congestive heart failure (usually when the jugular venous pressure is over 10 cm) and following pulmonary hypertension in mitral stenosis or in ostium primum atrial septal defect.
Endocarditis in drug addicts.
Giant 'v' waves are present in the jugular venous pulse and there may be jaundice from hepatic congestion (pages 46–47).

Pulmonary stenosis *Congenital* 10% of all congenital heart disease (second in frequency to atrial septal defect) and may follow maternal rubella.
Rheumatic }
Carcinoid } very rare

Symptoms Fatigue and syncope occur if stenosis is severe.

Signs Cyanosis, low volume pulse and a large 'a' wave in the jugular venous pressure. The heart may show right ventricular hypertrophy. There is a systolic thrill and murmur in the pulmonary area (second left intercostal space). The pulmonary component of the second sound is quiet and late.

Congenital heart disease (CHD)

Congenital heart disease may present as an isolated cardiac abnormality or as part of a systemic syndrome.

Maternal rubella

It is dangerous in the first 3 months of pregnancy (particularly the first month—50% of fetuses are affected). The cardiac lesions are in three groups:
— patent ductus arteriosus
— septal defects: ASD, VSD, Fallot's tetralogy
— right-sided outflow obstruction: pulmonary valve, artery or branch stenoses

The systemic syndrome includes cataract, nerve deafness and mental retardation.

If a pregnant woman is in contact with rubella, she should be given γ-globulin and serum taken for antibody levels to rubella. If raised, this is evidence of previous infection and there is little or no risk to the fetus. If the titre is not raised, a repeat sample is measured 3–4 weeks later (or if symptoms appear in the mother) and if the titre has risen significantly, this is evidence of recent infection. The earlier the pregnancy the greater the risk to the fetus.

Mongolism (21-trisomy)

Associated with septal defects, particularly ventricular.

Turner's syndrome (XO)

Associated with coarctation of the aorta.

Marfan's syndrome

Associated with coarctation of the aorta, AI, ASD, MI, aortic aneurysms and aortic dissection.

Working classification

An asterisk denotes the most frequent.

Stenosis

Semilunar valves: AS (supra- and sub-valvar and valve stenoses), PS*
Atrioventricular valves: MS, TS, Ebstein
Major arteries: coarctation of aorta*, pulmonary artery stenosis

Incompetence

Semilunar valves: AI, PI
Atrioventricular valves: MI, TI

Shunts

Left to right: ASD*, VSD*, PDA*, anomalous pulmonary venous drainage, aorta-pulmonary window
Right to left (cyanotic): transposition of the great vessels (frequent but die at birth), Fallot's tetralogy*, Eisenmenger's syndrome

Atrial septal defect (ASD)

Twenty per cent of congenital heart disease. Associated with Marfan's syndrome.
Ostium secundum (95% of ASDs) is usually uncomplicated. Compared with congenital heart defects, there is a high (late) incidence of atrial fibrillation (20%) and an extremely low incidence of endocarditis.
Ostium primum (5% of ASDs) is often complicated

because it tends to involve the atrioventricular valves and produces mitral and tricuspid incompetence and even an associated VSD. In most respects (embryology, cardiodynamics, complications and prognosis) it is quite different from ostium secundum ASD.

Symptoms

In simple lesions there are usually no symptoms though bronchitis occurs in 10% of cases. Symptoms usually occur for the first time in middle age. It is usually detected at routine chest X-ray.

Signs

The precordium may be deformed. The pulse volume may be small. There may be a left parasternal lift of right ventricular hypertrophy and a palpable pulmonary artery. Flow through the defect does not itself produce a murmur but increased right heart output may give a flow murmur of pulmonary stenosis (louder on inspiration). Characteristically there is a fixed wide split of the second sound. In ostium primum there may be signs of the associated lesions (TI and MI) and a mitral diastolic murmur is not uncommon.

ECG Ostium secundum: right axis deviation and right ventricular hypertrophy with partial right bundle branch block. Atrial fibrillation may occur. Ostium primum: there is usually left axis deviation with evidence of right ventricular hypertrophy. Conduction defects and nodal arrhythmias may occur.

Chest X-ray Enlargement of the right atrium and ventricle with enlarged pulmonary arteries and plethoric lung fields (evidence of increased right-sided flow). The aorta is hypoplastic (evidence of decreased left-sided blood flow).

Complications

Pulmonary hypertension may lead to flow reversal through the defect (Eisenmenger's syndrome).
Atrial fibrillation.
Tricuspid incompetence (from right ventricular enlargement).
Infective endocarditis occurs in ostium primum defects.

Management

Ostium secundum: operate if pulmonary-systemic flow ratio is more than 2:1.
Ostium primum: operate for symptoms or for cardiac enlargement with mitral incompetence.
NB Eisenmenger's syndrome contraindicates surgery.

Patent ductus arteriosus (PDA)

Ten per cent of all congenital heart disease. It is associated with the rubella syndrome. It is commoner in females.

Symptoms

Usually there are none. Bronchitis and dyspnoea on exertion occur with severe lesions.

Signs

The pulse may be collapsing (waterhammer). The left ventricle may be hypertrophied. There is a continuous (machinery) murmur with systolic accentua-

tion maximal in the second left intercostal space and posteriorly. This continuous murmur must be distinguished from other causes, i.e. jugular venous hum, MI plus AI, VSD plus AI, pulmonary arterio-venous fistulae.
ECG: normal or there may be left ventricular hypertrophy.
Chest X-ray: left ventricle may be enlarged. The pulmonary artery is enlarged and there is pulmonary plethora.

Complications

'Endocarditis' (of the shunt).
Heart failure (Eisenmenger's syndrome following pulmonary hypertension and shunt reversal).

Management

Surgical ligation (8–12 years). Cyanosis contraindicates surgery.

Ventricular septal defect (VSD)

Eight per cent of congenital heart disease, occurring as an isolated lesion.
Small defect Maladie de Roger, i.e. just the murmur with a normal sized heart, chest X-ray and ECG.
Large defect The clinical importance depends on pulmonary vascular resistance which determines how much shunting is present and its direction of flow.

Symptoms

None unless the VSD is large when there may be dyspnoea and bronchitis.

Signs

There may be a small volume pulse. Left ventricular hypertrophy may be present (and right ventricular hypertrophy if there is pulmonary hypertension). A pansystolic murmur (and thrill) is present in the fourth left intercostal space. A flow murmur of MS may be present, and of PI occurs in the presence of pulmonary hypertension.
ECG: left ventricular hypertrophy.
Chest X-ray: enlargement of the left atrium and ventricle may be present. The pulmonary arteries may be enlarged in pulmonary hypertension.

Complications

Endocarditis in 20–30% with emboli into the pulmonary circulation.
Eisenmenger's syndrome.

Management

Chemoprophylaxis to prevent endocarditis.
Small VSD: these may close spontaneously. Surgery is not indicated for the endocarditis risk alone.
Large VSD: surgery is indicated in most cases to prevent pulmonary hypertension developing. It is contraindicated once Eisenmerger's syndrome has developed.

Fallot's tetralogy

Ten per cent of congenital heart disease and 66% of cyanotic congenital heart disease.

There is a VSD in which the shunt is from right to left because of pulmonary stenosis (infundibular or valvar). The load on the right ventricle results in right ventricular hypertrophy. There is associated dextraposition of the aorta so that it sits over the septum in the defect.

Symptoms

Syncope (20%)
Squatting (this may help to decrease the right to left shunt by increasing systemic resistance)
Dyspnoea
Retardation of growth

Signs

Cyanosis and finger clubbing
The typical murmur is of pulmonary stenosis. P_2 is quiet. There is no VSD murmur.
ECG: usually moderate right atrial and ventricular hypertrophy.
Chest X-ray: there is a large aorta with a small pulmonary artery and pulmonary oligaemia.
Polycythaemia is common.

Complications

Cyanotic and syncopal attacks (sometimes fatal)
Cerebral abscesses (10%)
Endocarditis (10%)
Paradoxical emboli
Strokes (thrombotic—polycythaemia)
Epilepsy is commoner than in the general population.
NB Only 1 in 10 reach 21 years if untreated.

Management

Total correction on cardiopulmonary bypass.
Blalock shunt (uncommonly performed now), i.e. anastomosis of the left subclavian to the left pulmonary artery to increase pulmonary blood flow.

Pulmonary stenosis (PS)

Ten per cent of congenital heart disease. It is usually acyanotic unless it is part of a Fallot's tetralogy (central cyanosis) or is very severe (peripheral cyanosis). The stenosis is usually valvar but may be subvalvar (infundibular).

Symptoms

Even with considerable stenosis there may be no symptoms. Severe stenosis may give dyspnoea, fatigue, angina and syncope.

Signs

The characteristic sign is a pulmonary systolic murmur with or without a thrill. Classically its intensity increases with deep inspiration. Moderately severe stenosis produces a large a wave in the jugular venous pulse, signs of right ventricular hypertrophy and a wide split of the second sound (delayed P_2). Severe stenosis results in a reduced cardiac output with a small volume arterial pulse, peripheral vasoconstriction (with peripheral cyanosis) and P_2 becomes soft.
Chest X-ray: poststenotic dilatation of the pulmonary artery with pulmonary oligaemia when the stenosis is moderately severe or worse.
ECG: degrees of right atrial hypertrophy (P pulmonale) and right ventricular hypertrophy (with 'strain pattern') corresponding to the degree of stenosis (a better guide than the symptoms).

Complications — Endocarditis
Right heart failure

Management — If mild or moderate (right ventricular systolic pressure less than 70 mmHg) observe; if severe, valvotomy (or infundibular resection) is indicated.

Coarctation of the aorta — Ten per cent of congenital heart disease. It is associated with berry aneurysms, Marfan's and Turner's syndromes. Ninety-eight per cent are distal to the origin of the left subclavian artery.

Symptoms — Sixty per cent have none. Forty per cent have symptoms including those of hypertension, stroke, endocarditis and occasionally intermittent claudication.

Signs — There may be radiofemoral delay with a small volume femoral pulse. Blood pressure may be raised in the arms and may be different on the two sides and low in the legs. Asymmetry of radial pulses may be present.
Visible and/or palpable scapular collaterals.
Left ventricular hypertrophy may be present.
The following murmurs may be heard:
— a stenotic murmur at front and back of the left upper thorax
— collateral murmurs over the scapulae
— an aortic systolic murmur (of an associated bicuspid valve in 70% of cases) is usually obscured by the coarctation murmur
ECG: 50% have left ventricular hypertrophy.
Chest X-ray: double aortic knuckle due to stenosis and poststenotic dilatation, rib notching (and at the scapular margin), left ventricular enlargement.

Associations — Bicuspid aortic valve, cerebral artery aneurysms (berry aneurysms), and patent ductus arteriosus.

Prognosis — Ninety per cent die by the age of 40 years from endocarditis, heart failure or cerebrovascular haemorrhage.

Management — Surgical resection. The operative mortality is 5%.

Eisenmenger's syndrome — This refers to the situation in which there is reversal of a left to right shunt (e.g. VSD, ASD, PDA) due to pulmonary hypertension. With left to right shunts there is a pulmonary circulatory overload and an increase in pulmonary vascular resistance may follow with the development of pulmonary hypertension. When the pressure on the right side of the shunt exceeds that on the left side, the shunt flow reverses. The patient becomes cyanosed and deteriorates rapidly with symptoms of dyspnoea, syncope and angina. The lesion must be surgically corrected before this stage is reached.

Infective endocarditis

Acute

This is a rare disease in which the heart valves are infected as part of an acute septicaemia of which the features are swinging fever, rigors, delirium and shock. Healthy valves may be affected. This may follow infection with staphylococcus usually from primary infection of the lungs or skin. *Streptococcus pneumoniae*, *Haemophilus influenzae*, gonococcus and meningococcus may be responsible.

The prognosis is that of the generalised septicaemia unless valve destruction leads in addition to acute intractable cardiac failure.

Subacute

This is usually bacterial and subacute in onset (SBE).

Predisposing abnormalities

Congenital Ventricular septal defect, patent ductus arteriosus, coarctation of the aorta and bicuspid aortic valves may be infected.

NB Atrial septal defect of the secundum (common) variety do not develop endocarditis although the rare primum lesion where the mitral valve is also involved may become infected.

Acquired Any rheumatic valve may be affected, the mitral more than the aortic and mitral incompetence more frequently than mitral stenosis. Syphilitic aortic incompetence and calcified aortic stenosis predispose to endocarditis. It may occur postoperatively following cardiac catheterisation or surgery. The normal tricuspid valve may become involved in mainlining drug addicts.

Organisms

Streptococcus viridans (non-haemolytic) is still the commonest in Britain and the most usual source is the teeth.

Staphylococcus aureus and *albus*.

Streptococcus faecalis especially in young women (abortion) and old men (genitourinary surgery and catheterisation). Other bacteria include gonococcus, brucella and proteus.

Coxiella burnetii (Q fever).

Fungi (monilia, aspergillus, histoplasma).

The origin of infection varies with the infecting organism and includes the teeth and tonsils (*Strep. viridans*), urinary tract (*Strep. faecalis*), cardiac catheterisation (staphylococcus), and the skin (staphylococcus).

Clinical features

The disease classically affects young adults (20–30 yr) with rheumatic valve or congenital heart disease, but is now more commonly recognised in the over fifties.

The symptoms and signs may be considered in three groups:

Signs of general infection Lethargy, malaise, anaemia and low-grade fever are frequent but not invariable (fever is occasionally intermittent or persistently absent). Clubbing of the fingers (50% of cases) and splenomegaly are fairly late signs (6–8 weeks). Occasionally there is transient myalgia and/or arthralgia. 'Café au lait' complexion is now exceedingly rare since it occurs only in the neglected late stage. The white cell count may be raised, normal or low.

Signs of underlying cardiac lesions must be sought. New lesions are highly suggestive as are changing murmurs—the patient must be examined at least daily, and the intensity of the murmurs recorded.

Embolic phenomena Large emboli may travel to the brain and viscera or cause occlusion of peripheral arteries. Emboli from left to right shunts (VSD and PDA) and on the right-sided heart valves (TI and PS) go to the lungs giving pleurisy and lung abscesses. Small emboli may travel to:

— the finger pulp to produce Osler's nodes (pathognomonic)
— the nail bed to produce splinter haemorrhages
— the kidney to produce microscopic haematuria and proteinuria.

The renal lesion in SBE appears to be of two kinds:

— a diffuse acute proliferative glomerulonephritis. The changes are not necessarily associated with streptococcal SBE and also not specifically diagnostic of SBE
— a focal 'embolic' glomerulonephritis in which only a part of the glomerulus is involved. The tissue is sterile on culture

Both the above may be due to precipitation of immune complexes: complement levels are reduced. Rheumatoid factor is present in up to 50%.

Diagnosis

The diagnosis should be considered in any patient with a predisposing cardiac lesion who becomes ill. It may have to be made on the basis of the clinical picture even when unconfirmed by the isolation of the organism from blood culture. The most efficient way to make the diagnosis is:

— repeated examination particularly for changing heart murmurs
— blood culture (at least 6 samples)
— mid-stream urine examination for microscopic haematuria

NB Endocarditis may present with atrial fibrillation in the elderly.

Prognosis

The mortality is 95% in untreated cases. It is still 30% even with modern therapy. One of the commoner complications is valve perforation or incompetence giving rise to heart failure.

Management

Prophylaxis Antibiotics must be given during intercurrent infections and any dental procedures to those at risk. Parenteral benzylpenicillin 1 megaunit ½h preoperatively and then oral penicillin V 250 mg 4 times daily for 3 days. If the patient is on prophylactic penicillin (for rheumatic heart disease) either cephaloridine (0·5 g i.m.) or vancomycin may be given. Good dental hygiene is essential. Prophylactic dental extraction is not indicated in the absence of dental disease.

Chemotherapy It is essential to obtain blood cultures before starting chemotherapy but it should not be delayed longer than 1 week in the presence of good clinical evidence even if cultures are negative. Penicillin G, 10–20 megaunits (6–12 grams) parenterally with or without probenecid, is the drug of first choice. When the results of bacterial sensitivities are available, therapy is guided by this, an attempt being made to achieve serum levels of the antibiotic at least three times the minimal inhibitory concentration (MIC) of the organism. Therapy should be continued for 8 weeks. The patient should be carefully followed for recurrence. Emboli may occur for up to 1–2 months after 'cure'.

Indications for surgery

Surgery must be considered early for intractable cardiac failure, resistant infection particularly of a valve prosthesis, and if the organisms are drug resistant.

'Culture-negative endocarditis'

This diagnosis is considered after 12 successive negative cultures when culture technique is known to be good. The following should be considered:

— unsuspected organisms, e.g. Rickettsiae (Q fever)—especially if the aortic valve is diseased. The diagnosis is dependent upon finding a rise in antibody titre. Bacteroides—anaerobic culture is required (and kept for up to 3 weeks). Fungi—monilia, aspergillus, histoplasma

— partly-treated bacterial cases, including L-forms in those treated only with penicillins

— right-sided endocarditis

— polyarteritis nodosa and atrial myxoma

Acute pericarditis

Aetiology

Pericarditis is common within the first week of acute myocardial infarction. Dressler's syndrome is uncommon and occurs 2 weeks to 2 months after myocardial infarction or cardiac surgery. It is characterised by fever, pleurisy, pericarditis and the presence of antibodies to heart muscle.

Infective pericarditis is usually a complication of chest infection. 'Acute benign pericarditis' affects young men, often follows a respiratory infection and is probably viral. A rising antibody titre to Coxsackie B virus is sometimes found. Suppurative pericarditis is rare. It results from infection with the staphylococcus or occasionally haemolytic streptococcus. Tuberculous pericarditis is very rare and non-suppurative.

Pericarditis may be part of a systemic syndrome: rheumatic fever, severe uraemia, local extension of carcinoma of the bronchus and following trauma. It may be the first indication of systemic lupus erythematosus.

Clinical features

There is central, poorly localised tightness in the chest which varies with movement, posture and respiration. There may be pain referred to the left shoulder if the diaphragm is affected. A pericardial rub is usually present which varies with time, position and respiration.

Pericardial effusion may develop and produce toxaemia (if it is purulent) or cardiac tamponade. The signs of pericardial effusion, without tamponade are an 'absent' apex beat, a 'silent' heart, and disappearance of the rub.

Tamponade, which is rare, produces:

— pulsus paradoxus. The pulse volume decreases in the normal person on inspiration. This is more marked with tamponade and is then known as pulsus paradoxus. The paradox which Kussmaul noted was that the heart continued to beat strongly whilst the peripheral arterial pulse virtually disappeared during inspiration.

— a rise in the jugular venous pressure on inspiration (Kussmaul's sign). Both may be the result of decreased cardiac filling on inspiration due to the descending diaphragm stretching the pericardium and increasing the intrapericardial pressure.

ECG: there is raised concave elevation of the ST segment in all leads (especially II and V_{3-4}) and later T wave inversion. The voltage is low in the presence of effusion.

Chest X-ray: it is unchanged in the absence of effusion. Effusion classically produces an enlarged pear-shaped cardiac shadow with loss of the normal contours.

Management

Aspirate for tamponade (if the systemic pressure falls below 90–100 mmHg). Treat the underlying condition. Steroids are used for lupus erythematosus and in acute benign pericarditis if it is severe or prolonged.

Constrictive pericarditis

It is now very rare in Britain.

Aetiology

Some are due to tuberculosis following spread from the pleura or mediastinal lymph glands. Others follow acute viral or pyogenic pericarditis. Haemopericardium, irradiation and carcinoma account for the rest. It never follows acute rheumatic fever. It may be simulated by cardiomyopathy (page 241).

Clinical features

Symptoms appear from a few weeks to 30 years after a primary tuberculous infection. They result from cardiac constriction with decreased filling and a low cardiac output. Fatigue and ascites with little or no ankle swelling are characteristic, but dyspnoea and ankle swelling may occur later. Pulmonary oedema and paroxysmal noctural dyspnoea are rare.

Examination

The pulse is rapid and the volume is small. Atrial fibrillation is present in 30% of cases. The jugular venous pressure is raised and rises further on inspiration (Kussmaul's sign). There is diastolic collapse of the jugular venous pressure (steep y descent). The liver is enlarged and ascites may be present. Ventricular contraction may cause localised indrawing of the chest wall at the apex. The heart sounds are quiet and a third (ventricular) sound may be present. There is no rub.

ECG: there may be widespread ST changes or low voltage complexes.

Chest X-ray: there is calcification of the pericardium (seen best in the lateral film) in 50% of the cases which are secondary to tuberculosis.

Management

No action is needed if the patient is symptom-free and the tuberculosis inactive. Pericardiectomy may be required if severe constriction is present. Diuretics and salt restriction are given for ascites and oedema.

Syphilitic aortitis and carditis

It is now very rare in Britain. Acquired syphilis affects the aorta, the aortic ring to produce dilatation or aneurysm, and aortic incompetence, and the coronary artery orifices to cause angina.

NB Congenital syphilis does not produce aortitis.

Pathology

Endarteritis and occlusion of the vasa vasorum of the aortic muscle wall which becomes degenerate and fibrotic. Atheromatous plaques form over the damaged areas.

Aortic incompetence

The symptoms are similar to those of rheumatic aortic incompetence (see above for differential diagnosis). It is often gross with no haemodynamic stenosis (though there may be a systolic murmur).

Syphilitic angina

Fifty per cent of patients with syphilitic aortitis are affected. The angina is severe, attacks are long, often nocturnal, and respond poorly to glyceryl trinitrate.

Syphilitic aneurysms

Ascending aorta This is the 'aneurysm of signs' with evidence of gross aortic incompetence, local pulsation and systolic bruit and thrill in the second or third right interspace, marked carotid pulsation in the neck, signs of superior vena cava obstruction if the aneurysm is sufficiently large, and dilatation and calcification of the ascending aorta.

Arch of aorta This is the 'aneurysm of symptoms' as it compresses the trachea and recurrent laryngeal nerve to produce cough, the left bronchus to produce collapse of the left lower lobe, the vertebrae producing erosion and pain, and occasionally the oesophagus causing dysphagia. Horner's syndrome may result from compression of the sympathetic trunk, and the left radial pulse may be absent due to compression of the left subclavian artery.

Abdomen These are usually atheromatous and rarely due to syphilis. They present as pulsating abdominal masses.

Cardiomyopathy

This word means 'disorder of heart muscle'. It is usually used to describe two clinical syndromes. (NB Some physicians restrict the use of the word to primary cardiomyopathies, i.e. to those cardiomyopathies 'of unknown cause or association'.)

Hypertrophic cardiomyopathy

Previously known as HOCM or hypertrophic obstructive cardiomyopathy. It is sometimes familial. It appears to be a single specific disease entity in which there is an abnormality of the myocardial cell resulting in:

— loss of left ventricular distensibility which leads to symptoms of dyspnoea, pulmonary oedema and syncope. Some patients develop angina.

— hypertrophy particularly of the left ventricle which leads to a subvalvar aortic stenosis and mitral incompetence. This may disappear with progression of the disease in some patients as the heart muscle fails.

Signs

When aortic outflow obstruction is present, there is a steep-rising jerky pulse (unlike the slow-rising plateau pulse of aortic valve stenosis), cardiac hypertrophy and a late systolic aortic ejection murmur, usually heard best in the left third and fourth intercostal spaces. There may be associated signs of mitral incompetence. Complications include atrial fibrillation, systemic embolism and congestive heart failure.

Management

β-adrenergic blockade may be very effective in reducing outflow obstruction. If the patient develops atrial fibrillation, anticoagulants and digoxin may be added. (NB Digitalis may exacerbate any obstruction by increasing the efficacy of contraction.) Surgical relief of obstruction is probably now seldom indicated. Patients are at risk from endocarditis.

Congestive cardiomyopathy

Previously known as COCM. This is very rarely familial.

The label 'congestive cardiomyopathy' covers a large group of aetiologically unrelated disorders which tend to present as low-output congestive heart failure. By convention the more common and more easily diagnosed myocardial disorders are excluded, i.e. ischaemic, hypertensive and rheumatic heart diseases.

Angina (10%), conduction defects and arrhythmias occur.

Aetiology

Unknown (idiopathic): this is determined by the elimination of the following causes.
Alcoholism and thiamine deficiency (beri-beri).
Infections: viruses, e.g. influenza A_2, Coxsackie B, toxoplasma, diphtheria.
Infiltrations: sarcoidosis, amyloidosis (primary and secondary to myeloma), haemochromatosis.
Collagen disease: systemic lupus erythematosus, polyarteritis nodosa, diffuse systemic sclerosis.

Muscular dystrophies and Friedreich's ataxia.
Endocrine: hyper- and hypo-thyroidism.

Management

Bed rest, digitalis and diuretics form the basis of treatment of the cardiac failure. Any underlying pathology (e.g. thyroid disease, collagen disease) should be treated appropriately.

Hypertension

Introduction

There is no 'normal' blood pressure except in the statistical sense of those which fall within a certain distance of the mean of a 'normal' population. However, even within this 'normal' range (down to 100/60) the complications normally regarded as characteristic of hypertension have an incidence related to the height of the diastolic pressure.

About 20% of the adult population of the United Kingdom have blood pressures above 160/95.

Hypertension is the most significant risk factor in strokes and heart failure, and in ischaemic heart disease is as important as smoking, obesity or hypercholesterolaemia.

Aetiology

'Essential': 90% of all cases and diagnosed as such by elimination of the following.
Renal disease: chronic glomerulonephritis, chronic pyelonephritis, renal artery stenosis, polycystic disease, polyarteritis nodosa.
Endocrine disease: Cushing's syndrome, Conn's syndrome, phaeochromocytoma, acromegaly.
Eclampsia and pre-eclamptic toxaemia.
Coarctation of the aorta.

Symptoms

The patients are usually symptom-free. There may be a family history of hypertension in essential hypertension.

Signs

There may be no abnormal signs other than the raised blood pressure.

In the heart there may be left ventricular hypertrophy with an aortic ejection murmur and a loud aortic second sound. There may also be signs of coarctation of the aorta.

The optic fundi may show retinopathy. Grades I and II indicate atherosclerosis.

Grade I: arterial narrowing
Grade II: arteriovenous nipping
Grade III: haemorrhages and exudates
Grade IV: grades I–III and papilloedema

In the abdomen there may be the enlarged kidneys of polycystic disease and a bruit from renal artery stenosis.

Complications

Left ventricular failure
Strokes and hypertensive encephalopathy
Renal failure
Myocardial infarction

Retinopathy
Complications of treatment (postural hypotension, hypokalaemia)

Investigation

The degree to which a doctor investigates a patient with hypertension varies with the facilities available, with the patient's age and the degree of hypertension. Any factors pointing to the aetiology will determine some special investigations (e.g. endocrine disease). Otherwise routine investigations are aimed at detecting treatable renal disease, and assessing cardiac and renal function. Repeated measurements of blood pressure are necessary except in severe cases: few physicians will treat a single moderately-raised pressure reading.
Chest X-ray and ECG.
MSU × 2–3 (for cells, casts, proteinuria and evidence of infection).
Blood urea, and electrolytes, and calcium in the presence of renal failure.
24-hour urine sample for creatinine clearance and protein (if proteinuria has been found).
IVP: some physicians would restrict this to those patients who are young and with considerably raised pressures, those who do not respond to drug therapy and those with evidence of renal disease. Rapid sequence films may demonstrate unilateral renal artery stenosis. Contrast medium appears more slowly on the affected side because of a reduced glomerular filtration rate and becomes more concentrated on that side because of the increased tubular water reabsorption.
Radioactive renography (and scan) where available is a simple technique which may give evidence of renal artery stenosis or of outflow obstruction.
Renal arteriography is indicated if surgery might be performed, e.g. in patients with evidence of unilateral renal disease aged under 35 years.
Blood renin and aldosterone levels.

Management

Secondary hypertension

Treat the underlying condition:
— pyelonephritis with antibiotics
— endocrine disease and coarctation surgically
— renal artery stenosis is not often successfully corrected surgically, but this should be considered in patients under 35–40 years of age, particularly if control of the hypertension is difficult

Primary (essential) hypertension

Men develop more hypertensive complications than women. In uncomplicated hypertension, most physicians would always start therapy when repeated diastolic readings are above 100 mmHg in men and 105 mmHg in women. Many would start at 95 mmHg and 100 mmHg respectively.

Treatment may be indicated at lower pressures in the presence of ECG and radiological evidence of cardiac enlargement, or in the presence of other complications.

Hypotensive drugs Methyldopa, bethanidine, guanethidine and debrisoquine are often the drugs of first choice, though they produce variable degrees of postural hypotension and impotence. Reserpine, clonidine and β-blockers are chiefly useful in the young male patient because they do not produce impotence, but reserpine may produce severe depression, and the β-blockers potentiate heart failure and asthma. Hydrallazine produces peripheral vasodilatation and may be useful together with β-blockade or adrenergic nerve blockade.

Diuretics Thiazide diuretics are used to potentiate the action of hypotensive agents. Potassium chloride supplements or potassium-retaining diuretics (e.g. amiloride, spironolactone, triamterene) are usually needed and the serum potassium monitored especially in renal failure. Salt restriction ('no added salt') seems logical in these circumstances and a more severe restriction may be necessary in unresponsive hypertension.

While paying attention to the treatment of hypertension to reduce the risks of cardiovascular disease, it should not be forgotten that there are a number of other risk factors often of equal or greater statistical importance. These include obesity, blood lipid values (cholesterol and triglycerides), cigarette smoking and glucose intolerance. However it is not proven that modification of anything but hypertension and obesity has any definite effect on mortality.

Malignant (accelerated) hypertension and hypertensive encephalopathy

Very rapid reduction of blood pressure (within minutes) is seldom indicated. Bethanidine 10–20 mg, guanethidine 10–20 mg, methyldopa 0·5 g and reserpine 1–5 mg intramuscularly will work within 1–3 hours. Rapid reduction (i.e. in the presence of fits or a rapidly rising blood pressure) may be achieved with diazoxide (150 mg i.v. rapidly repeated up to 600 mg if necessary), hydrallazine (20 mg i.v.) or pentolinium (0·1 mg i.v. slowly, which may be doubled at 5-minute intervals until the desired effect is achieved. The patient should be tilted head-up as blood pressure becomes posture-dependent under the effects of ganglionic or postganglionic blockade). It is best to become familiar with one or two standard drugs.

Prognosis

Mortality from strokes and uraemia is decreased if hypertension is treated. The incidence of myocardial infarction is unaffected. It is better in women than men.

Peripheral arterial disease

There are four common clinical syndromes:

Intermittent claudication

Ninety per cent are males over 50 years of age. The disorder is associated with smoking, very occasionally with hyperlipidaemia (types III and IV) and occasionally precipitated by anaemia. Obstruction may be femoropopliteal (80%), aortoiliac (15%), or distal (5%).

Diagnosis

The history is of pain in the calf on effort with rapid relief by rest. The Leriche syndrome is buttock claudication with impotence. The major peripheral arterial pulses are reduced or absent. There may be arterial bruits over the femoral arteries. The tissues of the leg atrophy (muscle bulk is reduced) and hair loss is common. There may be cyanosis, pallor or redness, oedema, ulcers or gangrene.

(In the reactive hyperaemia test, the legs are elevated 45 degrees with the patient lying down for about 2 minutes and the degree of pallor noted. The patient then sits with the feet hanging down and the time taken for a normal pink colour to reappear is noted. In normal people this occurs within 10 seconds but in those with arterial disease it takes 15 to 60 seconds, the time depending roughly on the severity of the disease. The time taken for the veins to fill in the same test is another indicator of blood flow. In patients with ischaemic disease, a vivid redness may appear perhaps due to vasodilators released in response to the unusual degree of ischaemia produced by raising the legs.)

Prognosis

The symptom indicates generalised vascular disease and 80% die from cardiovascular disease. The prognosis is similar to that of angina or myocardial infarction. Leg gangrene is uncommon.

Management

Exercise within the effort tolerance to help to develop collateral vessels.
Stop smoking.
Treat obesity, hypertension and hyperlipidaemia, despite the lack of firm evidence that this affects the prognosis: a positive attitude to therapy is itself reassuring.
Check for diabetes, polycythaemia and anaemia and treat if necessary.
Keep the body and arms warm, and the legs cool.
Attend carefully to foot hygiene.
Surgery. Disobliteration is indicated if there is a high block with good distal vessels on angiography. Bypass (vein graft) surgery may be indicated if angiography shows the vessels to be satisfactory distal to the block. Sympathectomy is rarely successful in relieving symptoms of muscle ischaemia.

Acute obstruction
(90% in the legs)

This may be due to thrombosis or to embolism (usually blood clot in atrial fibrillation).

Diagnosis

Pain (usually severe) is associated with numbness, paraesthesiae and paresis. There is pallor and coldness of the limb below the obstruction followed by cyanosis. The limb becomes anaesthetic and the arterial pulses weak or absent.

Management

Maintain the limb at room temperature or below to decrease local cell metabolism and therefore its oxygen demand.

Assess early for surgical disobliteration which is the treatment of choice. The muscles are probably viable if firm and tender and resist movement. The skin is probably not viable if it is densely cyanosed and anaesthetic.

Hyperbaric oxygen, if available, may be helpful, and anticoagulants, thrombolytic agents, vasodilators and low molecular weight dextrans may be tried if surgery is contraindicated or delayed.

Ischaemic foot

This is caused by chronic arterial obstruction distal to the knees, and is most commonly seen in diabetes.

Symptoms

Areas of necrosis and ulceration.

Pain in the foot (often not present in diabetics because of associated peripheral neuropathy).

Intermittent claudication.

Signs

Pallor and/or cyanosis, empty veins in the feet with trophic changes in nails and absence of hairs. The feet are cold and the pulses diminished or absent.

Management

Foot hygiene is especially important in diabetes. Pain may be severe and require morphine. Sympathectomy may improve skin blood supply.

Raynaud's phenomenon

Definition

Intermittent, cold-precipitated, symmetrical attacks of pallor and/or cyanosis of the digits without evidence of arterial obstructive disease. The digits become white (arterial spasm), then blue (cyanosis) and finally red (reactive arterial dilatation).

Aetiology

Idiopathic and familial usually in young women (Raynaud's disease).

Collagen disease, especially systemic lupus erythematosus and scleroderma.

Arterial obstruction, e.g. cervical rib.

Trauma, usually in occupations involving vibrating tools.

Management

Treatment is disappointing. The hands and feet should be kept warm and free from infection. The patient is reassured about the long-term prognosis (usually good) and advised to stop smoking. Reserpine, griseofulvin and thyroxine are of unproven value as is α-blockade with thymoxamine. Sympathectomy is sometimes successful as a last resort particularly in the presence of recurring skin sepsis.

Dermatology

The commonest diseases are eczema, contact eczema, psoriasis, acne vulgaris, drug eruptions and athlete's foot.

Primary skin disorders

Psoriasis

This affects about 1% of the population and may be inapparent, trivial or chronic. Partial remissions are characteristic. It is familial.

Psoriasis may present acutely in children who develop multiple small round silver-scaly lesions on the body, limbs and scalp (guttate psoriasis). This tends to remit spontaneously over 2–4 months, but some patients subsequently develop chronic psoriasis.

In adults, chronic skin lesions occur mainly on the extensor surfaces (back, elbows, knees) and scalp, but any area of skin may be affected and symmetry is a feature. Removal of the plaques produces multiple small haemorrhages.

The rare psoriatic arthropathy resembles sero-negative rheumatoid arthritis and is associated with thimble-pitting in the nail beds (page 121).

Treatment

Preparations containing tar (coal tar ointment, coal tar and salicylic acid for scalp lesions) often produce improvement. Sunlight may increase the benefit. Dithranol (0·25–1%) is particularly useful for severely thickened lesions on extensor surfaces—it is irritant to the eyes. Local steroids (betamethasone) may be required for mucosal and perineal psoriasis, but should not be used in widespread cases.

Methotrexate acts as an antifolate and still probably has a place in treatment. It may cause marrow suppression and has caused death, and should only be used in otherwise resistant psoriasis under expert supervision.

Lichen planus

A disorder usually of adults who present with an irritating rash affecting the flexures of the wrist and forearms, the trunk and the ankles. The rash consists of discrete purple, shiny, polygonal papules with fine white lines passing through them (Wickham's striae), often occurring in scratch marks and other sites of injury (Koebner's phenomenon). Lichen planus involves the buccal mucosa and resembles leukoplakia. The lesions may be diffuse or confined to one or two papules. Lesions may occur on the buccal mucosa or in the nails without other lesions on the skin.

The disorder usually resolves within 6 months but recurrences may occur. It is relatively rare.

Treatment

Local antipruritic agents may be sufficient to suppress symptoms until resolution has occurred. Local steroids under occlusion (betamethasone) will usually heal localised lesions. Systemic steroids may be required to suppress the pruritus of widespread lichen planus if therapy with antihistamines is unsuccessful.

Pityriasis rosea

The rash is preceded by a 'herald patch'—a solitary red, scaly oval lesion on the abdomen or over the scapular area. This is followed after 3–4 days by a mildly itching maculopapular rash which may cover the entire trunk, the upper thighs and upper arms. The macules tend to be aligned along the natural skin creases. The disorder occurs in small outbreaks in schools and families and may be caused by a virus.

The disorder is self-limiting usually within 6 weeks.

Treatment

Local application of calamine lotion is usually sufficient to suppress itching. Oral antihistamines may also be required.

Eczema

Clinically the term describes a patchy diffuse irritating lesion with vesicles which rupture to leave a raw weeping surface. Secondary infection is common. In early lesions scaling may be present and in chronic lesions the skin may become thickened and itchy (lichenification).

Histologically the initial abnormality is oedema of the epidermis and this finally results in vesicle formation. Vesicles or oedema dominate depending upon the thickness of the corneal layer, i.e. in eczema of the face and genitalia oedema is marked, but on the palms and soles vesicles are more prominent.

Contact eczema

Eczema usually results from contact with local irritants and commonly follows skin sensitisation at the initial contact. Subsequent contact causes eczema. This involves the part of the body usually in contact but often the hands and arms, face and genitalia are also affected. Chromates, nickel, rubber, dyes, plastics, lipsticks, perfumes, antibiotics (topical), detergents, some plants and antiseptics are frequent sensitisers.

Constitutional eczema

This term applies to situations where no local irritant or sensitiser can be implicated. The disorder increases with age suggesting that dryness of the skin may be an important factor.

The lesions are characteristically discoid, multiple, often symmetrical and distributed over the limbs and trunk (*cf.* contact eczema). Occasionally lesions follow ingestion of eggs, milk, penicillin or sulphonamides.

Treatment

The local irritant or sensitiser must be removed.

Avoid soap which may be locally irritant and wash in water alone.
Calamine lotion for early acute lesions.
Zinc paste is useful for dry skin and for eczema in the healing stage.
Topical steroids (0·5–1% hydrocortisone) may be required and is usually effective.

NB Dermatitis means inflammation of the skin which may or may not be eczematous. Confusion arises because the terms 'contact eczema' and 'contact dermatitis' are often used synonymously. However, 'eczema' is a more precise descriptive term.

Atopic eczema (infantile eczema) and flexural eczema differ from other forms of eczema in that they usually begin in infancy or childhood, there may be a family history of allergy and usually a history of hay fever or asthma. The disorder results from hypersensitivity to many agents, particularly foodstuffs (milk, eggs) and inhaled dusts (feathers, wool, pollen). Circulating antibodies may be found in the serum. Hypersensitivity is seldom restricted to one substance alone making specific desensitisation frequently impossible. The eczema may persist into childhood (Besnier's prurigo).

Acne vulgaris

A disease of puberty in which plugging of hair follicles by keratin causes retention of sebum producing the characteristic comedo ('blackhead'). These may become secondarily infected with skin staphylococci. The comedos are distributed on the face—particularly the chin—the shoulders and upper thorax. The skin is usually greasy. It is associated with increased androgens and usually disappears in early adult life often with residual scarring. Acne is seen in Cushing's syndrome (page 134).

Treatment

Frequent washing with soap and water or local detergents (e.g. cetrimide) to degrease the skin.
Sulphur-containing pastes (e.g. resorcin and sulphur applied nightly) to produce desquamation and remove keratin plugs. Ultraviolet light is useful if local applications are ineffective.
Low-dose tetracycline (250 mg daily) is given for 1–3 months and is sometimes effective.

Rosacea

A disorder, more common in women, beginning usually after 30 years of age, with episodic blotchy flushing of the face. This settles spontaneously but tends to recur over weeks or months leaving a permanent erythematous rash over the cheeks, nose, chin and forehead. Keratitis and corneal ulceration are rare important complications. Finally the lesion may become papular and telangiectatic.

Treatment

Avoid precipitating factors (e.g. hot drinks, sunlight, alcohol).
Local sulphur creams to improve seborrhoea.
Low-dose tetracycline may be effective when given long-term.

Fungus infections

Candidiasis (monilia, thrush)

In general medical practice this should raise the suspicion of underlying diabetes mellitus (and the rare hypoparathyroidism), or other factors which suppress normal immune mechanisms, e.g. leukaemia, Hodgkin's disease, steroid therapy.

The nail beds are commonly involved, sometimes producing obvious paronychia. Thrush occurs frequently in the vagina, and on the oral mucosa which may spread to affect the entire gastrointestinal tract especially after antibiotics.

NB Oesophageal moniliasis has a characteristic radiological appearance with barium adhering to the patches of monilia.

Treatment

Nystatin as a topical ointment and, if necessary, orally (500,000 units 6-hourly) is the drug of choice but may be ineffective if the underlying disorder does not respond to specific therapy.

Ringworm

The ringworm fungi are a group of related organisms (Trichophyton, Microsporum, Epidermophyton) which live in the keratin layer of the skin. The disorders produced are described after their site on the body, viz. tinea pedis, tinea cruris and tinea capitis. Diagnosis is confirmed by observing fungal hyphae in skin scrapings treated with potassium hydroxide.

Tinea pedis (athlete's foot)

The most common of the group, affecting the interdigital skin usually between the fourth and fifth toes. The nails may be involved. The lesion is irritating and the skin appears white and macerated. Secondary infection is common. The infection tends to be recurrent or chronic. The disorder must be distinguished from simple skin maceration and footwear (contact) dermatitis.

Topical therapy with Whitfield's ointment (benzoic and salicylic acids) is the treatment of choice. Griseofulvin is not usually prescribed for a lesion confined to the interdigital cleft of the fourth and fifth toes as it may require therapy for 6 months to 1 year and tends to recur when treatment is stopped.

Tinea cruris

This may result from spread of infection from the feet. The lesion affects the upper inner thighs and tends to be symmetrical, raised and with a scaly margin. In contrast, monilia is asymmetrical, with ill-defined edges and small satellite lesions. Tinea is extremely irritating. Local application with Whitfield's ointment, $\frac{1}{4}$–$\frac{1}{2}$ strength, may be of value if the lesions are not widespread. The feet should also be treated. Oral griseofulvin is usually started when the diagnosis has been confirmed. Treatment may need to be continued for 3–6 months.

Tinea capitis

A disease of prepubertal children who present with an area of baldness containing 'clubbed' hairs. The hair stumps reveal fungal spores after treatment with potassium hydroxide. They show characteristic fluorescence when viewed under Wood's light. The underlying scalp is scaly and may become secondarily infected. Griseofulvin is usually effective within 1–2 months.

Drug eruptions

Many drugs can produce skin eruptions which may be erythematous, maculopapular, urticarial or purpuric. The pattern for any one drug may not always be the same and most drugs may at times produce one or other type of reaction, i.e. virtually any drug can produce any eruption—an overstatement but necessary to consider in any patient with a rash. Barbiturates are in common use and it is always worth enquiring about night sedation. Topical antibiotics, particularly the sulphonamides, penicillins and the neomycin group frequently produce skin sensitivity.

Urticarial reactions

The penicillins are probably the most common group of drugs which produce urticaria. Of all patients receiving a penicillin, 1–2% have adverse reactions, and many of them (if asked) give a history of previous sensitivity. Reactions are more frequent in adults, probably a measure of previous exposure. Sensitivity to one penicillin may mean sensitivity to all, and cephaloridine sensitivity in about 1 in 10 patients. The common drug rash of ampicillin may be specific to it, and due to an impurity. (It is almost universal in patients with infectious mononucleosis.) The urticarial eruption usually occurs 3–7 days after therapy is started. Rarely, an acute hypersensitivity reaction occurs within minutes and is associated with serum-sickness-like features of fever, wheezing, arthralgia and hypotension. Chronic cases should avoid dairy produce as antibiotics are generously used in farming.

Other drugs which produce urticarial reactions include barbiturates, salicylates, streptomycin, sulphonamides, tetracyclines, phenothiazines and chloramphenicol.

Purpura
(page 69)

This may be a feature of any severe drug reaction and results from capillary damage. Bone marrow suppression by gold, carbimazole, or phenylbutazone may cause thrombocytopenic purpura (page 74).

Other disorders

Light sensitivity (sulphonamides, thiazides, chlorpropamide, tolbutamide, griseofulvin, chlorpromazine).

Fixed drug eruption. This describes an eruption which has the same character and occurs in the same site when the causative drug is taken. Phenolphthalein, used in some laxatives is frequently incriminated. Other drugs include penicillin, phenylbutazone, aspirin and sulphonamides.

Lichen planus (gold, phenylbutazone, mepacrine, quinidine).

Exfoliative dermatitis (gold, barbiturates, phenytoin, chlorpropamide).
Erythema multiforme (page 254).
Lupus erythematosus (page 111).

Management of drug eruptions

Stop all drugs.
Oral antihistamines for local irritation.
Systemic steroids may be required in severe reactions and may be life saving in acute hypersensitivity reactions including shock and angioneurotic oedema.

Skin manifestations of systemic disease

Erythema nodosum

Clinical presentation

Tender, red, raised lesions usually on the shins and less frequently the thighs and upper limbs. The lesions pass through the colour changes of a bruise.

Aetiology

Sarcoidosis is probably the most common cause in this country.
Streptococcal infection and hence rheumatic fever.
Tuberculosis.
Drugs (particularly sulphonamides and including penicillin and salicylates).
Other causes include ulcerative colitis, Crohn's disease, leprosy, and fungal infections. Erythema nodosum occasionally occurs as an isolated, sometimes recurrent, disorder.

Haemolytic streptococcal infection

Skin lesions frequently occur as a sign of streptococcal sensitivity and present as erythema nodosum, erythema marginatum (very rare but virtually diagnostic of rheumatic fever), erythema multiforme (also occurs in rheumatic fever), erysipelas (slightly raised, well circumscribed, acutely painful bright red lesion of half to one hands–breadth diameter. The elderly are more commonly affected and the legs and face the most common sites. There may be generalised symptoms of headache, fever and vomiting. Response to parenteral penicillin is usually rapid). The classical endotoxin rash of scarlet fever is now rarely seen.

Malignancy

Generalised pruritus is associated with tumours of the reticuloendothelial system such as Hodgkin's disease.

Herpes zoster ('shingles')

Although it usually occurs in isolation, herpes zoster may occur in any debilitating disease and particularly with Hodgkin's disease, the leukaemias and patients on steroids. The lesion consists of ringed vesicles on an inflamed base. Pain precedes the lesions in nerve root distributions. Postherpetic neuralgia may be severe and virtually intractable. The virus (herpes zoster) is identical with the virus of chickenpox and denotes earlier clinical or subclinical infection in childhood. The virus appears to remain latent within dorsal root ganglia until diminished resistance allows reactivation.

Dermatomyositis (see page 113)

Fifty per cent of adult cases occur in association with carcinoma usually of bronchus, stomach, breast, ovary or kidney.

Acanthosis nigricans

Brown pigmented warts or plaques most marked in the axilla are associated with underlying carcinoma particularly of the bronchus, gastrointestinal tract, prostate, breast and uterus. It is very rare.

Other manifestations

These include acquired ichthyosis (Hodgkin's disease), vitiligo, mycosis fungoides (chronic myeloid leukaemic skin infiltration), secondary skin metastases, and exfoliative dermatitis.

Xanthomatosis

Dull yellow plaques commonly in the inner angles of the eyelids. Xanthelasmata may indicate hyperlipidaemia with raised serum cholesterol (types II and IV) and are associated with myxoedema, diabetes and primary biliary cirrhosis. Eruptive xanthomata may occur with greatly elevated serum lipid levels.

Other rare manifestations

The following conditions are rare but well recognised:

Necrobiosis lipoidica in diabetes mellitus.
Pretibial myxoedema in thyrotoxicosis.
Lupus pernio (a purple macular eruption) in sarcoid.
Lupus vulgaris and erythema induratum (Bazin's disease) in tuberculosis.
'Café au lait' spots and multiple neurofibromata of neurofibromatosis (von Recklinghausen's disease).
Light sensitivity and blistering in porphyria (page 149).

Mucosal ulceration

These may be localised to the buccal mucosa or associated with generalised disease. Causes include aphthous ulcers, herpes simplex ulceration, herpangina (Coxsackie virus type A), agranulocytic ulcers in aplastic anaemia usually drug induced or leukaemic, erythema multiforme and Stevens-Johnson syndrome, Behçets syndrome, and under dental plates (often monilia).

Bullous lesions

Drugs may produce bullous eruptions. There are four other primary bullous skin disorders which are well recognised. All are rare.

Dermatitis herpetiformis

This usually occurs in association with gluten-sensitive enteropathy, though this is often subclinical. The skin of the limbs and trunk is affected.

Clinical presentation

Symmetrical clusters of itching urticarial lesions on the occiput, interscapular and gluteal regions and extensor aspects of the elbows and knees. Vesicles follow and only rarely become bullous as skin trauma is provoked by the itching. There are seldom lesions in the mouth and there is no fever.

Prognosis and management

The disease starts acutely and may remit spontaneously, but tends to become chronic. Secondary bacterial infection is common. Dapsone is the drug of choice, and a gluten-free diet may be curative (if gluten-induced enteropathy is present).

Pemphigus vulgaris

Clinical presentation

A disease mainly of middle age in which crops of bullae (and eroded bullae) appear in the mouth and/or on the limbs and trunk. The surrounding skin is normal. Degeneration of the cells of the epidermis (acantholysis) is seen on skin biopsy. The superficial skin layer can be moved over the deeper layers (Nikolski's sign) and tends to disintegrate. Lesions appear at sites of pressure and trauma and are extremely painful. There is fever and severe constitutional disturbance.

Complications and management

Secondary bacterial infection is common and septicaemia may result. Protein loss from weeping skin may occur in widespread disease. Prednisone (100–200 mg daily) may be required to control the eruptions. The prognosis is poor and hopeless without treatment.

Pemphigoid

A disease of the extremes of age, presenting with bullae on the limbs and trunk. Mucosal ulceration is rare and acantholysis does not occur, hence the bullae are large and tense. The lesion is in the dermis and the bullae are not easily broken. Nikolski's sign is negative. Secondary infection is common.

Management

The disease is usually self-limiting but steroids (prednisone 40–60 mg daily) may be required to control the eruption. An underlying neoplasm may be suspected if steroids produce no benefit within 2–3 weeks.

Erythema multiforme

Clinical presentation

A generalised disease sometimes with prodromal symptoms of fever, sore throat, headache, arthralgia and gastroenteritis. These are followed by a pleomorphic erythematous eruption which may become bullous. The forearms and legs are commonly affected but the rash may involve the entire body. The buccal mucosa is commonly involved. Target lesions—concentric rings of differing shades of erythema—are characteristic. The disease remits spontaneously in 5–6 weeks but may recur.

'Stevens-Johnson syndrome' is a severe form of erythema multiforme characterised by lesions in the mouth, conjunctiva and genital regions.

Aetiology	The disease sometimes follows drug therapy (sulphonamides, penicillin, salicylates and barbiturates). The aetiology is usually unknown.
Management	Withdraw drugs. Local treatment with calamine for pruritus. Stevens-Johnson syndrome may require steroids to suppress the eruption.

Recommended reading

Journals

Leading articles and annotations in the *Lancet*, *British Medical Journal* and *New England Journal of Medicine*.
Quarterly Journal of Medicine.
Hospital Update.
Medicine—monthly add-on series.
British Journal of Hospital Medicine.

General texts

Comprehensive textbooks

Beeson P.B. & McDermott W. ed. (1975) *Cecil–Loeb's Textbook of Medicine*, 14th edn. Saunders, Philadelphia.
Bodley Scott Sir R.B. ed. (1973) *Price's Textbook of the Practice of Medicine*, 11th edn. Oxford University Press, London.
Wintrobe M.M. *et al.* ed. (1974) *Harrison's Principles of Internal Medicine*, 7th edn. McGraw-Hill, New York.

Concise textbook

Davidson S. & MacLeod J. ed. (1974) *The Principles and Practice of Medicine*, 11th edn. Churchill Livingstone, Edinburgh.

Special textbooks

Campbell E.J.M., Dickinson C.J. & Slater J.D.H. ed. (1975) *Clinical Physiology*, 4th edn. Blackwell, Oxford.
Davies I.J.T. (1972) *Postgraduate Medicine*, 2nd edn. Lloyd-Luke, London.
Matthew H. & Lawson A.A.H. (1974) *Treatment of Common Acute Poisonings*, 3rd edn. Churchill Livingstone, Edinburgh.
Robinson R.O. (1970) *Medical Emergencies*. Heinemann, London.
The Medical Annual. John Wright, Bristol.
Symposium on Advanced Medicine (annually). Pitman, London.

Specialist texts

Chest disease

Crofton J. & Douglas A. (1975) *Respiratory Diseases*, 2nd edn. Blackwell, Oxford.

Cardiology

Oram S. (1971) *Clinical Heart Disease*. Heinemann, London.
Schamroth L. (1971) *An Introduction to Electrocardiography*, 4th edn. Blackwell, Oxford.

Endocrinology

Hall R., Anderson J., Smart G.A. & Besser M. (1974) *Fundamentals of Clinical Endocrinology*, 2nd edn. Pitman, London.

Stanbury J.B. *et al.* (1972) *The Metabolic Basis of Inherited Disease*, 3rd rev. edn. McGraw-Hill, New York.

Williams R.H. ed. (1974) *Textbook of Endocrinology*, 5th edn. Saunders, Philadelphia.

Diabetes

Malins J. (1968) *Clinical Diabetes Mellitus*. Eyre and Spottiswoode, London.

Oakley W.G., Pyke D.A. & Taylor K.W. (1975) *Diabetes and its Management*, 2nd edn. Blackwell, Oxford.

Kidney disease

Berlyne G.M. (1974) *A Course in Renal Disease*, 4th edn. Blackwell, Oxford.

Black Sir D.A.K. ed. (1972) *Renal Disease*, 3rd edn. Blackwell, Oxford.

De Wardener H.E. (1973) *The Kidney*, 4th edn. Churchill Livingstone, Edinburgh.

Strauss M.B. & Welt L.G. (1972) *Diseases of the Kidney*, 2nd edn. Williams and Wilkins, Baltimore.

Gastroenterology and liver disease

Avery Jones F., Gummer J.W.P. & Lennard-Jones J.E. (1968) *Clinical Gastroenterology*, 2nd edn. Blackwell, Oxford.

Sherlock S. (1975) *Diseases of the Liver and Biliary System*, 5th edn. Blackwell, Oxford.

Truelove S.C. & Reynell P.C. (1972) *Diseases of the Digestive System*, 2nd edn. Blackwell, Oxford.

Haematology

De Gruchy G.C. (1970) *Clinical Haematology in Medical Practice*, 3rd edn. Blackwell, Oxford.

Thompson R.B. (1970) *Short Textbook of Haematology*, 3rd edn. Pitman, London.

Immunology

Roitt I.M. (1974) *Essential Immunology*, 2nd edn. Blackwell, Oxford.

Dermatology

Levene G.M. & Calnan C.D. (1974) *Colour Atlas of Skin Diseases*. Wolfe, London.

Neurology

Bickerstaff E.R. (1973) *Neurological Examination in Clinical Practice*, 3rd edn. Blackwell, Oxford.

Lord Brain & Walton J.N. (1969) *Brain's Diseases of the Nervous System*, 7th edn. Oxford University Press, London.

Matthews W.B. (1975) *Practical Neurology*, 3rd edn. Blackwell, Oxford.

Matthews W.B. & Miller H. (1972) *Diseases of the Nervous System*, 2nd edn. Blackwell, Oxford.

Walton J.N. (1971) *The Essentials of Neurology*, 3rd edn. Pitman, London.

Psychiatry

Tredgold R.F. & Wolff H.H. ed. (1970) *U.C.H. Notes on Psychiatry*. Duckworth, London.

Willis J.H.P. (1974) *Lecture Notes on Psychiatry*, 4th edn. Blackwell, Oxford.

Rheumatology

Boyle J.A. & Buchanan W.W. (1976) *Clinical Rheumatology*. 2nd edn. Blackwell, Oxford.

Mason M. & Currey H.L.F. (1975) *Introduction to Clinical Rheumatology*. 2nd edn. Pitman, London.

Radiology

Kreel L. (1971) *Outline of Radiology*. Heinemann, London.

Sutton D. (1976) *Radiology for General Practitioners and Medical Students*, 3rd edn. Churchill Livingstone, Edinburgh.

Infectious diseases

Christie A.B. (1974) *Infectious Diseases: Epidemiology and Clinical Practice*, 2nd edn. Churchill Livingstone, Edinburgh.

Warin J.F. & Ironside A.G. (1975) *Lecture Notes on Infectious Diseases*, 2nd edn. Blackwell, Oxford.

Wright F.J. & Baird J.P. (1975) *Tropical Diseases* (supplement to *The Principles and Practice of Medicine*, 5th edn). Churchill Livingstone, Edinburgh.

Pharmacology

Blacow N.W. ed. (1972) *Martindale's Extra Pharmacopoeia*, 26th edn. Pharmaceutical Press, London.

Goodman L.S. & Gilman A. ed. (1975) *The Pharmacological Basis of Therapeutics*, 5th edn. Macmillan, London.

Laurence D.R. (1973) *Clinical Pharmacology*, 4th edn. Churchill Livingstone, Edinburgh.

Statistics

Smart J.V. (1970) *Elements of Medical Statistics*, 2nd edn. Staples, London.

Swinscow T.D.V. (1976) *Statistics at Square One*. British Medical Journal, London.

Clinical biochemistry

Zilva J.F. and Pannall P.R. (1975) *Clinical Chemistry in Diagnosis and Treatment*. Lloyd-Luke, London.

Clinical Genetics

Fraser G. and Mayo O. *Textbook of Human Genetics* Blackwell Scientific Publications, Oxford.

SI units conversion table

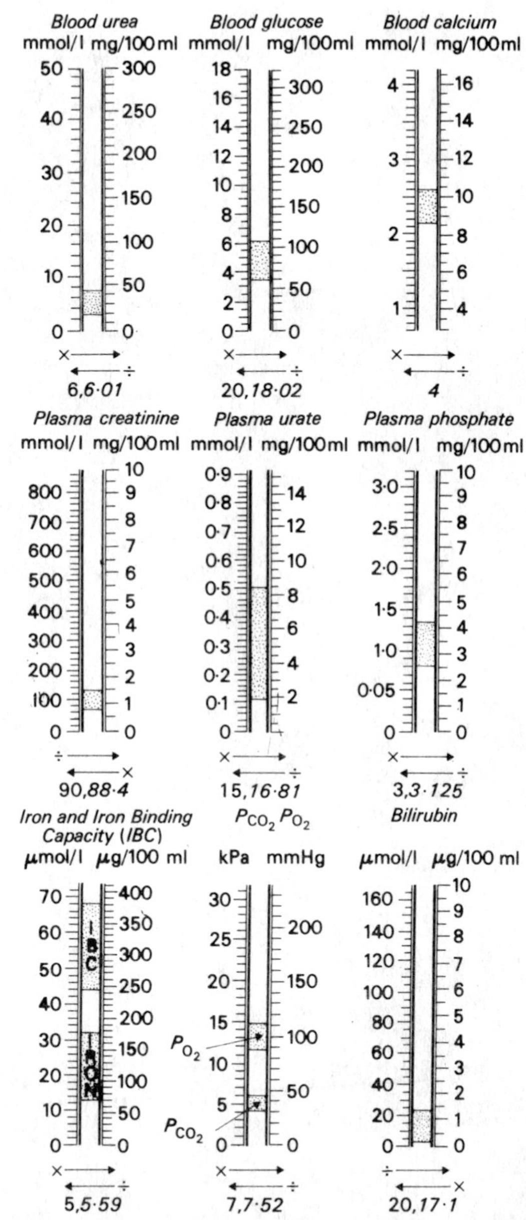

Figures in italics give the exact conversion factor, those in roman give a rough approximation.

Index